Seventh Edition

A Cancer Source Book for Nurses

Edited by

CLAUDETTE VARRICCHIO, DSN, RN, OCN, FAAN
Program Director/Nurse Consultant
National Cancer Institute
Bethesda, Maryland

Associate Editors

MARGARET PIERCE, RN, CS, MPH, MS, AOCN
Assistant Professor
University of Tennessee, College of Nursing
Knoxville, Tennessee

CAROLYN L. WALKER, RN, PHD, CPON
Professor
San Diego State University, School of Nursing
San Diego, California

TERRI B. ADES, RN, MS, OCN, FNP-C
Director, Detection and Treatment/Nursing
American Cancer Society
Atlanta, Georgia

American Cancer Society
Professional Education Publication

Editorial, Sales, and Customer Service Offices
Jones and Bartlett Publishers
40 Tall Pine Drive
Sudbury, MA 01776
(508) 443-5000
(800) 832-0034
info @ jbpub.com
http://www.jbpub.com

Jones and Bartlett Publishers International
Barb House, Barb Mews
London W6 7PA
UK

The American Cancer Society, Inc., Atlanta, GA 30329

Library of Congress Cataloging-in-Publication Data
A cancer source book for nurses. — 7th ed. / American Cancer Society.
    p. cm.
    Includes bibliographical references and index.
    ISBN 0-7637-0424-0
    1. Cancer—Nursing.   I. American Cancer Society.
    [DNLM: 1. Neoplasms—Nursing.   2. Oncologic Nursing. WY 156
C2198 1997]
RC266.C3564   1997
610.73'698—dc20
DNLM/DLC
for Library of Congress   96-29088
                                     CIP

Printed in the United States of America

00 99 98 97 96   10 9 8 7 6 5 4 3 2 1

Contents

Preface   *vi*
    Terri B. Ades

Contributors   *viii*

UNIT 1   INTRODUCTION TO CANCER NURSING   **1**
    Susan B. Baird

UNIT 2   OVERVIEW OF CANCER   **11**

1   Incidence and Mortality   **13**
    Karen Smith Blesch

2   The Nature of Cancer   **27**
    Jan Ellerhorst-Ryan

3   Cancer Prevention and Risk Assessment   **35**
    Karen Billars Heusinkveld

4   Cancer Screening and Early Detection   **43**
    Marilyn Frank-Stromborg

5   Special Populations   **56**
    Janice Phillips, Anne Belcher, and J. Anne O'Neil

UNIT 3   TREATMENT APPROACHES   **67**

6   Cancer Clinical Trials   **69**
    Mary S. McCabe

7   Surgical Oncology   **80**
    Cindy Stahl

8   Radiation Therapy   **91**
    Ryan R. Iwamoto

9   Chemotherapy   **103**
    Margaret Barton Burke

10   Biotherapy   122
Elizabeth Abernathy

11   Hematopoietic Stem Cell Transplantation   139
Cynthia R. King

12   Alternative and Complementary Methods of Cancer
Management   152
Nancy E. Kane

UNIT 4   NURSING MANAGEMENT OF PATIENT
RESPONSES   159

13   Myelosuppression   161
Paula Trahan Rieger

14   Common Clinical Problems   174
Anna R. Du Pen and Joan T. Panke

15   Vascular Access Devices and Ambulatory Pumps Used in
Cancer Treatment   185
Dawn Camp-Sorrell

16   Nutritional Support   200
Gail M. Wilkes and Tracy Yemma

17   Oncologic Emergencies   214
Brenda K. Shelton

18   Sexuality, Sexual Dysfunction, and Cancer   231
Margaret Barton Burke

19   Psychosocial Responses to Disease and Treatment   245
Ginette G. Ferszt and Ruth C. Waldman

20   Rehabilitation   253
Frances K. Barg

21   Palliative Care   260
James C. Pace

UNIT 5   SITE-SPECIFIC CANCERS   269

22   Cancers of the Head and Neck   271
Darlene W. Mood

23   Lung Cancer   284
Elizabeth J. White

24   **Breast Cancer   295**
     Karen Hassey Dow

25   **Colorectal Cancer   307**
     Marlyn D. Boyd

26   **Urinary Tract Cancers   316**
     Julena Lind

27   **Male Genital Cancers   327**
     Debra L. Brock

28   **Gynecologic Malignancies   335**
     Virginia R. Martin

29   **Central Nervous System Cancers   349**
     Betty Owens

30   **Skin Cancers   359**
     Anne Marie Maguire

31   **Cancers of the Bone   372**
     Michele V. Bennett

32   **Leukemia   379**
     Colette N. Chaney and Patricia Jassak

33   **Lymphomas   390**
     Margie Graff Anderson

34   **Multiple Myeloma   401**
     Bonny Libbey Johnson

35   **Other Cancers   410**
     Deborah Lowe Volker

36   **Childhood Cancers   423**
     Marcia Rostad and Ki Moore

APPENDICES

I   **Resources in Cancer Care   439**
     Marilyn Frank-Stromborg

II   **American Cancer Society:
     Who We Are and What We Do   453**
     Terri B. Ades

Glossary   457
     Linda Yoder

Index   475

Preface

The American Cancer Society is dedicated to improving the quality of care for individuals with cancer and their families and those at risk for cancer. To fulfill this mission, the American Cancer Society has established a long history of anticipating and responding to the educational needs of professional nurses who are involved in providing care to people with cancer.

The first edition of *A Cancer Source Book for Nurses* was published by the American Cancer Society in 1950. At that time, oncology care was provided by public health nurses in the home. Usually, the patient was dying. Since then the field of oncology has burgeoned, and there are now more than 10 million cancer survivors. Nurses in every practice setting are involved in providing care to such survivors, to individuals with cancer, and to those at risk for cancer: the family nurse practitioner providing primary health care to the woman with a history of breast cancer; the home care nurse visiting the man recovering from a radical prostatectomy; the pediatric ambulatory care nurse evaluating a little one with bruising and bleeding; the staff nurse providing supportive care to the cancer patient with pain; and the nursing student making a first, tentative visit to a patient with cancer. This seventh edition of *A Cancer Source Book for Nurses* was written for them and for other health care professionals.

Often referred to as the *Source Book*, this work has evolved from a book written by a physician who provided the "basic knowledge of the facts about cancer" to a book written by nurses for nurses. The seventh edition is a comprehensive, basic reference covering the continuum of oncology care: what is known today about cancer prevention and how to reduce one's risk for cancer; early detection tests to diagnose potentially curable cancers; current treatment modalities for cancer, with information on some of the newer therapies and clinical trials; advances in symptom control; and issues related to survivorship. In addition to information on the most common cancers and treatments, specific strategies for nursing care have been detailed by nurse specialists experienced in providing care to people with cancer. Several new chapters on vascular access devices, special populations, childhood cancers, bone marrow transplantation, clinical trials, biological therapies, and alternative therapies have been added to reflect advances in treatment and care, as well as changes in health care delivery.

The *Source Book* is intended to provide a quick, yet practical and comprehensive reference for nurses and other health professionals. For individuals who would like more in-depth reading, a bibliography is provided at the end of each chapter. Resources for individuals with cancer and their families are identified. An extensive glossary defines terms commonly used in oncology care. These glossary terms are set in **boldface** type as they first appear in the text.

The American Cancer Society is grateful to the authors, reviewers, and editors for their generous contribution of time and the expertise, talent, and leadership they shared. We believe that this seventh edition reflects the excellence of their unsparing commitment to the fields of oncology and nursing and to the well-being of people with cancer. Without them, this timely work could not have been written.

ACKNOWLEDGMENTS

Many people lent their expertise to this book by contributing content or by reviewing chapters for accuracy and relevancy to practice. Their valuable suggestions and careful reviews added immeasurably to the final text. The time they gave is greatly appreciated.

Nancy Agee
Mary Ann Anglim
Margaret Barton Burke
Jean K. Brown
Caroline Burnett
Victoria Champion
Marylin Dodd
Karen Hassey Dow
Lynn Erdman
Genevieve Foley
Marcia Grant
Pat Grimm
Shirley Gullo

Darlene Hall
Laura Hilderley
Judy Holcombe
Casey Hooke
M. Tish Knobf
Susan McMillan
Janice Post-White
Judy Rivers
Linda Sarna
Marguerite Schlag
Diana Wilkie
Penelope Wright

Terri B. Ades

Contributors

Elizabeth Abernathy, RN, MSN
Assistant Professor
School of Nursing
UNC, Chapel Hill
Chapel Hill, North Carolina

Margie Graff Anderson, RN, MN
Instructor
Seattle Central Community College
Seattle, Washington

Susan B. Baird, RN, MPH, MA
Director of Nursing and Patient Services
Nursing Administration
Fox Chase Cancer Center
Philadelphia, Pennsylvania

Frances K. Barg, MEd
Coordinator
Cancer Control Education
University of Pennsylvania
School of Nursing
Philadelphia, Pennsylvania

Anne Belcher, PhD, RN, FAAN
Associate Professor and Chair
Department of Acute and Long-Term Care
University of Maryland, School of Nursing
Baltimore, Maryland

Michele V. Bennett, RN, MA, ONC,
  OCN
Clinical Nurse Specialist
Orthopaedics
New York University Medical Center
New York, New York

Karen Smith Blesch, RN, PhD
Post-Doctoral Fellow
School of Public Health
Department of Epidemiology and
  Biostatistics
University of Illinois at Chicago
Chicago, Illinois

Marilyn D. Boyd, PhD, RN, CHES
Research Professor
College of Nursing
University of South Carolina
Columbia, South Carolina

Debra L. Brock, MSN, RN, CS
Nurse Practitioner
Nashville Family Medicine
Nashville, Indiana

Margaret Barton Burke, RN, PhD
  (candidate), OCN
Consultant in Oncology Nursing
Oncology Consulting Services
West Roxbury, Massachusetts

Dawn Camp-Sorrell, RN, MSN, FNP,
  AOCN
Oncology Nurse Practitioner
University of Alabama at Birmingham
  Hospital
Birmingham, Alabama

Colette N. Chaney, RN, BSN
Research Nurse Clinician
RUSH University
Chicago, Illinois

Karen Hassey Dow, RN, PhD, FAAN
Associate Professor
School of Nursing, University of Central
  Florida
Orlando, Florida

Anna R. Du Pen, ARNP, MN
Nurse Practitioner
Swedish Pain Management Services
Seattle, Washington

Jan M. Ellerhorst-Ryan, RN, MSN, CS
Primary Care Nurse
Vitas Health Care Corporation of Ohio
Cincinnati, Ohio

Ginette G. Ferszt, MSN, RN, CS
Psychiatric Clinical Specialist
College of Nursing, University of Rhode
  Island
Kingston, Rhode Island

Marilyn Frank-Stromborg, EdD, JD,
  ANP, FAAN
Professor and Acting Chair
School of Nursing, Northern Illinois
  University
DeKalb, Illinois

Karen Billars Heusinkveld, RN,
  DrPH
Associate Professor
Director, RN to BSN Program
University of Texas at Arlington
School of Nursing
Arlington, Texas

Ryan R. Iwamoto, RN, MN
Clinical Nurse Specialist
Radiation Oncology
Virginia Mason Medical Center
Seattle, Washington

Patricia Jassak, MS, RN, OCN
Administrative Director
Illinois Masonic Cancer Center
Chicago, Illinois

Bonny Libbey Johnson, RN, MSN,
  OCN
Clinical Research Coordinator
University of Connecticut Health Center
Farmington , Connecticut

Nancy E. Kane, MS, RN, OCN
Director of Oncology Services
Optima Health
Manchester, New Hampshire

Cynthia R. King, RN, NP, MSN, CNA
PhD Candidate, University of Rochester
School of Nursing and
Nurse Consultant, Special Care
  Consultants
Rochester, New York

Julena Lind, MN, RN
Assistant Professor of Clinical Nursing
USC Center for Health Professions
Los Angeles, California

Anne Marie Maguire, ARNP, MN, OCN
Hospice Coordinator
DVA Puget Sound Health Care System
Seattle VA Medical Center
Seattle, Washington

Virginia R. Martin, MSN, RN, AOCN
Clinical Director, Ambulatory Care
Fox Chase Cancer Center
Philadelphia, Pennsylvania

Mary S. McCabe, BA, BS
Special Assistant to the Director
Division of Cancer Treatment, Diagnosis,
  and Centers
National Cancer Institute
Bethesda, Maryland

Darlene W. Mood, PhD
Professor
College of Nursing
Wayne State University
Detroit, Michigan

Ki Moore, RN, DNS, FAAN
Associate Professor, Interim Director
Division of Nursing Practice
College of Nursing
Tucson, Arizona

J. Anne O'Neil, RN, PhD
Clinical Instructor
University of Maryland
Baltimore, Maryland

Betty Owens, RN, MS
Division of Neurosurgery
University of Colorado
  Health Sciences Center
Denver, Colorado

James C. Pace, DSN, MDiv, ANP-CS
Associate Professor of Adult Health
  Nursing
Emory University
Nell Hodgson Woodruff School of
  Nursing
Atlanta, Georgia

Joan T. Panke, BSN
Research Nurse
Pain Management Services
Swedish Medical Center
Seattle, Washington

Janice Phillips, PhD, RN
American Cancer Society Professor of
   Oncology Nursing
Assistant Professor
School of Nursing, University of
   Maryland
Baltimore, Maryland

**Paula Trahan Rieger, MSN, RN, OCN,
CS, ANP**
Nurse Practitioner
University of Texas, M. D. Anderson
   Cancer Center
Houston, Texas

Marcia Rostad, RN, MS, OCN
Clinical Nurse Specialist
College of Nursing
Tucson, Arizona

**Brenda K. Shelton, MS, RN, CCRN,
OCN**
Critical Care Clinical Nurse Specialist
The Johns Hopkins Oncology Center
Baltimore, Maryland

Cindy Stahl, RN, BSN, OCN
Clinical Educator
City of Hope Medical Center
Duarte, California

Deborah Lowe Volker, RN, MA, OCN
Director of Nursing Staff Development
University of Texas, M. D. Anderson
   Cancer Center
Houston, Texas

Ruth C. Waldman, MS, RN, OCN
Assistant Dean, College of Nursing
University of Rhode Island
Kingston, Rhode Island

Elizabeth J. White, RN, MN
Community Health Nurse
VA Puget Sound Health Care System
Seattle, Washington

Gail M. Wilkes, RN, MS, AOCN
Clinical Nurse Specialist/Nurse Manager
Boston City Hospital
Boston, Massachusetts

Tracy Yemma, RD
Outpatient Dietician
Boston City Hospital
Boston, Massachusetts

Linda Yoder, RN, MBA, PhD, OCN
Lieutenant Colonel, Army Nurse Corps.
Director, Nursing Research
Nursing Research Service
Brook Army Medical Center
Fort Sam Houston, Texas

Unit 1

Introduction to Cancer Nursing

Introduction to Cancer Nursing

Susan B. Baird

Cancer care offers tremendous challenges to nurses regardless of the setting in which they practice or their role within the setting. Throughout the history of nursing there have been poignant examples of valuable and substantial contributions to the care of patients with cancer. A body of knowledge has been built through years of experience and research that now provides a solid foundation for a dynamic specialty.

Nurses specializing in cancer care can use the existing knowledge base and help in its continuing development. Cancer poses challenging opportunities for clinical problem solving and for helping patients and families along the cancer care continuum. From prevention and detection to rehabilitation and continuing care, the interested nurse will find a range of patient care concerns that can be addressed through skilled intervention. Each chapter in this book is testament to the complexity of cancer and its treatment. Nurses are clearly essential members of multidisciplinary teams working together, pooling their interests and experience for the benefit of patients and families.

When examining this challenging and rewarding field of specialization, several fundamental concepts come to mind. First, every nurse has a role and responsibility in cancer care and can make a valuable contribution. Second, there is infinite variety in the types of opportunities that exist for nurses—opportunities that continue to evolve as the knowledge base expands. Third, the complexity of the disease provides nurses with both the opportunity and the challenge to make a tangible difference in patients' and families' lives. Finally, nurses convey a message of hope in their caring—hope for comfort, for quality of life, and for the continuing development of effective treatment.

OPPORTUNITIES FOR NURSES

Every nurse can make a valuable contribution to cancer care. Some opportunities arise naturally, because nursing is a helping and resourceful profession. Continually expanding opportunities present themselves as changes occur in the health care arena and along the disease continuum.

The Community

In family and community settings, people naturally turn to nurses for information about cancer much as they turn to them for advice about many other aspects of health care. They may ask about cancer risk, early detection methods, or treatment options. Their inquiries may stem from personal experience, something they heard or were told, or perhaps a headline they saw in a tabloid at the grocery checkout line. Surveys have shown that the public places trust in nurses as providers of health care information. Nurses can take advantage of casual inquiries to dispel myths, update information, provide health counseling, or direct people to needed resources.

Volunteer activities in the community through organizations such as the American Cancer Society, schools, and churches provide additional avenues for nurses to participate in cancer education. Organizations frequently need nurses to participate in health fairs or screening activities, where a few hours of time can be a valued contribution to others and a rewarding experience. An example of developing community outreach for nurses is parish nursing, a primarily volunteer activity aimed at identifying individuals within the parish who are at risk for various diseases.

The Disease Continuum

Nurses have traditionally identified themselves with the active, treatment phase of disease. The majority of nurses have been employed in acute care settings, working with patients who are newly diagnosed, receiving primary therapy, or being treated for recurrence. Nurses have also been involved in the continuation of care through home care or long-term care when the patient's needs can no longer be met at home. The re-emergence of hospice over the past 2 decades as an organized approach to palliative care for terminally ill patients has presented a challenging role for nurses.

Increased emphasis on earlier detection for many cancers creates opportunities for nurses to participate in prevention and detection functions. Forecasts for changing health care roles frequently cite prevention and detection as especially appropriate for nurses who are moving into community-based settings. Identifying populations at high risk for specific cancers and helping to develop surveillance programs are potentially important roles for nurses and other health care providers as the emphasis on prevention increases. Genetic screening and counseling for individuals and families at high risk for cancer are also emerging nursing roles.

Finally, the patterns of disease have changed substantially over time. Many patients today live longer with their disease than was previously possible. As this pattern continues, nurses will find that they will work with some patient populations that have acute disease episodes interspersed with periods of general wellness. They will work with patients who are returning to school, work, or family responsibilities, and they will be able to facilitate comprehensive rehabilitation plans for these populations.

Health Care System Changes

Nurses are practicing within a rapidly and erratically changing health care environment. The hope for health care reform, a major impetus in the past decade, has clearly not been realized. The depth and breadth of change, however, are pervasive and have many implications for cancer nursing opportunities.

The most notable aspect of change is probably the shift away from acute care hospitals as the major site for care delivery and decreased lengths of hospital stay. These changes mean that acute care is compressed; therefore, care and teaching must be organized and efficient. More diagnostic and staging activities occur on an ambulatory basis. Patients scheduled for surgery most often arrive at the hospital on the day of surgery, and patients in the hospital tend to be more acutely ill than in the past. With patients leaving the hospital more quickly, home care has become the most rapidly expanding health care setting. The range of services that can be delivered at home has also been expanded, with home infusion an especially important service in cancer care.

Ambulatory care settings are the focal point of care delivery, where brief, intermittent visits require careful planning and integration of services to avoid unnecessary visits and gaps in care. Chemotherapy infusions, many of which until recently required inpatient admissions, are routinely done in ambulatory settings. Ambulatory surgery has also expanded, with a variety of complex procedures done on an outpatient or same-day basis.

The increased prevalence of managed care is exerting substantial influence on what services will be covered through third-party payers and where services are to be offered. Nurses will find challenges in trying to coordinate care components and in working with patients to understand the limitations of their coverage. As Medicare and Medicaid plans also move into managed care, this need will be even more acutely experienced by people who may find it difficult to understand restrictions and make appropriate choices.

Cancer Care Settings

Cancer care is delivered in a variety of institutions—in general hospitals and in specialized centers. The number of cancer centers and cancer programs within hospitals continues to increase. Many cancer centers have extensive affiliative networks with community hospitals, facilitating referrals and education processes. Cancer outreach programs aimed at rural areas or areas with large underserved populations are increasing. These setting changes and the proliferation of telecommunication systems promoting collaborative care delivery increase the likelihood that patients will receive state-of-the-art care.

Decreasing the number of hospital beds and reconfiguring services within hospitals may affect dedicated oncology units. After a steady increase in the number of dedicated oncology beds over the past decade, oncology units are now frequently being merged with similar services. Careful planning and quality improvement monitoring are essential tools in ensuring that the quality of care available through specialized units does not suffer. As hospitals merge into larger networks, services are frequently consolidated to avoid duplication and reduce costs. Well-defined standards of care, clinical pathways, and outcome measures will help ensure quality care. There has never been a greater need for nurses skilled in oncology care to develop and update these tools and to ensure consistent implementation. The need to interest other nurses in cancer care and its challenges is also acute, given the shifts in settings for care delivery.

NURSING ROLES IN CANCER CARE

In General Practice

All nurses should know the signs and symptoms of cancer and why they occur. They should know the risk factors for specific cancers, the guidelines for cancer check-ups, and how to perform self-examination techniques and teach them to others. Nurses are often in advantageous positions in their own families and in the community to teach lifestyle changes that can prevent cancer and increase the likelihood of early detection. The American Cancer Society encourages nurses to participate in prevention and early detection activities at the community level and provide frequent training programs and materials for these purposes.

In addition, nurses in every area of practice should be familiar with general cancer treatment modalities and be able to identify both the usual and the untoward effects of the disease and its treatment. Nurses should be familiar with the cancer-related resources available at the community, state, and national levels and know how patients can gain access to these services. Coordinating care with other care providers and organizations is a valuable service to patients and families.

Cancer Care in Other Specialty Areas

Despite forecasts suggesting that specialization within nursing is decreasing as an educational and practice focus, nurses do function within a wide variety of specialties that are oriented by disease site, such as oncology or cardiovascular care, or by setting, such as emergency room or occupational health nursing. Almost every specialty has some direct connection with cancer care. A school nurse may help a child with cancer get reintegrated into the classroom or prepare classmates for the appearance of a recovering child. An emergency room nurse may encounter patients experiencing oncology emergencies or treatment complications. Regardless of the specialty, it is important for nurses within that area to identify ways they may be involved in cancer care or with cancer patients or families and define the knowledge base they need to build. Keeping up to date with the nursing literature within their own specialty and within cancer nursing and also taking advantage of cancer continuing education programs are helpful approaches.

Specializing in Cancer Care

There are many opportunities for nurses who want to focus on cancer care. Nurses can work on special units in hospitals or ambulatory care facilities. Some units are organized by treatment modality, such as chemotherapy or radiation clinics; others specialize in a certain type of cancer, such as a gynecological oncology unit. Nurses can also combine their interests and experiences in subspecialties, such as pediatric oncology.

Cancer centers with prevention and detection programs frequently employ nurse practitioners or clinical educators for screening and the development of education programs. Programs targeted at specific populations, such as women's centers or survivor services, are also being developed.

The rapid growth in home care and home infusion services has created a growing need for nurses with excellent intravenous and infusion skills. Nurses who have specialized skills in other areas frequently can combine these with oncology skills to meet the needs of specialized programs, such as enterostomal therapy or endoscopy. Case management at both the provider and the reimbursement levels is a fast-growing area of specialization for nurses with good experiential backgrounds.

Education and Research

Within the cancer specialization there are many opportunities in education and research. Staff development in cancer centers is an important component because this is a rapidly changing field. Both orientation and skill building are important components of this area. Many cancer centers also use nursing educators for patient education programs and for continuing education. Oncology specialization in master's programs as well as doctoral programs for clinical nurse specialists and nurse practitioners provide opportunities for nurses prepared at advanced levels.

The greater emphasis on scientifically based practice throughout the nursing profession has prompted nurses to use research methods to test care approaches and to increase the understanding of many facets of cancer care. Nurses have successfully competed for research funds and have disseminated their findings through publications and presentations. Nursing opportunities are frequently available in medical research as well. Nurses who have a good grasp of cancer, cancer care, and research methods can be valuable members of the research team. They can actively assist in the informed consent process, in providing information to patients, and in data collection and monitoring of clinical trials.

SPECIALTY PREPARATION

Education

Both formal academic preparation and continuing education programs can provide nurses with the knowledge needed to work in cancer care. Continuing education programs are readily available in most geographic areas through the American Cancer Society Divisions and Units, through Oncology Nursing Society programs offered nationally and through its local chapters, and through most cancer centers. Basic offerings, such as comprehensive cancer courses or chemotherapy certification programs, are valuable for nurses starting in this specialty. Updates or programs on specific aspects of cancer care, such as pain or psychosocial aspects, are good ways to expand basic knowledge.

Cancer organizations and oncology nursing groups have made efforts to increase the cancer content of undergraduate courses so that graduating nurses have a basic knowledge of cancer and have had the opportunity to provide care to this patient population. Programs offering a clinical specialization in oncology nursing or nurse practitioner preparation at the master's level are now available in almost every state. Specialization at the doctoral level is also available at many leading universities. The American Cancer Society and the Oncology Nursing Society (see Appendix I) are good sources of information about current programs and available financial assistance.

Resources

A tremendous advantage nurses have today is a wealth of readily available resources in numerous formats. Several cancer nursing journals are available, as are journals in subspecialties of interest, such as pain, palliative care, and hospice. Multidisciplinary journals are also available. In the general nursing literature, the topic of cancer is covered regularly. The same is true in some of the other specialties. Both professional and patient education materials of high quality are available from the American Cancer Society, the Oncology Nursing Society, the National Cancer Institute, and several pharmaceutical companies. Materials in other formats are developed and released regularly. These include audio- and videotapes, programmed instruction, and computerized programs. Databases, newsletters, and interactive learning opportunities increase in availability every day. Standards of Care and guidelines for many technical aspects of treatment delivery, such as chemotherapy and infusion management, are available through the Oncology Nursing Society. Excellent texts are available on every aspect of cancer care.

Certification

Certification in oncology nursing is available at both the general level and the advanced level through the Oncology Nursing Certification Foundation. Biannual testing is available for the general level at many sites across the country. The advanced level testing is relatively new, and the availability of testing sites will increase. Review materials and courses are offered through a variety of sources.

THE CHALLENGES AND REWARDS OF CANCER CARE

Meeting Support Needs

Whether a nurse has chosen to focus exclusively on cancer care or to deliver cancer care as part of a broader spectrum of responsibilities or is involved in the care of a friend or family member with cancer, the role is multifaceted and challenging. Because nurses spend a considerable amount of time directly with the patient and family while providing care, they are in an ideal position to provide support in a variety of ways. Patients and families may express concerns and fears, and the nurse can interpret information, explain what may not be clearly understood, and explore alternatives. Nurses can promote cooperation and communication by helping patients and family members develop trust in their care providers and by identifying questions they want to ask the doctor or other provider.

Rapid Changes in Care

Nurses are challenged to keep current with rapid changes in all aspects of cancer care. They need to have current information for planning and evaluating care. Continuing changes in the health care arena only increase the need for remaining current. Knowing what care options are available and helping patients make the best use of those resources are valuable nursing functions. Nurses can help patients differentiate among standard care approaches, experimental treatments, and unproven methods of treatment. They can also help patients understand adjuncts to treatment, such as massage, therapeutic touch, and nutrition.

Community Resources

A major focus in cancer nursing is to identify sources of support and to encourage helpful relationships while helping the patient and family preserve their energy and independence as much as possible. Information about community resources, such as equipment loan closets or transportation, can be particularly useful. Nurses can frequently coordinate care among settings and providers, a vital function for families with limited resources who are trying to understand competing choices. Nurses can also help families locate the appropriate place to take questions about finances and reimbursement, rehabilitation, and reemployment.

Rewards of Cancer Nursing

Nurses working in cancer care frequently express the satisfaction they feel in working in this demanding field. Nurses working in prevention are rewarded when someone makes lifestyle changes or choices that promote health. Participation in screening efforts that detect cancer at an earlier stage, when treatment efforts are the most beneficial, can also be fulfilling.

Relationships that develop among nurses, patients, and families are special. Nurses accompany the patients on their journey as they make progress and when they face difficulties. When working closely with a person facing life-threatening challenges, the skilled nurse tailors knowledge, experience, creativity, and caring to that individual. Gratification comes from sharing the patient's joys, hopes, and sorrows within professional boundaries and from recognizing that the care and support given are meaningful and appreciated.

BIBLIOGRAPHY

American Nurses' Association and Oncology Nursing Society. (1987). *Standards of oncology nursing practice*. Kansas City, MO: Author.

Clark, Robert T. (1995). Preparing your hospital for managed care. *Oncology Issues, 10*(2), 28–29.

McCorkle, R., Grant, M., Frank-Stromborg, M., & Baird, S. B. (Eds.). (1996). Cancer nursing as a specialty. In *Cancer nursing: A comprehensive textbook* (2nd ed., pp. 1–11). Philadelphia: W. B. Saunders.

Nielsen, B. B., Scofield, R. S., Mueller, S., Tranin, A. S., Moore, P. & Murphy, C. M. (1996). Certification of oncology nurses: A history. *Oncology Nursing Forum, 23*(4), 701–708.

Oncology Nursing Society. (1995). *Graduate programs in cancer nursing*. Pittsburgh: Author.

Oncology Nursing Society. (1990). *Standards of advanced practice in oncology nursing*. Pittsburgh: Author.

Spitzer, R. B., & Davivier, M. (1987). Nursing in the 1990s: Expanding opportunities. *Nursing Administration Quarterly, 11*(2), 55–61.

Unit 2

Overview of Cancer

1

Incidence and Mortality

Karen Smith Blesch

In 1996 it was estimated that there would be 1,359,150 new cases of cancer and 554,740 deaths due to cancer in the United States. Over 8 million Americans alive today have a history of cancer, and 5 million of those were diagnosed over 5 years ago. Approximately one out of three Americans will experience cancer in his or her lifetime. Approximately one out of five deaths in the United States is due to cancer.

Cancer incidence and mortality data help quantify the impact of cancer and cancer control efforts on the population. High cancer incidence and mortality rates in a population suggest directions for future cancer control efforts; declining cancer incidence and mortality rates help researchers evaluate the effectiveness of cancer control efforts already in place. This chapter acquaints the reader with basic concepts regarding cancer incidence and mortality and with factors that influence the risk of developing and/or dying of cancer.

CANCER INCIDENCE

Cancer **incidence** refers to the number of new cases of cancer. Since simple enumeration of cases does not provide enough information to assess the risk of developing cancer in different populations, cancer incidence is often expressed as an **incidence rate**: the number of new cases of cancer in the population divided by the number of people in the population for a given period of time (usually 1 year). Because this division usually results in a very small number, the results may be multiplied by 100,000 or any other number that is convenient. Cancer incidence and mortality rates are usually expressed in terms of 100,000 population.

Cancer incidence rates reflect the probability or risk of developing cancer in the population. Comparing cancer incidence rates from one population to another (e.g., African Americans compared to Caucasians), helps identify groups

TABLE 1–1   Age-Adjusted Cancer Incidence Rates per 100,000 Population, All Sites, by Race and Sex, United States SEER Program, 1991

White		African-American	
Male	Female	Male	Female
494.5	347.8	597.9	334.0

Source: Data from Gloeckler Ries, L. A., Miller, B. A., Hankey, B. F., Kosary, C. L., Harras, A., & Edwards, B. K. (Eds.). (1994). *SEER cancer statistics review, 1973–1991*. (NIH Pub. No. 94-2789). Bethesda, MD: National Institutes of Health.

that are at highest and lowest risk of developing cancer. Table 1–1 gives *age-adjusted* cancer incidence rates by race and gender for 1991. It shows that African-American males are at higher overall risk of developing cancer (597.9 per 100,000) than Caucasian males or females or African-American females.

CANCER MORTALITY

Cancer **mortality** refers to the number of deaths due to cancer. As with cancer incidence, mortality may be expressed as a **mortality rate** (number of deaths per 100,000), so that comparisons can be made between populations. Cancer mortality rates reflect the overall risk of dying of cancer in a population. Table 1–2 shows **age-adjusted cancer mortality rates** by race and gender in the United States for 1991. African-American males are at higher risk of dying of cancer (317.4 per 100,000) than any other group represented on the table.

Comparing Table 1–1 to Table 1–2 reveals that the risk of developing cancer is higher than the risk of dying of cancer. This is an important consideration. Differences between cancer incidence and mortality rates are influenced by cancer detection and treatment efforts, as well as by tumor biology. The difference is also an indicator of the **prevalence** of cancer in a population, and it suggests directions for allocation of resources for persons with cancer.

Cancer incidence and mortality rates are useful for estimating the probability of developing cancer. However, for assessing the magnitude of the cancer problem and planning resource allocation, numbers of cases and deaths are also useful. Figure 1–1 shows estimated cancer incidence and mortality by site for males and females in 1996. Breast cancer comprises the largest proportion of female cancer cases (184,300/594,850, or 31%), while prostate cancer comprises the largest proportion of male cancer cases (317,100/764,300, or 41%). However, the largest proportions of cancer deaths in both sexes are due to lung cancer (25% of female cancer deaths and 32% of male cancer deaths). These numbers suggest that breast, prostate, and lung cancer should receive priority in allocation of cancer control resources.

TABLE 1–2 Age-Adjusted Cancer Mortality Rates, per 100,000 Population, All Sites, by Race and Sex, United States, 1991

White		African-American	
Male	Female	Male	Female
213.3	140.6	317.4	169.9

Source: Data from Gloeckler Ries, L. A., Miller, B. A., Hankey, B. F., Kosary, C. L., Harras, A., & Edwards, B. K., (Eds.). (1994). *SEER cancer statistics review, 1973–1991.* (NIH Pub. No. 94-2789). Bethesda, MD: National Institutes of Health.

FACTORS THAT INFLUENCE CANCER RISK AND MORTALITY

Cancer incidence and mortality are most frequently described in terms of person, place, and time. *Person* refers to characteristics of the population such as age, race, gender, ethnicity, socioeconomic status, occupation, level of education, lifestyle, and genetic make-up. *Place* refers to geographic location of the population. *Time* refers to the population's position in time. Comparing cancer incidence and mortality among populations with different person, place, and time characteristics provides clues to better understanding of the risk factors for developing and dying of cancer.

Person Characteristics

Advancing age is the most powerful risk factor for developing and dying of cancer. Cancer incidence and mortality rates rise dramatically with age (Table 1–3). Persons over age 55 comprise approximately 21% of the population, but they account for 79% of cancer incidence and 66% of all deaths due to cancer.

Race and ethnicity are also important predictors of cancer risk. Cancer incidence and mortality rates are generally higher for African Americans than for white Americans. Cancer sites for which African Americans have significantly higher incidence and mortality rates include the esophagus, uterine cervix, stomach, liver, prostate, and larynx, and multiple myeloma also presents a greater risk for this population. Incidence and mortality rates for other minority groups, such as Hispanics, are often lower than those for white Americans or African Americans. Because cancer risk is strongly associated with lifestyle and behavior, differences between ethnic and cultural groups can provide clues to factors involved in the development of cancer, such as dietary patterns, alcohol use, and sexual and reproductive behaviors. Table 1–4 shows the number of cancer deaths reported in 1991 among various racial and ethnic groups in the United States.

Cancer incidence and mortality statistics for broad racial classifications such as "white," "black," "Hispanic," or "Asian" overlook the fact that many racial

Cancer Cases by Site and Sex

Male

Prostate
317,100

Lung
98,900

Colon & Rectum
67,600

Bladder
38,300

Lymphoma
33,900

Melanoma of the Skin
21,800

Oral
20,100

Kidney
18,500

Leukemia
15,300

Stomach
14,000

Pancreas
12,400

Liver
10,800

All Sites
764,300

Female

Breast
184,300

Lung
78,100

Colon & Rectum
65,900

Corpus Uteri & Unspecified
34,000

Ovary
26,700

Lymphoma
26,300

Melanoma of the Skin
16,500

Cervix Uteri
15,700

Bladder
14,600

Pancreas
13,900

Leukemia
12,300

Kidney
12,100

All Sites
594,850

Cancer Deaths by Site and Sex

Male

Lung
94,400

Prostate
41,400

Colon & Rectum
27,400

Pancreas
13,600

Lymphoma
13,250

Leukemia
11,600

Esophagus
8,500

Liver
8,400

Stomach
8,300

Bladder
7,800

Kidney
7,300

Brain
7,200

All Sites
292,300

Female

Lung
64,300

Breast
44,300

Colon & Rectum
27,500

Ovary
14,800

Pancreas
14,200

Lymhoma
11,560

Leukemia
9,400

Liver
6,800

Brain
6,100

Corpus Uteri & Unspecified
6,000

Stomach
5,700

Multiple Myeloma
5,100

All Sites
262,440

*Excluding basal and squamous cell skin cancer and in situ carcinomas except bladder.

FIGURE 1–1 Leading Sites of New Cancer Cases and Deaths—1996 Estimates.*

Source: American Cancer Society. (1996). *Cancer facts and figures.* Atlanta: Author.

TABLE 1–3 Cancer Incidence and Mortality Rates, All Sites, per 100,000 Population at Age 25, 65, and 85 and Over, All Races, Both Sexes, 1987–1991.

	25 Years	*65 Years*	*85 Years and Over*
Incidence	57.1	1,702.4	2,494.0
Mortality	8.7	754.3	1,712.3

Source: Data from Gloeckler Ries, L. A., Miller, B. A., Hankey, B. F., Kosary, C. L., Harras, A., & Edwards, B. K., (Eds.). (1994). *SEER cancer statistics review, 1973–1991.* (NIH Pub. No. 94-2789). Bethesda, MD: National Institutes of Health.

groups are composed of numerous subpopulations with diverse genetic, geographical, and cultural origins. Cancer incidence and mortality data for immigrants living in the United States may not be entirely accurate, because immigrants with cancer may come to the United States for treatment or may leave the United States and return to their homeland when cancer is diagnosed.

Socioeconomic status is linked to education, occupation, lifestyle, diet, race, ethnicity, and other factors such as access to health care, health insurance, or transportation. Cultural values and belief systems can affect attitudes about seeking medical care or following screening guidelines. Some of these factors can lead to increased risk for developing cancer, while others contribute to late diagnosis, high mortality, and shorter survival times.

Place Characteristics

Geographic differences in cancer incidence and mortality may reflect population differences in many variables such as age, population density, lifestyle, culture, health practices, access to health care, occupational risks, or environmental contaminants. Figure 1–2 shows the distribution of new cancer incidence in the 50 states in 1996. The states with the highest numbers of cancer cases (California, Florida, and New York) are those that have dense populations and high proportions of elderly people in their populations.

Time Characteristics

Cancer incidence and mortality change over time. Comparing these changes provides clues to causes of cancer and reflects the effectiveness of cancer control efforts. Some increases in cancer incidence over time can be attributed to improved cancer detection practices (e.g., breast cancer) or overall aging of the population (e.g., prostate cancer and breast cancer). Other increases over time may be due to the presence of risk factors in the environment. The increased incidence and mortality rates of lung cancer in the second half of this century are due to the fact that Americans began smoking cigarettes in large numbers in the first half of the century. Reductions or stability in cancer mortality that are not accompanied by similar reductions or stability in cancer incidence reflect

TABLE 1-4 Reported Cancer Deaths, 10 Leading Causes of Cancer Death and Percent of Total Cancer Deaths, by Race, US, 1992

	White	African American	Native American [1,2]	Asian & Pacific Islander [2]	Hispanic [3]
	All sites 454,516 (100%)	All sites 58,401 (100%)	All sites 1,473 (100%)	All sites 6,173 (100%)	All sites 15,218 (100%)
1	Lung 128,704 (28.3%)	Lung 15,472 (26.5%)	Lung 381 (25.9%)	Lung 1,371 (22.2%)	Lung 2,674 (17.6%)
2	Colon & rectum 50,516 (11.1%)	Colon & rectum 6,073 (10.4%)	Colon & rectum 119 (8.1%)	Colon & rectum 668 (10.8%)	Colon & rectum 1,466 (9.6%)
3	Female breast 37,797 (8.3%)	Prostate 5,485 (9.4%)	Female breast 105 (7.1%)	Liver & other biliary 653 (10.6%)	Female breast 1,297 (8.5%)
4	Prostate 28,430 (6.3%)	Female breast 4,889 (8.2%)	Liver & other biliary 87 (5.9%)	Stomach 523 (8.5%)	Liver & other biliary 913 (6.0%)
5	Pancreas 22,519 (5.0%)	Pancreas 3,180 (5.4%)	Prostate 87 (5.9%)	Female breast 387 (6.3%)	Stomach 885 (5.8%)
6	Lymphoma 20,074 (4.4%)	Stomach 2,213 (3.8%)	Stomach 67 (4.5%)	Pancreas 309 (5.0%)	Prostate 873 (5.7%)

18

7	Leukemia 17,045 (3.8%)	Esophagus 1,897 (3.2%)	Pancreas 63 (4.3%)	Lymphoma 263 (4.3%)	Lymphoma 851 (5.6%)
8	Ovary 12,142 (2.7%)	Leukemia 1,587 (2.7%)	Leukemia 55 (3.7%)	Prostate 238 (3.9%)	Pancreas 850 (5.6%)
9	Liver & other biliary 11,283 (2.5%)	Multiple myeloma 1,543 (2.6%)	Kidney 53 (3.6%)	Leukemia 225 (3.6%)	Leukemia 739 (4.9%)
10	Brain & CNS 11,132 (2.4%)	Liver & other biliary 1,476 (2.5%)	Ovary 41 (2.8%)	Oral cavity 156 (2.5%)	Ovary 454 (3.0%)

Note: Since each column includes only the top 10 cancer sites, site-specific numbers and percentages do not add up to the All Sites totals.
[1]Includes American Indians and Native Alaskans.
[2]Numbers are likely to be underestimates due to underreporting of Asian, Pacific Islander, and Native American race on death certificates.
[3]Persons classified as of Hispanic origin on death certificates may be of any race. Hispanic origin is reported for all states except New Hampshire and Oklahoma. In 1990, the 48 states from which data were collected accounted for about 99.6% of the Hispanic population in the United States.

Source: American Cancer Society. (1996). *Cancer facts and figures*. Atlanta: Author.

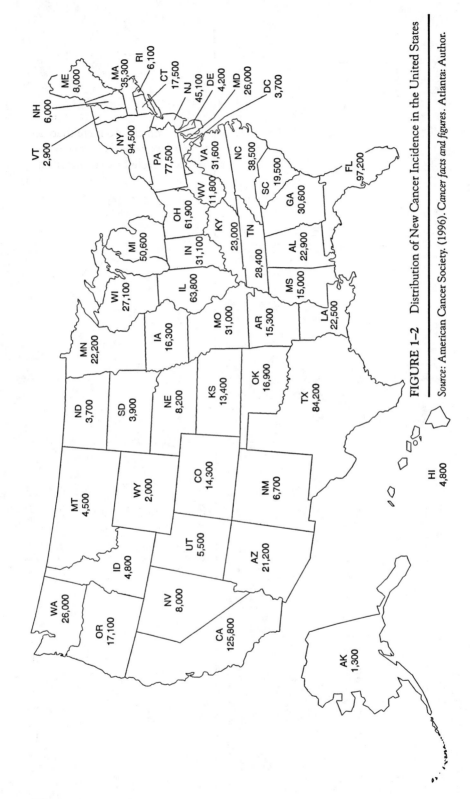

FIGURE 1–2   Distribution of New Cancer Incidence in the United States

Source: American Cancer Society. (1996). *Cancer facts and figures.* Atlanta: Author.

improved screening and treatment efforts. Examples include cervical, breast, colorectal, and testicular cancer.

Figure 1–3 shows the amounts of increase and decrease in the incidence of cancer originating in various sites for men and women from 1973 to 1991. The incidence of prostate cancer and malignant melanoma in men more than doubled in this time period. The risk of lung cancer for women also more than doubled. Figure 1–4 shows time trends in cancer mortality rates. For women, mortality from stomach, uterus, and colorectal cancer has declined dramatically during this century, while breast cancer mortality has increased slightly. Stomach cancer mortality has declined dramatically in men, while prostate and pancreatic cancer mortalities have increased. The most striking rise in cancer mortality in this century in both sexes has been for lung cancer. ,

SURVIVAL

Cancer survival is the reciprocal of cancer mortality: When cancer mortality rates decline, cancer survival rates increase. Cancer survival is reported as a **survival rate:** the proportion of a cohort with cancer that is still alive after a defined time interval. Approximately 40% of patients diagnosed with cancer in 1996 will be alive 5 years after diagnosis, an **observed survival rate** of 40%. Because some patients with cancer die of causes unrelated to cancer (e.g., heart disease, accident), observed cancer survival rates are adjusted for other causes of death. This adjusted rate is called the **relative survival rate,** and it is higher than the observed cancer survival rate because it reflects the probability of surviving cancer alone as a cause of death. The 5-year observed survival rate of 40% increases to 54% when it is adjusted for other causes of death.

Cancer survival rates vary along with the person, place, and time characteristics of the population. Table 1–5 shows time trends in 5-year cancer relative survival rates by race. Although both African Americans and white Americans have made gains in cancer survival over the years, whites still hold a survival advantage over African Americans. Much of this survival advantage is thought to be due to racial and ethnic differences in socioeconomic status, education, and access to health care.

CONCLUSION

By documenting observed differences in cancer incidence, mortality and survival among different populations, it is possible to identify cancer risk factors, suggest future directions for cancer control efforts, and evaluate current cancer control efforts. It is essential that nurses involved in cancer control efforts (prevention, detection, diagnosis, and treatment) understand trends in cancer incidence, mortality, and survival rates and numbers and be able to interpret them to others.

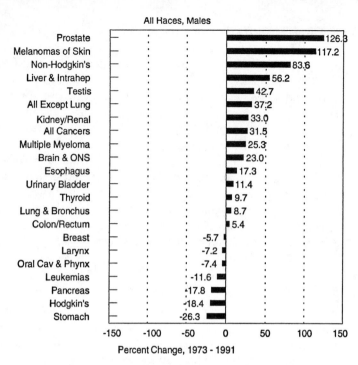

All Races, Males

Site	Percent Change, 1973 - 1991
Prostate	126.3
Melanomas of Skin	117.2
Non-Hodgkin's	83.6
Liver & Intrahep	56.2
Testis	42.7
All Except Lung	37.2
Kidney/Renal	33.0
All Cancers	31.5
Multiple Myeloma	25.3
Brain & ONS	23.0
Esophagus	17.3
Urinary Bladder	11.4
Thyroid	9.7
Lung & Bronchus	8.7
Colon/Rectum	5.4
Breast	-5.7
Larynx	-7.2
Oral Cav & Phynx	-7.4
Leukemias	-11.6
Pancreas	-17.8
Hodgkin's	-18.4
Stomach	-26.3

Percent Change, 1973 - 1991

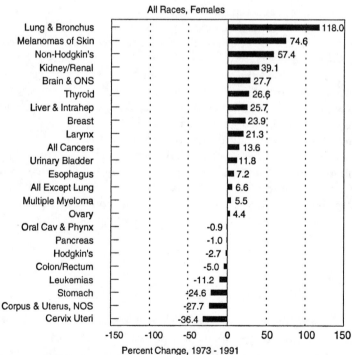

All Races, Females

Site	Percent Change, 1973 - 1991
Lung & Bronchus	118.0
Melanomas of Skin	74.6
Non-Hodgkin's	57.4
Kidney/Renal	39.1
Brain & ONS	27.7
Thyroid	26.6
Liver & Intrahep	25.7
Breast	23.9
Larynx	21.3
All Cancers	13.6
Urinary Bladder	11.8
Esophagus	7.2
All Except Lung	6.6
Multiple Myeloma	5.5
Ovary	4.4
Oral Cav & Phynx	-0.9
Pancreas	-1.0
Hodgkin's	-2.7
Colon/Rectum	-5.0
Leukemias	-11.2
Stomach	-24.6
Corpus & Uterus, NOS	-27.7
Cervix Uteri	-36.4

Percent Change, 1973 - 1991

*Surveillance, Epidemiology, and End Results

FIGURE 1–3 Trends in SEER* Incidence Rates by Primary Cancer Site 1973–1991

Source: Data from Gloeckler Ries, L. A., Miller, B. A., Hankey, B. F., Kosary, C. L., Harras, A., & Edwards, B. K. (Eds.) (1994). *SEER cancer statistics review, 1973–1991*. (NIH Pub. No. 94-2789). Bethesda, MD: National Institutes of Health.

Age-Adjusted Death Rates, *Females by Site, US 1930-1992

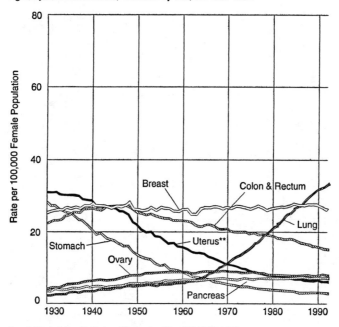

Age-Adjusted Death Rates, *Males by Site, US 1930-1992

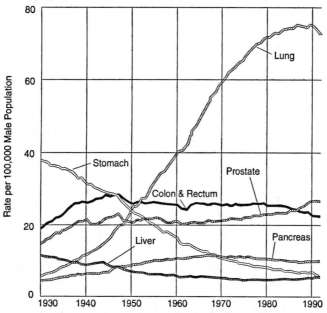

*Rates are per 100,000 and are age-adjusted to the 1970 standard population.
**Uterine cancer death rates are for cervix and corpus combined.
NOTE: Due to changes in ICD coding, numerator information has changed over time. Rates for cancer of the liver are particularly affected by these coding changes. Denominator information for the years 1930-1967 and 1991-1992 is based on intercensal population estimates, while denominator information for the years 1968-1990 is based on postcensal recalculation of estimates.

FIGURE 1–4   Time Trends in Cancer Mortality Rates

Source: National Center for Health Statistics, U.S. Department of Health and Human Services. Vital statistics of the United States, 1995. Washington, DC: U.S. Government Printing Office.

TABLE 1–5 Trends in Cancer Survival by Race (Cases Diagnosed in 1960–63, 1970–73, 1974–76, 1980–82, 1986–91)

	White					Black				
	Relative 5-Year Survival Rate (Percent)					Relative 5-Year Survival Rate (Percent)				
Site	1960–63[1]	1970–73[1]	1974–76[2]	1980–82[2]	1986–91[2]	1960–63[1]	1970–73[1]	1974–76[2]	1980–82[2]	1986–91[2]
All sites	39	43	50	52	58*	27	31	39	40	42*
Oral cavity & pharynx	45	43	55	55	55	—	—	36	31	33
Esophagus	4	4	5	7	11*	1	4	4	5	7*
Stomach	11	13	15	16	19*	8	13	16	19	20
Colon	43	49	50	56	62*	34	37	45	49	53*
Rectum	38	45	49	53	60*	27	30	42	38	52*
Liver	—	—	4	4	6*	—	—	1	2	5*
Pancreas	1	2	3	3	3*	1	2	3	5	5*
Larynx	53	62	66	69	68	—	—	58	59	52
Lung & bronchus	8	10	12	14	14*	5	7	11	12	11
Melanoma of skin	60	68	80	83	87*	—	—	66+	60++	70+
Breast (female)	63	68	75	77	84*	46	51	63	66	69*
Cervix uteri	58	64	69	68	71	47	61	64	61	56*
Corpus uteri & unspecified	73	81	89	83	85*	31	44	61	54	56
Ovary	32	36	36	39	44*	32	32	40	38	38
Prostate	50	63	68	74	87*	35	55	58	65	71*
Testis	63	72	79	92	95*	—	—	76+	90+	86+
Urinary bladder	53	61	74	79	82*	24	36	47	58	59*
Kidney & renal pelvis	37	46	52	51	59*	38	44	49	55	54

Brain & nervous system	18	20	22	25	28*	19	19	27	31	31
Thyroid gland	83	86	92	94	95*	—	—	88	95	91
Hodgkin's disease	40	67	71	75	81*	—	—	69	71	70
Non-Hodgkin's lymphoma	31	41	47	52	52*	—	—	48	51	45
Multiple myeloma	12	19	24	28	28*	—	—	27	29	29
Leukemia	14	22	35	39	41*	—	—	31	33	32

[1]Rates are based on End Results Group data from a series of hospital registries and one population-based registry.

[2]Rates are from the SEER program. They are based on data from population-based registries in Connecticut, New Mexico, Utah, Iowa, Hawaii, Atlanta, Detroit, Seattle-Puget Sound and San Francisco-Oakland. Rates are based on follow-up of patients through 1993.

*The difference in rates between 1974–76 and 1986–91 is statistically significant (p < 0.05).

†The standard error of the survival rate is between 5 and 10 percentage points.

††The standard error of the survival rate is greater than 10 percentage points.

—Valid survival rate could not be calculated.

Source: Cancer Statistics Branch, National Cancer Institute.

BIBLIOGRAPHY

American Cancer Society. (1996). *Cancer facts and figures—1996*. Atlanta: American Cancer Society.

Cartmel, B., & Reid, M. (1993). Cancer control and epidemiology. In S. L. Groenwald, M. H. Frogge, M. Goodman, & C. H. Yarbro (Eds.), *Cancer nursing principles and practice* (pp. 3–27). Sudbury, MA: Jones and Bartlett.

Frank-Stromborg, M., & Olsen, S. J. (Eds.). (1993). *Cancer prevention in minority populations: Cultural implications for health care professionals*. St. Louis: Mosby.

Fraumeni, J., Hoover, R. N., DeVesa, S. S., & Kinten, L. J. (1989). Epidemiology of cancer. In V. DeVita, S. Hellman, & S. Rosenberg (Eds.), *Cancer principles and practice of oncology* (pp. 196–235). Philadelphia: J.B. Lippincott.

Gloeckler Ries, L. A., Miller, B. A., Hankey, B. F., Kosary, C. L., Harras, A., & Edwards, B. K. (Eds.). (1994). *SEER cancer statistics review, 1973–1991*. (NIH Pub. No. 94-2789). Bethesda, MD: National Institutes of Health.

Jones, L. A. (Ed.). (1989). *Minorities and cancer*. New York: Springer-Verlag.

Lilenfeld, D. E., & Stolley, P. D. (1994). *Foundations of epidemiology* (3rd ed.). New York: Oxford University Press.

Oleske, D. M. (1991). Epidemiologic principles for cancer nursing practice: Assessing the cancer problem and planning its control. In S. B. Baird, R. McCorkle, & M. Grant (Eds.), *Cancer nursing: A comprehensive textbook* (pp. 91–103). Philadelphia: W. B. Saunders.

Parker, S. L., Tong, T., Bolden, S., & Wingo, P. A. (1996). Cancer statistics, 1996. *CA—A Cancer Journal for Clinicians, 46*, 5–28.

2

The Nature of Cancer

Jan M. Ellerhorst-Ryan

Although cancer is classified by organ system, it is actually a disease of cells. Every malignancy arises from one cell or a group of cells that were originally normal but have been altered in some way. The end result of the change, or transformation, is the loss of some or all of the cells' normal characteristics and the expression of abnormal characteristics. The changes that take place affect the cell's appearance, its surface membrane, and its growth characteristics (see Table 2–1).

CHARACTERISTICS OF MALIGNANT CELLS

Appearance

Each normal cell has a distinct and recognizable size, shape, and appearance, depending on the cell's degree of maturity. The space within the normal cell that is occupied by the nucleus is small compared to that containing the cytoplasm. When the cell has fully matured, or **differentiated,** it is ready to perform the specific function unique to its cell type. For example, a fully differentiated beta cell of the pancreas is able to manufacture insulin, while fully mature cardiac muscle cells are able to contract rhythmically.

Malignant cells have lost some, perhaps most, of the characteristic features of the normal cell's appearance. If the cancer cells appear fairly similar to their normal counterparts, the cancer is referred to as *well differentiated*. However, some malignant cells are so abnormal that their tissue of origin cannot be determined. These cells, referred to as **undifferentiated** or **anaplastic,** are usually more aggressive in their growth and behavior.

The nucleus of a cancer cell is often much larger than that of a normal cell, and occasionally more than one nucleus is present. Cancer cells are no longer

TABLE 2-1 Characteristics of Benign and Malignant Cells

Characteristic	Benign Cell	Malignant Cell
Shape, size	Regular, consistent	Irregular, pleomorphic
Differentiation	Well differentiated	Moderately differentiated to anaplastic
Nucleus	Single	Multiple
Nucleus-to-cytoplasm ratio	Small	High
Cell growth	Orderly, controlled	Random, uncontrolled
Mitoses	Rare	Frequent
Adherence	Present	Absent
Density-dependent growth inhibition	Present	Absent
Restriction point control	Present	Absent
Migration	Absent	Present

able to perform their designated function adequately, and they may sometimes assume functions of other cells. For example, **small-cell carcinoma of the lung** may begin to produce antidiuretic hormone, which is normally manufactured by the anterior pituitary gland.

Cell Surface

Normal cells manufacture cell surface components that enable the cells to bind closely and tightly together (adherence). A protein called fibronectin is particularly important in maintaining adherence between cells. Malignant cells produce surface components that are deficient in quantity and/or quality, so that the cells do not adhere well to each other.

Other components found on normal cell membranes are responsible for communication between one cell and another. These components enable cells to recognize the presence of another cell and to identify the tissue of origin. Cells that have the same tissue of origin will adhere to each other, but not to cells of different origin. Malignant cells often have fewer components attached to their surface, making it difficult to recognize and identify other cells in the vicinity. At the same time, some malignant cells may carry abnormal proteins on their surface, such as the alpha fetoprotein found on testicular cancer cells. These abnormal proteins, or **tumor markers,** are sometimes used to monitor the tumor's response to treatment or tumor recurrence.

Growth Characteristics

Normal cells reproduce in an orderly, controlled fashion. Under ordinary circumstances, normal cells divide for one of two reasons: to develop normal tissues, such as bone marrow, or to replace lost or damaged normal tissues, such as skin and intestinal mucosa. New cells are formed at a controlled rate, keeping the overall number of cells fairly constant.

TABLE 2–2 Common Carcinogens

Type	Example	Related Cancer
Chemical	Tobacco products	Lung, oral, bladder
	Alcohol products	Oral, esophageal
	Vinyl chloride	Angiosarcoma of the liver
Viruses	Human papilloma virus	Uterine cervix
	Human T-cell lymphotrophic virus type 1	Adult T-cell leukemia
	Hepatitis B virus	Liver
Radiation	Ionizing (diagnostic x-rays)	Almost any organ sufficiently exposed
	Ultraviolet (sunlight)	Skin, melanoma
Physical	Asbestos	Lung, peritoneum
	Wood dust	Nasal sinuses

Normal tissues recognize the presence of other cells and will not divide when there is inadequate space (density-dependent growth inhibition) or a lack of nutrients (restriction point control). With the exception of leukocytes and erythrocytes, normal cells do not wander from one tissue to another, but remain with other like cells within their designated organ or organ system (i.e., they are non-migratory).

Cells that have undergone **malignant transformation** have lost the ability to know when to stop dividing. Their growth pattern is random and disorganized. No longer respecting cell borders, the reproducing cells overlap, actually piling up as the malignancy grows. Cancer cells do not respond appropriately to poor environmental conditions; they continue to divide even when space and nutrients are lacking.

Cancer cells also have the ability to free themselves from the tumor or tissue of origin. By secreting enzymes that dissolve proteins binding normal cells together, cancer cells are able to migrate from one tissue or organ to another.

CARCINOGENESIS

Carcinogenesis is the process by which one or more normal cells undergoes genetic alterations that result in malignant transformation. It involves exposure of cellular DNA to **carcinogens,** substances or agents that can damage genetic material. Known carcinogens include chemical agents, viruses, ionizing and ultraviolet radiation, and physical substances. Specific examples of each category of carcinogen are listed in Table 2–2.

Malignant transformation occurs through a sequence of events: initiation, promotion, progression, and metastasis.

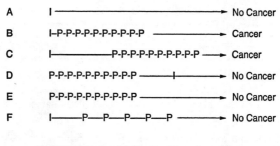

FIGURE 2–1 Malignant Transformation

Key: I = exposure to initiator; P = exposure to promotor

Initiation

Initiation is the direct exposure of DNA to a carcinogen resulting in irreversible changes that will permit malignant transformation. The initiated cell appears somewhat abnormal, perhaps referred to as *dysplastic* or *premalignant*, but it is still able to function normally.

Several factors are required for initiation to occur. The exposure must alter DNA structure—causing one or more breaks in the DNA chain, eliminating a genetic component, resulting in faulty DNA repair, or inserting new genetic information into the DNA strand. The change must be permanent and irreparable, and it must not inhibit the cell's ability to replicate itself. For malignant transformation to occur, the initiating event must precede promotion.

Promotion

Promotion occurs when the initiated cell is exposed to an agent that encourages or enhances cell growth. The promoting agent does not react directly with DNA; it reacts with other parts of the cell, such as cell surface receptors, to stimulate cell growth and activity.

Unlike those of initiators, the effects of promoters may be reversible if there are prolonged periods between exposures. Promoters have a definite threshold, a specific minimum required dose or exposure, before their effect occurs (Figure 2–1). Examples of promoting agents include certain hormones (e.g., prolactin), plant products, chemical agents (e.g., "Agent Orange"), and viruses.

A latency period typically exists between initiation and tumor development. The length of the latency period varies with individual genetic make-up and immune status, type of carcinogenic exposure, environmental considerations (e.g., occupation, alcohol and tobacco use, etc.), degree of exposure, and the type of cell exposed.

Progression

Progression is characterized by a series of changes in the transformed cell, including accelerated growth rate, enhanced invasiveness, and altered appearance and biochemical activity. Once the cluster of malignant cells has become a detectable mass (about 1 cm), it contains at least 1 billion cells.

Genetic instability within the colony of transformed cells results in the development of subpopulations that differ from each other in their growth properties, sensitivities to treatment modalities, and other such characteristics. Certain mutations will eventually provide to one or more subpopulations a *selection advantage*, a mutation that enables survival despite environmental changes that are unfavorable to other subpopulations.

Metastasis

Metastasis is the ability of transformed cells to relocate from their original population by direct extension, invasion, and/or establishment of remote sites. Metastasis is not the result of random survival of cells from the primary tumor; it represents the selective growth of specific cells or subpopulations with unique properties that equip them for survival and successful metastatic growth. Factors influencing metastatic potential include host immune defenses, mechanical factors (e.g., turbulence within the circulatory system), and the number of cells released by the primary tumor.

The term **metastatic cascade** is used to describe a multistep process for cancer spread beyond the primary tumor:

1. *Vascularization or angiogenesis.* The tumor progresses in size and develops internal vascularization. Tumor angiogenesis factor (TAF) stimulates growth and development of new blood vessels within the tumor; however, these newly formed vessels are often defective and easily invaded by tumor cells.

2. *Invasion.* The malignancy extends into surrounding tissue by producing enzymes that dissolve substances holding normal cells together. The tumor also manufactures motility factors, agents that facilitate encroachment of tumor cells into normal tissues.

3. *Intravasion.* The tumor penetrates through the basement membrane and into body cavities or blood vessels. Malignant cells produce enzymes that create holes the in capillary endothelium and allow transformed cells to escape.

4. *Embolization and transport.* Tumor cells are released to be carried to other body sites. En route, they will interact with platelets, lymphocytes, fibrinogen, and other host protective influences. It is estimated that only 1% of tumor cells reaching this stage will survive for 24 hours, with less than 0.01% establishing metastatic colonies.

5. *Arrest.* Tumor cells are eventually trapped in the capillary bed of the target organ. The cell or cell cluster adheres to the vascular epithelium, stimulating the intrinsic pathway of the coagulation cascade. Development of a fibrin meshwork around the malignant cell or cell cluster protects it from detection by the host's immune system.

6. *Extravasation*. The tumor cell releases enzymes that dissolve the basement membrane of the vascular endothelium and allow the cell to invade the surrounding tissues.

7. *Establishment*. The malignant cells manipulate the new environment to promote growth and development of the metastatic colony. If it is unable to establish its own vascular supply, the new colony will die.

GENETIC FACTORS IN CANCER DEVELOPMENT

Role of Oncogenes

Oncogenes are genes that, when activated, can enhance tumor progression. Often oncogenes are normal genes that should be permanently turned "off" but, because of chromosomal rearrangements caused by carcinogenic exposure, are switched "on" instead. One of the mechanisms thought to be linked to oncogene activation involves **anti-oncogenes,** or tumor suppressor genes. The purpose of these genes appears to be the regulation or suppression of oncogenes. If the tumor suppressor gene is damaged or removed, restriction of oncogene activity may be reduced or eliminated.

The results of oncogene activation may be qualitative (a defective protein is produced) or quantitative (the protein produced is normal but present in abnormally high amounts). In either event, the change in protein manufacture within the transformed cell accelerates neoplastic development.

An example of a well-known chromosomal rearrangement resulting in cancer progression is the **Philadelphia chromosome** associated with **chronic myelogenous leukemia (CML).** The oncogene known as *c-abl* is normally found on chromosome 22 but is moved, or translocated, to a specific site on chromosome 9 or, less frequently, chromosome 8. This rearrangement results in the production of an abnormal protein with markedly elevated enzyme activity (Figure 2–2).

Heredity and Cancer

Inherited cancers are those in which initiation occurs at conception. The genetic material in either the ovum or the fertilizing sperm contains a mutation that constitutes the first step in carcinogenesis. The mutation involved must be autosomal dominant—that is, the disease affects males and females equally and requires that only one parent pass on the defective gene. Examples include **retinoblastoma,** an intraocular malignancy that develops in infants and children; **Wilm's tumor,** a childhood cancer involving the kidney; and **familial adenomatous polyposis,** which leads to colorectal cancer in nearly 100% of those affected. More recently, genetic mutations responsible for hereditary breast and ovarian cancers have been identified.

Inherited cancers account for only about 1% to 2% of all malignancies; however, a significant percentage of certain tumors are inherited. For instance, up to 40% of retinoblastoma cases and 20% to 30% of Wilm's tumor cases involve

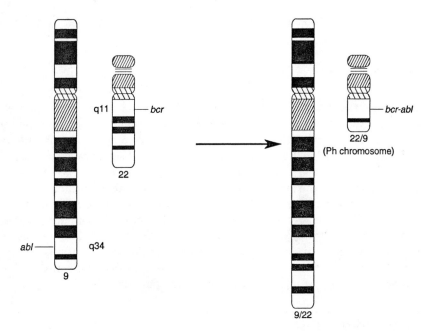

FIGURE 2–2 Reciprocal translocation between the long arms of chromosome 9 and 22 to generate the Philadelphia (Ph) chromosome. The *abl* proto-oncogene is translocated from 9q34 to the q11 region of chromosome 22, where a new fusion gene, *bcr-abl*, is formed. This leads to activation of *abl*.

inherited malignancies. On the other hand, only about 8% of all breast cancer cases and 5% to 10% of ovarian cancer cases are truly hereditary.

Inherited predisposition occurs when there is an indirect relationship between the genetic change and cancer development. Predisposition is inherited as autosomal recessive—that is, it affects both males and females but requires that both parents contribute altered genes. Examples include the syndrome of fragile chromosomes, marked by frequent chromosomal breakages and faulty DNA repair; xeroderma pigmentosa, an extreme sensitivity to sunlight (also associated with faulty DNA repair, particularly following ultraviolet damage to DNA); ataxia telangiectasia, characterized by progressive cerebellar ataxia, immune deficiencies, increased sensitivity to ionizing radiation, and higher incidence of leukemia; non-Hodgkin's lymphoma; and tumors of the breast, ovary, stomach, and pancreas.

Familial clustering, or *aggregation,* refers to those situations in which a pattern exists but the exact role of heredity is unclear. Multiple cancers presenting in one family may be the result of inherited susceptibility or of common exposures within the family, such as diet or environmental exposure. Most families having several members with breast cancer represent familial clustering rather than hereditary cancer.

CONCLUSION

Carcinogenesis is a multistep process by which a normal cell undergoes progressive changes and ultimately becomes malignant. Among the many differences between normal cells and their cancerous counterparts is cancer's lack of response to normal cell growth control mechanisms. Cancer cells continue to divide despite limited space and nutritional resources. They also have the ability to separate from the primary tumor and migrate to other body sites.

Recent cancer research findings have enhanced understanding about carcinogenesis, the metastatic cascade, and genetic factors that influence tumor growth and development. While much still needs to be known before improvements can be made in cancer treatment, nurses can play important roles in cancer prevention by educating consumers about known carcinogens in the environment and emphasizing the importance of reducing exposure.

BIBLIOGRAPHY

Garrol-Johnson, R. (Ed.). (1995). The genetic revolution: Promise and predicament for oncology nurses. *Oncology Nursing Forum, 22* (suppl.), 3–36.

Groenwald, S. L. (1993). Invasion and metastasis. In S. L. Groenwald, M. Frogge, M. Goodman, & C. Yarbro (Eds.), *Cancer nursing: Principles and practice* (3rd ed., pp. 59–70). Sudbury, MA: Jones and Bartlett.

Lind, J. (1992). Tumor cell growth and cell kinetics. *Seminars in Oncology Nursing, 8,* 3–9.

Mahon, S. M., & Casperson, D. S. (1995). Hereditary cancer syndrome: Part I: Clinical and educational issues. *Oncology Nursing Forum, 22,* 763–771.

McMillan, S. C. (1992). Carcinogenesis. *Seminars in Oncology Nursing, 8,* 10–19.

Weinberg, R. A. (1994). Oncogenes and tumor suppressor genes. *CA—A Journal for Clinicians, 44,* 160–170.

Workman, M. L. (1995). Altered cell development and growth. In D. D. Ignatavicius, M. L. Workman, & M. A. Mishler (Eds.), *Medical-surgical nursing: A nursing process approach.* (pp. 545–560). Philadelphia: W. B. Saunders.

Zbar, B. (1992). The biology and genetics of hereditary cancers. *Seminars in Oncology Nursing, 8,* 229–234.

3

Cancer Prevention and Risk Assessment

Karen Billars Heusinkveld

Cancer is the second leading cause of death in the United States, surpassed only by heart disease. However, it has been estimated that cancer will surpass heart disease as the number one cause of death by the year 2000. In 1996 alone, 1,359,150 individuals were expected to be diagnosed with cancer and 554,740 were expected to die from it. The best way to control cancer is to find ways of reducing the risk of cancer and potentially preventing it.

Researchers estimate that if everything known about cancer prevention were applied, up to two-thirds of cancers would not occur. Thus, cancer could be prevented in over 900,000 of the individuals expected to be diagnosed with cancer in 1996. Cancer evolves over time, and the pathological changes become less treatable or curable as the disease process continues. The ultimate aim of cancer prevention is to halt or reverse any *prepathogenesis*, or susceptibility of the individual to cancer. Yet, cancer prevention is not always possible.

LEVELS OF PREVENTION

The three-level model for intervention described in this chapter is based on the natural history of disease. The three levels of prevention are primary, secondary, and tertiary. The goal of intervention at each of the three levels is to prevent the pathogenic process from evolving further.

Primary Prevention

Primary prevention is aimed at intervention before pathological changes have begun. Primary prevention efforts include both general health promotion and specific protection.

General health promotion includes all activities that improve the physical environment, including the home, school, workplace, and outdoors, and those that favor healthy living. Health education aimed at informing the population about good nutrition, the harmful effects of smoking, and sun exposure is a form of general health promotion.

Specific protection refers to measures aimed at protecting individuals against specific agents such as infectious diseases. For conditions caused by noninfectious agents such as cancer, there may be no single agent. There is no inoculation, no onetime action, that can protect people from cancer. For example, lung cancer may result from tobacco use, air pollution, and hazardous substances in the workplace. Each of these potential agents must therefore be eliminated to ensure control of the disease. Specific protection measures such as removal of hazardous substances from the workplace will reduce occurrence óf the disease but will not eliminate it. Primary prevention depends upon the avoidance of cancer risks by individuals in their daily lives.

Secondary Prevention

Secondary prevention efforts seek to detect disease early and treat it promptly. The goal is to cure the disease at its earliest stage, or, when cure is impossible, to slow its progression, prevent complications, and limit disability. Thus, secondary prevention is focused primarily on presymptomatic disease or very early clinical disease.

Screening is the most common form of secondary prevention. It is estimated that 75% of all cancers in the United States could be cured if all the available early detection tests and self-examination methods were practiced routinely. Regular screening and self-examinations can detect cancers of the breast, tongue, mouth, colon, rectum, cervix, prostate, testis, and skin at an early stage, when treatment is more likely to be successful. If these cancers were detected early and treated promptly, the 5-year survival rate would be about 92%.

Tertiary Prevention

Tertiary prevention includes limitation of disability for individuals in the earlier stages of illness and rehabilitation for those who have already experienced residual damage. Preventing arm immobility after breast surgery and monitoring an individual's status for complications during chemotherapy are examples of tertiary prevention.

RISK FACTORS

Cancer is caused by both external factors (e.g., chemicals, radiation, and viruses) and internal factors (e.g., hormones, immune conditions, and inherited mutations). Causal factors may act together or in sequence to initiate or promote carcinogenesis. Ten or more years often pass between exposures and detectable cancers. Associations between disease and exposure to specific agents or factors are usually quantified in terms of different levels of risks. Knowledge of these risks plays a significant part in cancer prevention.

Risk is defined as the potential realization of unwanted consequences of an event—the probability of injury or death. A **risk factor** is an element of personal behavior, genetic make-up, or exposure to a known cancer-causing agent that increases a person's chances of developing a particular form of cancer.

Relative risk measures the strength of the association between a factor and the outcome. Relative risk of cancer is a ratio of the probability of developing cancer among a group having a particular characteristic or risk factor to the probability of developing cancer among a similar group without the characteristic or risk factor.

$$\text{Relative risk} \; = \; \frac{\text{Number with cancer in exposed population}}{\text{Number of exposed population}}$$

$$\div \; \frac{\text{Number with cancer in an unexposed population}}{\text{Number of unexposed population}}$$

If the relative risk is greater than 1, an individual with the characteristic or risk factor is more likely to develop cancer than an individual without that characteristic or risk factor. If the relative risk is less than 1, an individual with the characteristic or risk factor is less likely to develop cancer than an individual without it. If the relative risk is 1, the cancer and the characteristic or factor are not associated. The higher the relative risk, the greater the evidence of causation.

An example of relative risk assessment is found in a study of development of lung cancer in smokers and nonsmokers. In this study, 200,000 individuals, one-half of whom were smokers, were followed for 10 years. Of these, 1,300 smokers and 100 nonsmokers were diagnosed with lung cancer. The relative risk is calculated as follows:

$$\text{Relative risk} \; = \; \frac{1,300}{100,000} \; \div \; \frac{100}{100,000} \; = \; \frac{.013}{.001} \; = \; 13$$

The relative risk of 13 for lung cancer for smokers compared to nonsmokers indicates evidence of a causative link between smoking and lung cancer.

Tobacco use and exposure to ultraviolet radiation are known to be high risk factors for lung cancer and skin cancer respectively. Excessive alcohol consumption and a high-fat diet are also risk factors for development of cancer, but their associations are not as strong as those for tobacco use and ultraviolet radiation. Continued research is necessary to establish these associations.

Risk factors may be individual, family, or group attributes. A high-risk group is one that shares risk factors due to its members' common genetic make-up, socioeconomic status, occupation, habits, or ethnic background. Individuals who use tobacco are an example of a high-risk group, since their lung cancer incidence and mortality rates are significantly higher than the average. Individuals who practice the Mormon religion are an example of a low-risk group, since their cancer incidence and mortality rates are significantly below the average.

Risk factors can be classified into *exogenous* (environmental and lifestyle) and *endogenous* (genetic) factors. Much is known about the dangerous effects of lifestyle factors that are associated with certain cancers. Tobacco use, excessive alcohol use, and overexposure to the sun's rays are all factors indicating the need for a change in lifestyle to reduce the risk of developing cancer. Lifestyle changes are extremely difficult because personal choices must be made within a social context of values, attitudes, motivation, peer pressure, family, and community.

For some environmental risk factors, such as certain chemicals (benzene, asbestos, vinyl chloride) and ionizing radiation (x-rays, radon, cosmic rays), there is definite evidence of carcinogenesis in humans. Health protection strategies for these risk factors include regulatory measures that confer protection on large population groups. Both occupational and environmental safety regulations have been developed to reduce environmental risk factors.

In the field of genetics, profound advances have occurred relating to risk factors and cancer genes. Genetic changes may involve one or more gene mutations, gross chromosomal abnormalities, or changes in gene transcription involving altered growth properties of cells. **Oncogenes,** which play a role in normal cell growth and differentiation, can mutate and cause runaway cell growth associated with cancer. The presence of certain oncogenes can be used to identify family members at risk. Pre-symptomatic testing to determine susceptibility to common cancers such as those of the breast, ovary, colon, and prostate is a potentially substantial advance in cancer prevention.

Suppressor genes, which exist in normal cells to control cell growth, can become mutated and allow uncontrolled cell growth. The p53 suppressor gene is altered in more than 50% of cancers, including breast and lung cancers. A mutated gene, **BRCA1,** has been found to be associated with high lifelong risks for breast cancer and ovarian cancer. Some families show an unusually high incidence of cancer of all types. For example, for some families, the risk of developing breast cancer or colon cancer may be 20 to 30 times greater than that for the average-risk individual. However, clinical applications of genetic testing present a dilemma for health care professionals because appropriate medical care for individuals with genetic mutations has not yet been developed.

FACTORS RELATED TO CARCINOGENESIS

The following are areas in which certain health choices might reduce an individual's risk of cancer (see Table 3–1).

Tobacco

Use of tobacco is the most preventable cause of death in our society, and avoidance of tobacco is the best-known method of cancer prevention. Tobacco use is responsible for nearly one in five deaths in the United States. Cigarette smoking is responsible for 90% of lung cancer among men and 79% among women—about 87% over all. The risks of dying of lung cancer are 22 times higher for male

TABLE 3–1   High-Risk Factors for Selected Cancer Sites

Cancer Site	High-Risk Factor
Lung	Cigarette smoking Radiation exposure Secondhand smoke
Skin	Excessive exposure to sun Fair complexion Occupational exposure
Breast	Increasing age Personal/family history of breast cancer High-fat diet Early menarche/late menopause
Colon/rectum	Personal/family history of polyps High-fat and/or low-fiber diet History of ulcerative colitis Age: > 50
Prostate	African-American man Increasing age (after age 50) Family history of prostate cancer
Uterus/endometrial	Estrogen replacement therapy Early menarche/late menopause Age: > 50
Oral	Tobacco use (cigarette, cigar, pipe, smokeless tobacco) Excessive alcohol use

smokers and 12 times higher for female smokers than for people who have never smoked. In addition to being responsible for 87% of lung cancers, smoking is also associated with cancers of the mouth, pharynx, larynx, esophagus, pancreas, uterine cervix, kidney, and bladder.

This high-risk group has the following profile: Smoking prevalence is highest among people with incomes below the poverty level; over 70% of adults who have smoked started smoking daily before age 18; by age 18, about two-thirds of adolescents have tried smoking; and about 14% of high school students report frequent cigarette use.

Environmental tobacco smoke presents a serious problem in the United States. Each year about 3,000 nonsmoking adults die of lung cancer as a result of breathing the smoke of others' cigarettes. There has been a resurgence in the use of all forms of smokeless tobacco (plug, leaf, and snuff), but the greatest cause for concern is the increased use of "dipping snuff." When the snuff is placed between the gum and cheek, the highly addictive nicotine, along with a number of

carcinogens, is absorbed through the oral tissue. Oral cancer occurs several times more frequently among snuff dippers than among nontobacco users, and the risk of cancer of the cheek and gum may increase nearly fiftyfold among long-term snuff users. The use of smokeless tobacco is increasing among male adolescents and young male adults; in fact, 20% of male high school students use smokeless tobacco.

Nutrition and Diet

Research is showing the important role nutrition plays in preventing cancer. Individuals who are 40% or more overweight have an increased risk of cancer of the colon, breast, prostate, gallbladder, ovary, and uterus. Evidence indicates that diets that are high in fat may be a factor in the development of cancers of the breast, colon, and prostate. Diets that are high in salt-cured, smoked, and nitrite-cured foods have shown an association with cancer of the esophagus and stomach.

The risk of cancer can be lowered by eating a varied, low-fat diet: Daily consumption of at least five servings of a variety of vegetables and fruits can decrease the risk of lung, prostate, bladder, esophagus, colon/rectal, and stomach cancers. Diets that are high in fiber may reduce the risk of colon cancer.

Alcohol

Alcohol contributes to about 5% of all cancer deaths. High alcohol consumption has been associated with cancer of the buccal cavity, pharynx, larynx, esophagus, liver, large bowel, and breast. Because individuals tend to drink alcohol and smoke at the same time, it is difficult to calculate the role of alcohol consumption alone. Drinking alcohol and smoking together have a combined effect contributing to the high incidence of some cancers.

Estrogen

Estrogen treatment to control menopausal symptoms may increase the risk of endometrial cancer. However, including progesterone in estrogen replacement therapy helps to minimize the risk. The research is inconclusive on the association of estrogen use and breast cancer.

Ultraviolet Radiation

Skin cancer is the most common type of cancer among Caucasians in the United States. The most serious skin cancer is melanoma, and its incidence rate is increasing by about 4% per year. About 90% of skin cancer is thought to be related to sun exposure. About one in six individuals will develop skin cancer during the course of their lifetime. The sun's ultraviolet rays are strongest between 10 A.M. and 3 P.M. Exposure should be avoided at these times, and protective clothing should be worn. Sunscreens with an SPF (sun protection factor) of at least 30 should be used.

TABLE 3-2 Nursing Interventions for Prevention

Risk Factor	Nursing Intervention
Tobacco use	Educate minors on dangers of tobacco use Regulate for decreasing access to tobacco use for minors Regulate for smoke-free air Help smokers quit
Nutrition	Educate on low-fat, high-fiber diet Regulate for nutritional labels on food products
Sun exposure	Educate on sun exposure dangers Educate on use of sunscreens
Alcohol	Educate on alcohol use moderation
Estrogen	Counsel about risks versus benefits
Occupational hazards	Regulate for worker protection Regulate for prevention and removal of hazards
Increasing age	Educate that cancer incidence rises with age

Occupational Exposure

Exposure to several different industrial agents (e.g., nickel, chromate, arsenic, aflatoxin, benzine, asbestos, vinyl chloride) increases the risk of various cancers. Exposure to ionizing radiation and ultraviolet radiation have also been found to result in cancer in humans.

The federal government has developed health and safety regulations that must be followed, and firms have developed policies and procedures to protect their workers.

CANCER PREVENTION AND NURSES

In the past, little attention was given to cancer prevention and early intervention. The focus of health care providers was on providing more technology and services. With the shift in health care policy and priorities, however, changes are beginning to be seen, driven partly by economics and an aging population. Financial incentives are being created to prevent disease or detect it early. Educating individuals to adapt healthy lifestyles and change harmful behaviors is becoming increasingly important.

As a result, nurses now have an opportunity to take a leading role in reducing cancer mortality. We must make a concerted effort to encourage people to make appropriate lifestyle changes and to limit exposure to known carcinogens, for cancer prevention is the best defense against cancer (see Table 3-2).

There are three major approaches to cancer prevention: education, regulation, and host modification. Education is intended to reduce the cancer-causing behaviors of individuals. Educational programs must include messages to avoid tobacco use, avoid exposure to the sun and use sun blockers, modify the diet, and improve workplace practices to reduce exposure to carcinogens. Educational programs can be implemented on a one-to-one basis, be targeted to high-risk groups, or take the form of mass-media campaigns. All educational programs must be age and culture sensitive.

Some carcinogens cannot be avoided by means of individual behavior changes and educational programs. For some environmental carcinogens, a regulatory approach is needed. Regulations and guidelines are needed to prohibit the sale of tobacco to minors, to prohibit smoking in public places, to impose taxes on tobacco products, and to reduce workplace environmental carcinogens. Immunization and chemoprevention methods currently being explored show promise as risk-reduction techniques. With increasing knowledge about cancer genetics, nurses will be instrumental in educating the public and discussing the decisions that need to be made concerning appropriate use of genetic testing.

Nurses have an important responsibility and opportunity to help individuals, groups, and communities in cancer prevention activities. If we are willing to use the knowledge we now have about cancer prevention and risk reduction, we will be well on the road to the elimination of cancer. The time is right to increase our knowledge and skills and to integrate cancer prevention into nursing practice.

BIBLIOGRAPHY

Frank-Stromborg, M., Heusinkveld, K., & Rohan, K. (1996). Evaluating cancer risks and preventative oncology. In R. McCorkle, M. Grant, M. Frank-Stromborg, & S. Baird (Eds.), *Cancer nursing: A comprehensive textbook* (2nd ed., pp. 213–264). Philadelphia: W. B. Saunders.

Garfinkel, L. (1991). Nutrition and cancer. *CA—A Cancer Journal for Clinicians, 41,* 325–327.

Garfinkel, L. (1995). Perspectives on cancer prevention. *CA—A Cancer Journal for Clinicians, 41,* 5–7.

Heusinkveld, K. B. (1991). Preventative oncology. In S. Baird, R. McCorkle, & M. Grant (Eds.), *Cancer nursing: A comprehensive textbook* (pp. 143–154). Philadelphia: W. B. Saunders.

Loescher, L. J. (1995). Genetics in cancer prediction, screening, and counseling: Part I, genetics in cancer prevention and screening. *Oncology Nursing Forum, 22 (Suppl.),* 10–15.

U.S. Department of Health and Human Services. (1991). *Healthy people 2000: National health promotion and disease prevention objectives.* (DHHS Publication No. 91-50212). Washington, DC: Public Health Service.

U.S. Department of Health and Human Services. (1994). *Smoking and tobacco control monograph 5: Tobacco and the clinician.* (NIH Publication No. 94-3693). Washington, DC: Public Health Service.

4

Cancer Screening and Early Detection

Marilyn Frank-Stromborg

Secondary prevention, which consists of early screening, detection, and diagnosis of cancer, has become an important part of cancer care in the United States. By detecting cancer at the earliest stage possible, curing it or slowing its progression, preventing complications, and limiting disability, both length and quality of life can be maximized.

Cancer **screening,** the search for disease in persons without symptoms, is an organized effort to find cancer in its early stages in a defined population. Screening is conducted at intermittent time intervals and is usually site specific. Nurses frequently play an important role in educating the public about screening programs and in conducting screening tests. Once a person has had a positive screening test, or once signs or symptoms have been identified, further tests are considered diagnostic.

Early **detection** is the identification of disease in an individual—when it is still localized, curable, or manageable—or the identification of a precancerous lesion. The individual may or may not be asymptomatic, and identification is made through tests, examinations, and observations. Both cancer screening and early detection activities tend to focus on cancers that have a high incidence and in which early diagnosis contributes to increased survival.

In the secondary prevention of cancer, nurses' responsibilities may include assessment, counseling, teaching, screening and detection, planning, acting as an advocate, and acting as a role model. Nurses in advanced practice roles may conduct screening and detection tests, such as doing Pap smears, doing clinical breast examinations, and conducting physical examinations. In addition to fulfilling these roles, nurses provide support and guidance while performing these functions.

SCREENING ISSUES

There are multiple issues involved in screening a predetermined population (e.g., screening African-American men for prostate cancer), particularly in this era of cost containment. Questions raised about screening include the following: Can screening recommendations by the National Cancer Institute or the American Cancer Society decrease deaths from cancer? Are they cost effective? How can their performance be optimized?

An implicit assumption underlying any screening program is that early detection will lead to a more favorable prognosis, because treatment begun early in the disease course will be more effective than later treatment. This assumption holds true for some cancers, such as breast and testicular cancer, but it is not true for others such as lung cancer. Research has shown that using routine cytology and x-rays with heavy smokers has no effect in reducing lung cancer mortality. Thus, the American Cancer Society and other groups do not recommend that heavy smokers be screened yearly for lung cancer. Table 4–1 summarizes The American Cancer Society's recommendations for the early detection of cancer in a predetermined asymptomatic population. These should be incorporated into the regular physical examination as appropriate. The 1989 and 1990 federal legislation mandating Medicare coverage for cervical and breast cancer screening has enhanced compliance with the ACS recommendations. For women over the age of 65, Medicare currently covers a **Papanicolaou (Pap)** smear once every 3 years and a mammogram every 2 years. As a result of this coverage, many women are able to take advantage of national screening recommendations for this population.

Certain inherent characteristics must be present in a cancer for screening to be cost effective and efficient:

1. The cancer must have a poor prognosis when symptoms appear.
2. There must be a high prevalence of the cancer in the population being screened.
3. The cancer must be detectable in the presymptomatic stage.
4. There must be an improved prognosis when the cancer is found by screening.
5. There must be consensus on the efficacy of treatment for the early stages of this disease.
6. The test to detect the cancer must be available.

Another issue that arises with cancer screening concerns the sensitivity, specificity, and predictive value of the screening test itself. The screening test that is used should be able to detect cancer before the onset of signs and symptoms. **Specificity** is defined as the probability that a screening test will correctly classify an individual as negative for cancer when the individual does not have the disease. In contrast, **sensitivity** is defined as the probability that a screening test will correctly classify an individual as positive for cancer when that person actually does have the disease. The **predictive value** of a test refers to the per-

TABLE 4-1 Summary of American Cancer Society Recommendations for the Early Detection of Cancer in Asymptomatic People

Test or Procedure	Sex	Age	Frequency
			Population
Sigmoidoscopy, preferably flexible	M & F	50 and over	Every 3–5 years, based on advice of physician
Fecal occult blood test	M & F	50 and over	Every year
Digital rectal examination (DRE)	M & F	40 and over	Every year
Prostate-specific antigen blood test	M	50 and over	Every year
Pap test	F	All women who are or who have been sexually active, or have reached age 18	After a woman has had three or more consecutive satisfactory normal annual examinations, the Pap test may be performed less frequently at the discretion of her physician.
Pelvic examination	F	18–40	Every 1–3 years with Pap test
		Over 40	Every year
Endometrial tissue sample	F	At menopause, if at high risk*	At menopause and thereafter at the discretion of the physician.
Breast self-examination	F	20 and over	Every month
Breast clinical examination	F	20–40	Every 3 years
		Over 40	Every year
Mammography	F	40–49	Screening mammogram by age 40; then every 1–2 years
		50 and over	Every year
Health counseling and cancer checkup**	M & F	Over 20	Every 3 years
	M & F	Over 40	Every year

*History of infertility, obesity, failure to ovulate, abnormal uterine bleeding, or unopposed estrogen or tamoxifen therapy.
**To include examination for cancers of the thyroid, testicles, prostate, ovaries, lymph nodes, oral region, and skin.

Source: The American Cancer Society. (1996). *Cancer facts and figures—1996* (No. 5008.96). Atlanta: Author.

centage of persons with positive screening test results who actually have cancer. Presently there is no perfect test. Generally, the more sensitive a test is, the less specific it will be, and a balance must be struck between the two indices of sensitivity and specificity.

In tests with less than 100% sensitivity, a proportion of preclinical cancers will not be diagnosed at screening. A major problem with tests with low sensitivity is that they lead individuals to believe that they do not have cancer. In contrast, in tests with less than 100% specificity, false positives are expected. Tests with low specificity not only overwhelm diagnostic services and result in prohibitive follow-up costs, but also expose individuals to the risks of unnecessary diagnostic work-ups, resulting in potentially substantial physical and psychological morbidity and possible mortality.

The cost-benefit ratios are favorable for screening for cervical, breast, and colorectal cancers. Less is known about the cost-benefit ratios for screening for cancers of the stomach, esophagus, bladder, or liver.

It is known that sensitivity and specificity can vary from setting to setting. Factors that can influence these two indices include optimal laboratory practice and clinical expertise. Nurses can have a substantial impact on the accuracy of such screening techniques as the Pap smear, digital rectal examination for prostate cancer, and physical breast examination. For instance, nurses assisting with the collection of the Pap smear can make sure that (a) the patient is properly prepared for the examination and told not to douche or take a tub bath 24 hours prior to the examination; (b) the specimen taken from the patient is immediately fixed with fixative spray or put in the fixative solution; (c) the specimen is properly labeled; and (d) there is proper follow-up of positive results.

Effective screening practices should begin with a health history and physical examination. The accuracy and completeness of history taking and physical examination are essential to a differential diagnosis. Information gathered during history taking includes medical, family, social, occupational, and sexual background. When obtaining the health history, the nurse should make sure that every individual is asked whether he or she has experienced any warning sign or symptom that could indicate a cancer (see Figure 4–1). This is an excellent opportunity for the nurse to educate the individual about what to watch for. The nurse may also acquire information about exposure to certain cancer-causing agents, personal habits (e.g., smoking, chewing tobacco, excessive alcohol use), and membership in a particular racial or ethnic group (e.g., Hispanic, African American, Native American), all of which may place the individual in a high-risk category. The history may lead to detection of vague symptoms that the patient may be unaware of or be denying. This thorough history taking is followed by the physical examination of body systems, which includes inspection, palpation, percussion, and auscultation.

The screening process is more than a set of examinations and tests. It is an excellent opportunity for nurses to educate patients about self-examination techniques, stop-smoking programs, and personal and occupational health hazards. Patients can perform self-examination of breasts, testes, skin, and the oral cavity.

Change in bowel or bladder habits.
A sore that does not heal.
Unusual bleeding or discharge.
Thickening or lump in breast or elsewhere.
Indigestion or difficulty swallowing.
Obvious change in wart or mole.
Nagging cough or hoarseness.

FIGURE 4–1   The American Cancer Society's Seven
Warning Signs for Cancer

The American Cancer Society has excellent materials to teach self-examination techniques.

Nurses can receive specialized training in screening techniques such as oral examinations, pelvic examinations, rectal examinations, and breast examinations from the American Cancer Society and other organization-sponsored programs. Counseling, especially for high-risk individuals, is an integral part of care (see Chapter 3 for risk-related information). Nurses who provide screening services can also make an important contribution by educating employers and third-party payers about the benefits of screening.

EARLY DETECTION ISSUES

As defined at the beginning of this chapter, early detection refers to the application of screening and diagnostic tests that allow presumptive diagnoses of various cancers in asymptomatic persons. The process of cancer **diagnosis** involves the recognition of a complaint by the individual, its evaluation by a health care professional, and confirmation by laboratory tests or procedures (e.g., endoscopy).

One of the biggest issues concerning early detection of cancer is that the individual with the physical complaint or positive test result from a screening program is responsible for bringing himself or herself to the health care professional. It is not uncommon, once symptoms appear or the individual is told of the positive screening test, to delay for months before seeking medical attention. Nurses can have an important role in decreasing this delay by (a) contacting people who have been through a screening program and have positive test results, and (b) discussing the importance of follow-up. Follow-up phone calls allow individuals to discuss the fears, apprehensions, and misconceptions they have about follow-up for a positive screening test. Nurses can reduce the misconceptions about cancer by providing accurate information about follow-up procedures and providing an opportunity for individuals to verbalize their fears. There are many factors that influence whether or not individuals access screening programs or follow-up once they experience symptoms or have a positive screening test. These factors are listed in Table 4–2, along with suggested nursing activities to decrease the barriers to accessing screening and early detection programs.

TABLE 4-2 Factors Influencing Participation in Screening and Early Detection

Factor	Manifestation	Nursing Role
Delay	Individual may delay reporting symptom or follow-up on a positive test for months.	1. Phone follow-up on positive tests found during a screening program. 2. Educate the public about the Seven Warning Signs of Cancer. 3. Include questioning about the warning signs of cancer in every health history.
Lack of knowledge of the early warning signs	Research documents that both the public and health care professionals are not knowledgeable about cancer's warning signs. Ignorance results in lack of recognition that the symptom merits immediate attention.	1. Learn the Seven Warning Signs of Cancer. 2. Educate the public about the warning signs of cancer. 3. Encourage other health professionals to become familiar with the warning signs. 4. Post the Seven Warning Signs of Cancer in areas that the public would see.
Individual personality characteristics	Barriers to accessing screening programs or early detection: • Low self-esteem • Denial • Fear • Embarrassment	Discuss the personality characteristics that are barriers to both screening and early detection. Open discussion enables the nurse to present accurate information about the disease, tests, and value of early detection.
Confidence	Lack of confidence in the value of early detection. For instance, the public believes that detecting colorectal cancer early makes no difference in terms of survival.	1. Provide the individual with information and literature that documents the value of early detection. 2. Address misconceptions held about the value of early detection with the public.

Attitudes	Research has shown that individuals who participate in screening programs have positive attitudes about the value of preventive health practices, are better informed about serious illnesses, and are more optimistic and less frightened about cancer.	1. Provide patients with accurate information on the disease and the value of early detection. 2. Have an individual who exemplifies the value of early detection of cancer talk to individuals make or presentations at education programs designed for the public.
Age	The elderly are less likely to participate in screening programs or report suspicious symptoms.	1. Provide information, literature, and programs on the normal symptoms of aging and differentiate these from the warning signs of cancer. 2. Provide information affirming that age doesn't necessarily mean poor health. 3. When designing screening programs, keep in mind that the elderly are less likely to participate, and make special accommodations to encourage this group to participate.
Access to care	Lower socioeconomic status frequently results in lack of access to care and poorer survival.	1. Literature and community educational programs for individuals and groups from low socioeconomic backgrounds must reflect the reality of lack of access and specific suggestions for gaining access to health care services. 2. Special efforts must be made to reach lower socioeconomic groups in the community and bring screening and early detection programs to them only when follow-up health care is assured.
Socioeconomic status	Higher income positively impacts access to care, participation in screening programs, and less delay with suspicious symptoms.	See Access to Care above.
Race/ethnicity	1. African-Americans tend to know less about cancer than whites and delay longer than whites when confronted with suspicious symptoms. 2. Hispanics tend to be pessimistic about cancer, have language barriers, and have knowledge deficits.	1. Nurses need to be knowledgeable about the health beliefs and practices of the racial/ethnic group they work with and address these beliefs. 2. If language barriers exist, literature and all written information needs to be in the language the community members can read.

Compliance, a significant issue in any discussion of cancer self-examination practices and early detection, is another area that merits further attention. Nurses can increase compliance by addressing the issue in a forthright manner. To teach self-examination techniques (e.g., **breast self-examination [BSE]**, self-examination of the mouth) effectively, the nurse needs to spend time understanding how people feel about each technique, what barriers prevent them from practicing it, what is needed to help them practice it, and what benefits they feel are inherent in the procedure. These areas need to be discussed with the person learning the techniques, and consumer- (rather than health professional-) generated solutions should be encouraged.

SCREENING FOR AND EARLY DETECTION OF THE AMERICAN CANCER SOCIETY'S PRIORITY CANCERS

Skin Cancer

When obtaining the health history, the nurse needs to be sure to ask the following questions:

1. Have there been any skin sores that have not healed?
2. Have any new moles appeared?
3. Have there been any changes in any existing moles in terms of color, size, surface characteristics, sensation, areas around the mole, and elevation of the mole?
4. Does the individual sunbathe? Go to tanning booths? Spend significant amounts of time outside due to occupation or leisure activities?

When conducting the skin examination, the nurse must be sure to inspect the skin on the entire body using a good light. Areas that have been chronically exposed to the sun need to be assessed meticulously. If indicated, all moles should be mapped to serve as baseline data for future skin assessments. Signs and symptoms of skin cancer include the following:

- Loss of skin markings.
- Variegation in pigmentation.
- Irregular hyperkeratotic areas.
- Rough areas that scab over, rescab and fail to heal.
- Persistent ulcer.

Initial diagnosis is based on a physical examination and confirmed by the removal and biopsy of the skin and/or mole.

Education of the individual or the public should include information on decreasing risk factors for skin cancer, how to do routine skin self-examinations, and effective use of sun blockers. Since the elderly constitute the highest-risk group for skin cancer, they should be taught skin self-assessment and the importance of seeking medical attention for any change in the skin. The normal changes that occur with aging and how these normal changes differ from skin cancer should also be emphasized.

Breast Cancer

The health history should contain questions such as these:

1. Do you practice breast self-examination?
2. Have you ever had a mammogram? When was your last mammogram? What were the results?
3. Have you noticed any dimpling? Seen or felt any change in your breasts? Ever been told you have lumpy or cystic breasts?,
4. Have you ever felt a breast lump or been told you had a breast lump?
5. Do you have a family history of breast cancer?

The signs and symptoms of breast cancer include the following:

- Painless lump or mass.
- Unilateral serous nipple discharge.
- Bloody discharge.
- Dermatitis of nipple/areola.
- Dimpling of skin in breast.
- Nipple retraction.
- Change in the contour of the breast.
- Thickening of breast tissue.
- Fixation of a mass to the pectoral fascia/chest wall.
- Edema and erythema of breast skin.
- Axillary adenopathy.

Screening tests for asymptomatic women include BSE, clinical breast examination, and a mammogram.

It has been documented that women who practice regular BSE discover cancers at earlier stages than those who do not. However, the majority of American women do not practice regular BSE. Many factors contribute to not practicing BSE, including discomfort in practicing the examination, fear of finding cancer, and lack of confidence in the ability to detect cancers. The other issue with BSE is that there have been no prospective, controlled clinical trials to document the benefits of this technique in reducing mortality and increasing survival rates. Because there are no definitive data showing that BSE reduces mortality or increases survival rates, some national health groups do not make recommendations about whether or not to teach BSE during the periodic health examination. However, until there is definitive evidence on the existence or lack of long-term benefits of BSE, nurses should continue teaching this self-examination practice whenever possible.

There is also controversy surrounding mammography. There is no question that mammography detects the earliest cancer, but it is not as widely practiced as it could be. The American Cancer Society, National Cancer Institute, and American College of Radiology recommend that women between 40 and 49 years of age have a mammogram every 1 to 2 years. In fact, in randomized screening trials mammography and clinical breast examination have been shown to reduce mortality from breast cancer. Nurses are urged to inform all women about the known and proven benefits of mammography and emphasize that it is to their benefit to follow the national mammography recommendations. Information should be shared with women verbally, through printed materials, and through public education programs on breast cancer.

Prostate Cancer

The health history should contain the following questions:

1. Do you have to wait for your stream to begin?
2. Does your urine stream seem weak to you?
3. Do you have to strain to urinate?
4. Do you have the urge to urinate but find you cannot?
5. When was your last rectal examination? What were the results?
6. Have you noticed blood in your urine?
7. Do you dribble after urinating?

The signs and symptoms of prostate cancer include the following:

- Small asymptomatic nodule on rectal examination:
  Firm or stony consistency.
  Earliest palpable change.
  Probability of being neoplastic in about 50% of cases.
- Renal insufficiency and hematuria:
  Weak or interrupted flow of urine.
  Difficulty in starting and stopping urination.
  Need to urinate frequently (especially at night)—most common symptom.
  Painful burning urination.
- Blood in urine.
- Bone pain:
  Continuous pain in lower back, pelvis, or upper thighs.

Screening examinations include a **digital rectal examination** and **prostate-specific antigen (PSA)** blood test. If these two tests are suspicious, it is recommended that transrectal ultrasound be used as the follow-up test. There is controversy about how best to screen the general population, and some disagree over whether earlier detection will decrease mortality. However there seems to be general agreement that digital rectal examination combined with the PSA examination is the most effective screening technique for prostate cancer.

Cervical Cancer

The health history should contain the following questions:

1. When was your last Pap test? What were the results?
2. Have you ever been told you have herpes? Genital warts? Pelvic inflammatory infection? Sexually transmitted diseases? Have you received treatment for any of these conditions?
3. Do you have spotting between menstrual periods?
4. Do you have bleeding after intercourse? After douching?
5. When did you start sexual activity? Approximately how many sexual partners have you had?

The signs and symptoms of cervical cancer include the following:

- Abnormal uterine bleeding or spotting.
- Abnormal vaginal discharge.
- Pain and systemic symptoms are late manifestations.

The screening examination for cervical cancer is the Pap test and pelvic examination. If the Pap test is abnormal, **colposcopy, conization,** or biopsy will be recommended.

Colorectal Cancer

The health history should contain the following questions:

1. Do you have a history of cancer of the bowel or ulcerative colitis?
2. Have you been told you have polyps of the bowel? Did you receive any treatment?
3. Have you noticed a difference in your bowel habits?
4. Do you have diverticulosis? Ulcers? Nervous stomach?
5. Have you had gastrointestinal x-ray studies within the last 1 to 2 years? What were the results?
6. Do you have hemorrhoids or anal fissures?
7. Have you noticed any change in appetite? Loss of weight?
8. After you have a bowel movement do you still have to go to the bathroom and expel more stool? Do you experience pain with bowel movements?

The signs and symptoms of colorectal cancer include the following:

- Right side of cecum and ascending colon:
  Anemia.
  GI tract bleeding.

Vague pain.

Weight loss and anorexia.

Palpable mass.

- Transverse colon:

Change in bowel habits.

Blood in stool.

- Descending colon, rectosigmoid:

Change in bowel habits.

Increased use of laxatives.

Decrease in caliber of stools.

Bright red blood coating surface of stool.

Gas pains.

- Rectum:

Rectal pain.

Gross blood per rectal tenesmus.

Sense of incomplete evacuation.

Screening examinations include a digital rectal examination, stool blood test, and proctosigmoidoscopy. Because colorectal cancers have moved proximally over the last few decades, the digital rectal examination will not detect the large number of cancers that occur beyond the rectal area. Therefore, it is recommended that a test for stool blood also be done. There are several problems with the stool blood test, including (a) lack of compliance with the required dietary recommendations prior to obtaining the sample, (b) a high rate of false negatives and false positives, and (c) the high cost and inconvenience to the patient when there is follow-up because of a false positive test. The acknowledged problems with proctosigmoidoscopy include (a) the high cost, (b) patient discomfort, (c) physician reluctance to recommend the uncomfortable test, and (d) the risk of bowel perforation. If any of these tests are positive, a colonoscopy and barium enema may be recommended.

CONCLUSION

Secondary preventive efforts such as screening and early detection provide a very real and potent weapon against some cancers that only 20 years ago were considered incurable. Nurses need to understand the technical, psychological, and financial aspects of screening and early detection procedures in order to create an atmosphere of openness and trust that will encourage patients' participation in cancer prevention activities. Information on specific screening and early detection methods may be obtained from local units of the American Cancer Society. The nurse's primary responsibilities in cancer screening and early detection are to:

1. Be knowledgeable about the barriers to participation in screening and early detection programs.

2. Provide accurate information about cancer screening and early detection to individuals and the public.

3. Encourage individuals to discuss their perceptions and fears about cancer screening/early detection tests and clarify misconceptions.

4. Collect accurate information during the health history that includes questions about the seven warning signs of cancer and site-specific questions designed to identify the early signs and symptoms of cancer.

5. Assist in the collection of specimens during screening and early detection activities in a way that will ensure that they are as accurate as possible.

6. Perform screening examinations commensurate with the nurse's educational background.

BIBLIOGRAPHY

Cohen, R., & Frank-Stromborg, M. (1993). Cancer risk and assessment. In S. Groenwald, M. Frogge, M. Goodman, & C. Yarbro (Eds.), *Cancer nursing: Principles and practice* (3rd ed., pp. 102–123). Sudbury, MA: Jones and Bartlett.

Frank-Stromborg, M. (1988). Nursing's role in cancer prevention and detection. *Cancer, 62* (suppl.), 79–107.

Frank-Stromborg, M. (1991). Cancer screening and early detection. In S. Baird, R. McCorkle, & M. Grant (Eds.), *Cancer nursing: A comprehensive textbook* (pp. 190–218). Philadelphia: W. B. Saunders.

Frank-Stromborg, M. (1996). Evaluating cancer risk. In R. McCorkle, M. Grant, M. Frank-Stromborg, & S. Baird (Eds.), *Cancer nursing: A comprehensive textbook* (pp. 213–264). Philadelphia: W. B. Saunders.

Frank-Stromborg, M., & Cohen, R. (1993). Assessment and interventions for cancer prevention and detection. In S. Groenwald, M. Frogge, M. Goodman, & C. Yarbro (Eds.), *Cancer nursing: Principles and practice* (3rd ed., pp. 124–169). Sudbury, MA: Jones and Bartlett.

Frank-Stromborg, M., & Olsen, S. (1993). *Cancer prevention in minority populations: Cultural implications for health care professionals*. St. Louis: Mosby.

White, L. N. (1986). Cancer prevention and detection: From twenty to sixty-five years of age. *Oncology Nursing Forum, 13*(2), 59–64.

5

Special Populations

Janice Phillips
Anne Belcher
J. Anne O'Neil

Cancer respects no woman or man. It may be found in African Americans, Hispanics, Asians, and other ethnic and racial minorities as well as in white Americans. Cancer may afflict those who are otherwise healthy or persons already burdened with another disease or disability. Persons with cancer may also have diabetes, renal disease, or spinal cord injuries, have Down syndrome, or be blind or deaf. Persons with cancer may be highly educated or they may not have completed high school. They may be heterosexual or homosexual. They may have large supportive families or be alone in the world. Cancer is diagnosed in the young and the old, in the rich and the poor. Cancer comes to those with demanding jobs in large corporations that provide health insurance. It also comes to malnourished homeless people who have no insurance or access to health care. Any humans may at sometime in their lives be diagnosed with cancer.

Each of these groups may be considered a special population requiring attention to its individual needs for prevention, detection, and treatment. A **screening** program for early detection of prostate cancer in the African-American community will differ from a similar program directed toward an Asian community. Discussing radiation treatment schedules with a retiree diagnosed with lung cancer requires nurses to pay attention to different details than speaking with a young working mother with breast cancer. The elderly may be facing issues of who will care for them when they return from the hospital. Parents of a child with leukemia may be concerned about re-entry to school and the normal growth and development of their child. An African-American patient may be concerned about racial discrimination in his or her treatment. All special populations require nurses not only to be alert to the quality of their nursing skills, but also to be alert to the special needs any patient may have because of membership in one or more special populations. This chapter focuses on two large special populations, ethnic and racial minorities and the elderly. Special emphasis is placed on improving access to and use of early detection and screening services and state-of-the-art-treatment among these two special populations. The implications for nursing practice are also addressed.

CANCER AND MINORITIES

The American Cancer Society estimated that 1,359,150 cancers would be diagnosed in the United States in 1996. Of these, 136,380 cancers would be diagnosed among African Americans and 38,000 would be diagnosed among other minority groups. The four generally recognized minority groups in the United States include African Americans, Hispanics, Native Americans/Alaska Natives, and Asian/Pacific Islanders.

Recent population trends project a tremendous growth in minority populations by the year 2050. For example, by that year the U.S. population will include 71% whites, 23% Hispanics, 16% African Americans, 10% Asian/Pacific Islanders, and 1% Native Americans. The projected growth in minority populations, coupled with variations in cancer **incidence, mortality,** and **survival rates** noted among these groups, underscores the need to examine cancer patterns and cancer-related behaviors specific to minorities.

Ethnic/racial minorities show striking differences with regard to cancer incidence, mortality, and survival. For example, cancer incidence and mortality rates are usually higher for African Americans than for whites, while cancer incidence and mortality rates for other minority groups are often lower than those for both African Americans and whites. African Americans have significantly higher incidence and mortality rates for cancers of the esophagus, uterine cervix, stomach, liver, prostate, and larynx and for multiple myeloma. In contrast, Native Americans, Asian/Pacific Islanders, and Hispanics have lower incidence and mortality rates for cancers of the lung, female breast, prostate, colon, and rectum.

Table 5–1 shows the 10 leading causes of cancer deaths according to racial/ethnic identity. Because cancer deaths are based on recorded causes of death on death certificates, cancer statistics are likely to be underestimated due to underreporting of Asian/Pacific Islanders and Native Americans. More reliable data are available for African Americans.

When assessing the cancer profile and associated factors among racial and ethnic minorities, it is important to assess for distinct variations according to subgrouping. For example, Hispanics are further identified as the following five subgroups: Mexican Americans, Puerto Ricans, Cuban Americans, Central/South Americans or other Hispanics. Cancer incidence and mortality rates are lower for Mexican Americans than for most other subgroups. In contrast, Puerto Ricans have lower rates of breast, colon, lung, and prostate cancers, but higher rates of cancers of the larynx and esophagus. Interventions directed to reducing cancer mortality must take into account the diversity that exists within the subgroups of racial and ethnic minorities. Table 5–2 depicts the cancer

TABLE 5-1 Reported Cancer Deaths, 10 Leading Causes of Cancer Death and Percent of Total Cancer Deaths, by Race, US, 1992

	White	African American	Native American [1,2]	Asian & Pacific Islander [2]	Hispanic [3]
	All sites 454,516 (100%)	All sites 58,401 (100%)	All sites 1,473 (100%)	All sites 6,173 (100%)	All sites 15,218 (100%)
1	Lung 128,704 (28.3%)	Lung 15,472 (26.5%)	Lung 381 (25.9%)	Lung 1,371 (22.2%)	Lung 2,674 (17.6%)
2	Colon & rectum 50,516 (11.1%)	Colon and rectum 6,073 (10.4%)	Colon & rectum 119 (8.1%)	Colon & rectum 668 (10.8%)	Colon & rectum 1,466 (9.6%)
3	Female breast 37,797 (8.3%)	Prostate 5,485 (9.4%)	Female breast 105 (7.1%)	Liver & other biliary 653 (10.6%)	Female breast 1,297 (8.5%)
4	Prostate 28,430 (6.3%)	Female breast 4,788 (8.2%)	Liver & other biliary 87 (5.9%)	Stomach 523 (8.5%)	Liver & other biliary 913 (6.0%)
5	Pancreas 22,519 (5.0%)	Pancreas 3,180 (5.4%)	Prostate 87 (5.9%)	Female breast 387 (6.3%)	Stomach 885 (5.8%)
6	Lymphoma 20,074 (4.4%)	Stomach 2,213 (3.8%)	Stomach 67 (4.5%)	Pancreas 309 (5.0%)	Prostate 873 (5.7%)

7	Leukemia 17,045 (3.8%)		Esophagus 1,897 (3.2%)		Pancreas 63 (4.3%)		Lymphoma 263 (4.3%)		Lymphoma 851 (5.6%)
8	Ovary 12,142 (2.7%)		Leukemia 1,587 (2.7%)		Leukemia 55 (3.7%)		Prostate 238 (3.9%)		Pancreas 850 (5.6%)
9	Liver & other biliary 11,283 (2.5%)		Multiple myeloma 1,543 (2.6%)		Kidney 53 (3.6%)		Leukemia 225 (3.6%)		Leukemia 739 (4.9%)
10	Brain & CNS 11,132 (2.4%)		Liver & other biliary 1,476 (2.5%)		Ovary 41 (2.8%)		Oral cavity 156 (2.5%)		Ovary 454 (3.0%)

Note: Since each column includes only the top 10 cancer sites, site-specific numbers and percentages do not add up to the All Sites totals.
[1] Includes American Indians and Native Alaskans.
[2] Numbers are likely to be underestimates due to underreporting of Asian, Pacific Islander, and Native American race on death certificates.
[3] Persons classified as of Hispanic origin on death certificates may be of any race. Hispanic origin is reported for all states except New Hampshire and Oklahoma. In 1990, the 48 states from which data were collected accounted for about 99.6% of the Hispanic population in the United States.

Source: American Cancer Society. (1996). *Cancer facts and figures.* Atlanta: Author.

TABLE 5-2 Racial/Ethnic Populations Cancer Profile

Ethnic Group	Cancer Problems	Lifestyle Risk Factors	Barriers to Prevention	Possible Approaches
African American	Highest overall cancer incidence rate Highest overall cancer mortality rate Survival 30% lower than for whites Prostate cancer Breast cancer Lung cancer Colorectal cancer Cervical cancer Pancreatic cancer Esophageal cancer	Poverty Diet Smoking Hazardous occupational exposures Obesity Alcohol consumption Urban living	Low education & literacy levels Lack of credible messengers with whom community can identify For the poor, survival, not prevention, is priority Decreased access to health care and prevention	Use African American professionals for health care & as speakers Church-based information & speakers Forums at public housing sites Smoking cessation efforts directed to unique smoking habits of this group
Hispanic	Gallbladder cancer among New Mexico Hispanics of Native American ancestry Liver cancer among Mexican Americans Cervical cancer among women from Central and South America	Genetic tendency Possibly diet Young age of first sexual encounter	Low literacy, even in Spanish Fear of cancer General belief that cancer is God's will & only God can cure Modesty & sexuality issues associated with gynecologic exams	Public service ads, Hispanic media Speakers bureau of Hispanic health professionals Outreach via neighborhood stores, restaurants Spanish videotapes Footonovelas Use Hispanic professional for health care

Population	Cancer	Risk Factors	Barriers	Strategies
	Pancreatic cancer among Mexican Americans Prostrate cancer	Poverty and possibly associated alcohol use Dietary changes with associated acculturation	Lack of Spanish-speaking caregivers Male reluctance to have exams Decreased access to health care & prevention Decreased awareness of cancer warning signs & screening tests	Use of comadres and copadres as role models Advocate use of 1-800-4-CANCER number for Spanish translation & counseling
Asian/Pacific Islander Chinese	Nasopharyngeal cancer Liver cancer Esophageal cancer	Epstein-Barr virus Salt fish consumption Genetic predisposition Hepatitis B Consumption of salted foods, hot tea, & silica fiber contaminated grain Smoking	Low education & literacy in native languages "Prevention model" nonexistent Lack of trust in western health care Leaders lack health knowledge Decreased access to health care	Includes screening exams & prevention education crisis care visits Outreach with messages via stores Tie in with English as 2nd language classes
Native American	Lowest overall cancer incidence & mortality of all U.S. populations Survival rates are uniformly low Tribal cancer rate differences are important.		Inhospitable health care environment and insensitive personnel Lack of transportation to health clinic Low education & literacy levels Underfunded & overburdened health care system	Integrate cultural beliefs & practices Enlist support of key tribal leader and organizations Enlist support of tribal CHRS Perform exams with strict attention & concern for modesty, tribal customs, gender, & dress differences

Source: Olsen, S. & Frank-Stromborg, M. (1993). Cancer prevention and early detection in ethnically diverse populations. *Seminars in Oncology Nursing, 9,* 200–201. Reprinted by permission.

profile (cancer patterns, lifestyle, risk factors, barriers to prevention, and possible approaches) for minority populations.

Of all the factors influencing cancer incidence, mortality, and survival rates, perhaps most striking is the influence of socioeconomic status. Racial and ethnic minorities are disproportionately represented among the socioeconomically disadvantaged. The influence of socioeconomic status on cancer incidence and cancer outcome was perhaps best articulated in 1985 by the American Cancer Society's Subcommittee on Cancer and the Socioeconomically Disadvantaged. The committee reported that the economically disadvantaged have a higher incidence for several sites and lower survival rates for all cancer sites combined, with overall 5-year survival rates that are 10% to 15% lower than they are for the general population. Even with improved access to health care providers, there is evidence that there are fewer prevention services available to socioeconomically disadvantaged groups. Compliance with prevention-focused procedures, adherence to treatment protocols, and follow-up visits are difficult for economically disadvantaged individuals to manage.

The American Cancer Society committee cited a variety of factors responsible for the increased mortality and morbidity from cancer among the poor, including lack of employment, lack of education, inadequate housing and overcrowded conditions, lack of access to medical care, chronic malnutrition, lack of child care facilities, fatalism, feelings of powerlessness, and a focus on day-to-day survival that limits future-oriented health maintenance or preventive activities.

These and other reports challenge nurses to become actively involved in helping to ensure that all individuals, regardless of socioeconomic status, have access to cancer early detection services and state-of-the-art treatment.

Implications for Nursing Practice

In concert with other health care providers, policymakers, health care agencies, consumers, and others involved in providing cancer-related services, it is critical that nurses work to develop, implement, and evaluate prevention and early detection strategies that focus on reaching ethnic and racial minorities. In addition to improving the availability of cancer-related services such as early detection and treatment, the use of community leaders and peer role models within the target community has shown much promise in heightening awareness of these services. Programs such as the American Cancer Society's Tell-A-Friend program and the University of North Carolina's Save Our Sisters program use community lay individuals to provide education on cancer-related topics, resources for screening and treatment, and encouragement and support for the use of such services. Such programs not only promote early detection and treatment among racial and ethnic minorities or **underserved populations** through education, but also offer assistance with navigating the health care delivery system.

Strategies to promote cancer control among these populations must continue to include both primary and secondary activities that are culturally relevant, sensitive, and appropriate. Nursing interventions or strategies must include:

1. Individual and/or group education regarding cancer-related activities (i.e., prevention, early detection).

2. Cancer **risk** assessment incorporating cultural beliefs, values, and practices.

3. Counseling regarding risk status and risk reduction.

4. Program development (including outreach activities),implementation, and evaluation.

Nurses are challenged to become acquainted with the various cultural beliefs, values, and practices that may influence the development, early detection, and treatment of the various cancers. This cultural sensitivity is essential to assessing and transcending the various barriers that may interfere with achieving cancer control among racial ethnic minorities. As we approach the 21st century, nurses are encouraged to work toward achieving the cancer control objectives for racial and ethnic minorities outlined in the landmark document *Healthy People 2000: National Health Promotion and Disease Objectives*, published in 1991 by the U.S. Department of Health and Human Services. These objectives provide direction for reducing cancer mortality among minority populations and the underserved.

CANCER IN THE ELDERLY

More than 12% of Americans are over the age of 65; by 2010 approximately 39 million people will be "young-old," (65–74 years), "middle-old," (75–84 years), or "old-old" (85+ years). Age is the most important factor in determining cancer risk, since more than 50% of all cancers occur in people over the age of 65.

Special attention must be given to cancer prevention, detection, and treatment for the elderly, because cancer is increasingly a disease of aging. There are five theories of cancer causation that might explain this phenomenon:

1. Longer duration of exposure to carcinogens.

2. Increased cell susceptibility to carcinogens.

3. Decreased ability to repair damaged DNA.

4. Oncogene activation or amplification; tumor suppressor gene loss.

5. Decreased immune surveillance.

Myths and misconceptions held by both the elderly and the public in general are obstacles to prevention, early detection, and treatment of cancer in the elderly. In addition, health care providers may practice **ageism,** the stigmatizing effect of societal prejudices toward older persons. In each instance, the following beliefs may present barriers to cancer screening in the elderly:

- Older people are senile or demented and cannot give a reliable health history.

- Many elders are unhealthy and cannot care for themselves without assistance.

- The aging process is inevitable and results in general physical deterioration (see Table 5–3).

In reality, most elderly persons are not mentally disturbed, are able to carry on their preferred lifestyle, and have widely varying rates of declining organ and

TABLE 5–3   Examples of Altered Protective Mechanisms in the
Older Adult Patient with Cancer

Protective Mechanism	Alterations Secondary to General Aging Process	Alteration Secondary to Cancer-Related Etiologies
Hematologic	• Decreased bone marrow cellularity and reserve • Increased infection, anemia, fatigue	• Marrow-suppressive therapies (type, intensity, and duration) • Malignancies of lymphoreticular origins (e.g., chronic leukemias, myelomas)
Immunologic	• Thymic involution • Lymphocyte changes • Cellular and humoral immunity alterations • Decreased immuno-surveillance • Moderate immunodeficiency • Increased infection potential • Increased autoimmune disorders	• Immunosuppressive therapies (type, intensity, duration) • Malignancies of lympho-reticular origin
Skin and Mucous Membranes	• Decreased skin elasticity • Decreased subcutaneous tissue • Dermal/epidermal thinning • Increased wound-healing problems • Increased risk of skin break-down • Interplay of incontinence, immobility and nutritional deficiency	• Radiation-related skin changes • Treatment-related mucositis • Malignant cutaneous lesions • Prolonged immobility • Cancer cachexia
Neurosensory/ Perceptual	• Decreased cerebral blood flow • Decreased nerve conduction velocity • Decreased brain weight • Decreased peripheral nerve function • Sleep wake cycle changes • Decreased reaction time • Decreased visual, tactile, and auditory acuity • Increased confusion; altered mentation • Impaired mobility	• Anxiety-caused misperceptions • Polypharmacy-related acute confusion • Vinca alkaloid-induced neurotoxicity/parasthesias • Prolonged immobility • Primary or metastatic central nervous system tumor • Cranial irradiation • Prolonged hospitalization • Metabolic imbalances (e.g., hypercalcemia, hypo-magnesemia)

Source: Boyle, D. M., Engelking, C., Blesch, K. S., Dodge, J., Sarna, L., & Weinrich, S. (1992).
Oncology Nursing Society position paper on cancer and aging: The mandate for oncology nursing.
Oncology Nursing Forum, 19, 921. Reprinted by permission.

system function. There are, however, other barriers to prevention, early detection, and treatment of cancer in the elderly, some of which are based on their beliefs and behaviors:

- Taking their aches and pains for granted.
- Viewing ill health and disability as inevitable.
- Experiencing the gradual loss of friends and relatives to use as a support and referral system.
- Not having or using access to accurate health information.
- Being unable or unwilling to work or volunteer outside of the home, which lessens stimulation and incentives to stay healthy.
- Possessing negative and often fatalistic attitudes about cancer and about the value of early detection and the value of treatment.
- Experiencing the constraints of a fixed income and inadequate funds for preventive health care.

Cancer mortality is especially high in the elderly, particularly among the socioeconomically disadvantaged, because of a delay in diagnosis but also because of patients' coexisting diagnoses such as cardiovascular disorders, pulmonary alterations, renal and neurological changes, diabetes mellitus, and hypertension. These comorbidities, rather than chronological age, should be used by health care providers as guides to early detection and treatment decisions. For example, such factors as obesity, inadequate nutritional status, lung disease, complications of vascular and cardiac status, and impaired immunity may place older persons at additional risk with surgery, radiation therapy, and chemotherapy. In addition, the use of polypharmacy (multiple drug treatments) among the elderly may create individual problems with drug interactions and enhanced side effects in persons receiving chemotherapy. Elderly persons' experience with cancer may also be complicated by their increasing likelihood of living alone and losing supportive resources as they grow older. Poverty may intensify these changes in lifestyle. Out-of-pocket expenses associated with cancer and its treatment impact most severely on those with a fixed income. However, in spite of these potential constraints, many older persons can tolerate and benefit from standard or experimental treatment protocols.

Implications for Nursing Practice

Nurses must assist the elderly, the public, and other health care providers to avoid the assumption that a symptom or change in functional status is evidence of the aging process rather than a sign of a specific disease. Older individuals should be instructed in the value of adherence to the American Cancer Society's guidelines for screening procedures and the need to seek evaluation of signs and symptoms, whatever their nature and presumed cause. The elderly are known to accept as signs of aging such potential early warning signs of cancer as malaise, anorexia, weight loss, and alterations in bowel habits. Older persons have also been found to report lower intensity of such symptoms as pain, nausea, and vomiting. This often results in cancer being diagnosed at a later stage.

Cancer must be viewed as a chronic illness in the elderly. Not only does the disease occur more frequently in this age group, but persons live longer with the diagnosis. Thus, rehabilitation and survivorship issues are as important in this population as they are in younger persons. Nurses need to identify disease- and treatment-related factors that impact the older patient's quality of life. Assessment should focus on functional status, especially physical, social, and economic condition and spiritual well-being, as all of these affect the individual's ability to cope. In addition, cost containment measures and shortened length of hospitalization when resources and support may be inadequate raise complex psychosocial challenges for the patient and the care provider.

CONCLUSION

This brief discussion only partially highlights the cancer burden noted among racial and ethnic minorities and the elderly. For an in-depth discussion of cancer statistics, associated risk factors, and culturally sensitive and appropriate strategies for achieving cancer control and treatment among special populations, the reader is referred to the additional resources listed in the Bibliography. It is hoped that this beginning discussion will stimulate further inquiry and work in promoting cancer control among special populations. Most important, every nurse, while cognizant of the overall problems related to cancer prevention, detection, and treatment, must be aware of and attend to the needs of individuals in any special population group.

BIBLIOGRAPHY

American Cancer Society. (1991). *Cancer facts and figures for minority Americans 1991.* Atlanta: Author.

Blesch, K. (1988). The normal physiological changes of aging and their impact on the response to cancer treatment. *Seminars in Oncology Nursing, 4,* 178–188.

Boyle, D. M., Engelking, C., Blesch, K. S., Dodge, J., Sarna, L., & Weinrich, S. (1992). Oncology Nursing Society position paper on cancer and aging: The mandate for oncology nursing. *Oncology Nursing Forum 19,* 913–933.

Department of Health and Human Services. (1991). *Healthy people 2000: National health promotion and disease prevention objectives.* Washington DC: U.S. Government Printing Office.

Derby, S. E. (1991). Ageism in cancer care of the elderly. *Oncology Nursing Forum, 18,* 921–926.

Frank-Stromborg, M., & Olsen, S. J. (Eds.). (1993). *Cancer prevention in minority populations: Cultural implications for health care professionals.* St. Louis: Mosby-Year Book.

Jones, L. (1989). *Minorities and cancer.* New York: Springer-Verlag.

McGill, J. S., & Paul, P. B. (1993). Functional status and hope in elderly people with and without cancer. *Oncology Nursing Forum, 20,* 1207–1213.

McMillan, S. C. (1989). The relationship between age and intensity of cancer-related symptoms. *Oncology Nursing Forum, 16,* 237–241.

Unit 3

Treatment Approaches

6

Cancer Clinical Trials

Mary S. McCabe

Clinical research in cancer is focused on the evaluation of promising new modalities for the treatment, prevention, and diagnosis of cancer. Clinical trials are a critical component of this process. The **clinical trial** is a rigorous evaluation that is necessary to determine the efficacy of specific interventions, especially therapeutic ones. It is not directed toward new knowledge for its own sake; rather, it is directed toward knowledge that will lead to improvements in cancer treatment and care. Although they are not limited to treatment evaluation, the largest number of clinical trials in cancer are treatment trials that have as their primary focus increasing the efficacy of treatments, reduction of toxicity, and improvement in the quality of life of patients.

HISTORY OF CLINICAL TRIALS

A clinical trial is an experiment designed to evaluate the potential benefit of therapies in human subjects. Advances in medical treatments have come about through the knowledge gained from experiments, both formal and informal.

One of the earliest clinical trials was conducted by Lind in 1747. He evaluated the response of patients who had symptoms of scurvy and had been treated with various interventions. He found that those who had eaten oranges and lemons, natural sources of vitamin C, showed the most improvement in their symptoms. Later, in the 1800s, similar comparative studies were undertaken to evaluate the effects of new drugs and vaccines for the treatment of smallpox, diphtheria, and cholera. As comparisons between treatments became progressively more scientific, research focused on the treatment and prevention of infectious diseases. The prospective randomized controlled clinical trial became an important research standard, reducing bias and further assuring that valid conclusions could be drawn from the data. Since World War II, the prospective controlled randomized clinical trial has become the "gold standard" for evaluating new techniques and treatments.

Currently two important forces are active in maintaining and increasing the scientific rigor with which clinical research is conducted. The health professions—medicine and nursing—are focused on the scientific method as the proper approach to the development of new **therapies.** Patient advocates, as active participants in the research process, have become partners in ensuring the ethical conduct of clinical research activities.

The federal government, through the Department of Health and Human Services (DHHS) and the Food and Drug Administration (FDA), has established regulations for the conduct of all clinical trials in the United States. These guidelines include requirements that a clinical trial include scientifically valid research hypotheses and design, competent investigators, a favorable risk/benefit ratio, and an equitable selection of subjects. These regulations also include the requirement that a written informed consent document be provided to the participant that uses terms a layperson can comprehend and conveys the information necessary for the person to make an informed, voluntary decision about participation in the research. Also required by federal regulation is the review of a research protocol by an Institutional Review Board at the institution where the study is taking place.

In 1990 the National Institutes of Health (NIH) published a policy on the inclusion of women and minorities in clinical research. It mandates that no Public Health Service grant applications be approved unless women and minorities are adequately represented in the research proposed, unless the exclusion is justified (e.g., a prostate cancer study in which the patients are exclusively male).

THE CLINICAL TRIAL PROCESS

Once a drug compound or modality is thought to be of potential benefit, either through preclinical screening or preliminary testing, it is considered appropriate for clinical evaluation in humans. Such human evaluation in clinical trials is done in a stepwise progression that includes three separate phases. A Phase I trial is usually the first use of the agent or intervention in humans, and its goals are to determine the maximum dose that can be tolerated and the optimal schedule and mode of delivery of the therapy, and to identify and quantify the toxic effects of the therapy on the patient. The Phase II trial is designed (using the Phase I dose and schedule) to determine the activity of the treatment (usually measured as tumor reduction or alleviation of symptoms and defined in terms of response) in specific types of cancer. These studies are disease specific and are based on biochemical or pharmacologic data or antitumor activity seen in the Phase I studies. Treatments with known benefit, based on positive results in Phase II studies, are then taken to Phase III studies to compare the role of a new therapy (drug, drug combination, procedure, or device) to the standard therapy and are evaluated in terms of survival and quality of life.

This lengthy and complex process of clinical trial evaluation is the necessary and crucial approach to the development of better cancer therapies. It involves the care of many patients in all clinical settings and is dependent on the participation of qualified nurses in all aspects of the research endeavor (see Table 6–1).

CLINICAL TRIALS PROGRAMS

The design and conduct of clinical trials, care of patients, and reporting of clinical trials findings require an integrated, multidisciplinary effort of physicians, nurses, pharmacists, social workers, statisticians, and other health professionals. Because the conduct of these studies is a complicated process, most cancer clinical trials are conducted by three clinical trial programs in the United States— the National Cancer Institute (NCI)-sponsored cooperative oncology groups, the cancer centers, and the pharmaceutical industry.

Cooperative Oncology Groups

The NCI supports the research efforts of investigators at multiple institutions around the country. These researchers jointly develop and conduct studies at institutions that have the medical and nursing expertise to provide high-quality care and to collect research data. Each group is formally organized and receives financial support from the NCI to perform evaluations that relate to the national priorities for cancer treatment, prevention, and control research.

These groups were first conceived in 1955 when Congress appropriated funds for national chemotherapy testing. Currently there are 11 cooperative groups that focus on research in both children and adults (Figure 6–1). The major goals of the groups are first, and most important, to improve the survival and quality of life for cancer patients; second, to conduct basic science research on cancer biology, pathology, epidemiology, and supportive care; third, to serve as research bases for the conduct of cancer prevention and control studies; fourth, to conduct research on clinical trials methodology; and fifth, to conduct research in oncology nursing.

Cancer Center Program

The cancer center program was formally authorized through the National Cancer Act in 1971. This legislation allowed the NCI to develop institutions around the country that would serve as a comprehensive national resource for research; as a multidisciplinary approach to treatment, prevention, and control; and as a community resource through outreach programs. These institutions are among the best medical centers in the country. They must show that they have a critical mass of expert clinical and laboratory personnel, be able to quickly move new laboratory findings into the clinic, conduct continuing education for health professionals, and have active patient education programs.

Only a fraction of patients with cancer are treated at the university hospitals that make up these cancer centers; 80% of cancer patients are treated by community-based oncologists. Therefore, the NCI has made it a major goal to extend

TABLE 6-1 Clinical Trials of New Treatments

	Research Goals	Nursing Goals	Nursing Responsibilities
Phase I	Determine maximum tolerated dose with acceptable toxicity Define side effects Generate bioavailability and pharmacology data	Safety and comfort of patients Ethical issues Education	Knowledge of available preclinical data: rationale, mechanisms of action, routes of administration, animal toxicity
Phase II	Identify antitumor activity at given dose and schedule Elaborate and extend Phase I data on toxicity	Documenation of eligibility and availability of patient Full documentation of all benefits and side effects of treatment	Anticipation of adverse reactions and early recognition of toxicity Management of side effects Preparation for diagnostic procedures
Phase III	Prospectively compare the investigational therapy against an established form of treatment in order to determine impact on survival, identify prognostic factors, and assess quality of life	Confirmation and extension of toxicity data Delineation of management and education of the patient Continuity of care	Clinical skills: Supportive physical/emotional care Assessment of patient Knowledge about the disease and its national history, which enables the nurse to evaluate response and toxicity Use of clinical expertise to prevent or minimize treatment or disease-related toxicity, and education of patients to maximize personal control

Reprinted from *Clinical Cancer Update*, National Institute of Health.

Cancer and Leukemia Group B (CALGB)
Children's Cancer Group (CCG)
Eastern Cooperative Oncology Group (ECOG)
Gynecologic Oncology Group (GOG)
Intergroup Rhabdomyosarcoma (IRS)
National Surgical Adjuvant Breast and Bowel Project (NSABP)
National Wilm's Tumor Study Group (NWTS)
North Central Cancer Treatment Group (NCCTG)
Pediatric Oncology Group (POG)
Radiation Therapy Oncology Group (RTOG)
Southwest Oncology Group (SWOG)

FIGURE 6–1 NCI-Funded Clinical Cooperative Oncology Groups

research efforts into the community. It has done so through two programs, the Cooperative Group Outreach Program and the Community Clinical Oncology Program. The purpose of these programs is to bring research facilities to where patients actually get their treatment and to include a large network of community physicians in the clinical trials process.

The Pharmaceutical Industry

The NCI develops more new anticancer agents than any pharmaceutical company. It is the largest single sponsor of studies evaluating new drugs for use in cancer therapy. However, this pattern of the NCI alone developing cancer drugs has been changing in recent years. There has been an increase in cancer clinical trials done by drug companies. In fact, more and more drug development studies are done in conjunction with pharmaceutical and biotechnology companies. Because of this increasing interest, a complex three-way relationship exists among the investigator at the medical facility, the NCI staff, and the pharmaceutical company. Collaboration is essential for testing the agent, and a coordinated plan must be developed.

NURSING RESEARCH IN CANCER CLINICAL TRIALS

As the specialty role of oncology nursing developed, so did nurses' participation in research. Initially, the roles of nurses in clinical trials were almost exclusively as data managers and research nurses in support of the medical protocol, rather than as independent nurse researchers. However, today there is an increasing number of nurse investigators conducting independent research. This is a result of graduate nursing programs that provide training in research methodology for nurses.

There has been no shortage of important nursing research questions, including questions related to quality of life, long-term effects, symptom reduction, and patient education. These are among the areas in need of evaluation under the heading of *supportive care*. These types of evaluations can be independent, or they can be companion studies done in parallel with the medical protocol and requiring interdisciplinary collaboration. The "six C's" of collaborative research—contribution, communication, commitment, consensus, compatibility, and credit—are essential to the success of such studies.

Although clinical trials are rich with nursing research opportunities and there are skilled nurse researchers available to conduct these evaluations, it has been difficult for nurses to be the principal investigators because of the limited funds available and, often, the need to compete with physicians in the cooperative groups or cancer centers for funds. This problem is one that must be addressed. Any solution requires that nurses be very skilled at developing research proposals that can successfully compete for limited funds.

PROFESSIONAL ROLE FOR NURSES IN CLINICAL TRIALS

Oncology nurses have long played an essential role in the design and implementation of clinical trials. Nurses are crucial at each step of the clinical trial process in assisting patients directly with treatment and supportive care and in understanding the research protocol. The roles are varied and include that of clinical nurse, research nurse, nurse manager, nurse practitioner, and nurse researcher as principal investigator. Nurses in all these roles may interact with patients on clinical trials. Both an extensive research and clinical knowledge base are required to care for patients while following a research protocol and collecting data to evaluate the research hypothesis.

Part of the clinical role of the nurse is education of the patient and family about the proposed research. Many patients see a clinical trial as their only hope, or they are afraid of "experimentation." It is important that the patient fully understand the therapy being presented and have realistic expectations about the potential benefits and side effects. This information is essential to allay fears and at the same time allow the patient to make a fully informed decision about participation. Such an education process must begin as soon as the patient is seen for evaluation, and it is a collaborative effort of the nurses and physicians involved in the patient's care. This is a process that continues throughout the course of the clinical trial.

Nurses provide care to patients in clinical trials in a variety of settings, including the hospital, outpatient clinic, physician's office, and the home. Nurses in each of these settings may have different responsibilities at different phases of the treatment, but all are involved in assessment, planning, intervention, and evaluation. It is important for each of these nurses to know the protocol, the details of the intervention, and the anticipated side effects.

The oncology research team usually includes a nurse who participates in both the care of the patient and the medical research, but the professional activities vary depending on the institutional model of clinical practice and the patient population. This role has evolved over time to include extensive responsibilities related to patient education, symptom management, and toxicity identification.

Research nurses are often involved in the dissemination of research results through publications in journals, presentation of papers at meetings, and poster sessions. These nurses make important contributions to the generation of new knowledge about cancer that will benefit future generations of patients.

OBSTACLES TO PARTICIPATION IN CLINICAL TRIALS

Participation in clinical trials offers patients access to state-of-the-art therapy in a research context. Initially, clinical trials were conducted only at cancer centers and academic medical centers. But the National Cancer Institute has made it a major goal to offer trials in the community, where most patients are treated, receive their care, and prefer to remain. However, despite the success of general efforts to increase patient participation in clinical trials, the number of minority and economically disadvantaged patients participating in trials has not increased significantly. Inclusion of these patient groups is important, because not including such groups can affect the generalizability of the results and because all patients should have access to clinical trials without being restricted by race or economic status.

There are four major factors that influence access to clinical trials and should be considered when designing interventions to improve the access to these studies. These factors are availability, affordability, accessibility, and acceptability. They address obstacles that are tangible as well as those that are psychological. Outstanding among these factors are access and cost issues.

Availability

Availability of trials is related to having institutions geographically nearby that conduct such studies. It is important that trials be available not only in large urban centers but also in smaller community settings and rural locations. Having the study available at a treatment facility is only one part of the availability issue for the patient. There are other important factors such as transportation, child care, and temporary housing that determine whether the trial is a realistic option for the patient and the patient's family or caregivers.

Affordability

Significant indirect costs of participation in clinical trials are often overlooked. These include such things as time lost from work, travel to the treatment facility, and day care for children. For the economically disadvantaged patient, any or all of these factors present an overwhelming burden and may prevent participation.

Accessibility

With the enormous changes in health care delivery prompted by the organization of new managed care systems, access to clinical trials is becoming more restricted. Cost has become such an overriding issue that other considerations in the patient's best interest may not be given proper priority. This problem is becoming critical as health care payers are focused more and more on cost rather than on quality. Restricted access for insured individuals whose health plans do not cover clinical trials is unfortunately only one side of the access problem. There are approximately 35 million uninsured Americans who not only have no access to trials but have no access to consistent health care at all. This issue is one that needs national attention and a national solution, but, unfortunately, it is not being addressed comprehensively at this time.

Acceptability

There can be psychological barriers for patients who consider clinical trials. These include the fear of doctors and hospitals, fear of diagnosis and prognosis, and fear of experimentation. Many patients, when diagnosed with cancer, fear the worst and rely on incomplete or inaccurate information to guide their decisions. Among some groups, there also remains the perception that clinical trials are experimentation and that tests and procedures of unknown benefit or risk will be done to them without their consent. These types of barriers need to be addressed directly and in a culturally and community sensitive manner for a true understanding of clinical trials to develop.

ETHICAL ISSUES IN CLINICAL TRIALS

It is important that nurses involved in any aspect of cancer clinical trials understand the ethical issues related to the conduct of this type of research. Some important ethical issues for nurses to consider are (a) the established means for protecting the rights of research subjects; (b) the principle that clinical trials should be designed to generate useful knowledge with the benefits likely to outweigh the risks; and (c) the responsibility of health professionals to patients in clinical trials.

Protection of Research Participants

In considering the development of a clinical trial, the most important question to be asked is whether the needs and rights of the individual patient entering this study can be balanced and protected during participation in a clinical trial that is done for the common good. Clinical trials by their nature are not designed primarily to benefit the individual patient; rather, they are designed to evaluate therapies to be used by future groups of patients. However, individual patients may benefit from being in the trial because the intervention is successful. Simply stated, the question is, "Can the interests of the individual patient be maintained in a clinical trial that is being done to advance medical knowledge related to cancer therapy, diagnosis, and prevention?" This balance must exist for a clinical trial to be ethical. The balance must be monitored and maintained throughout the conduct of the trial.

The rights of patients in clinical trials have not always been protected. It was not until the experiments performed by Nazi physicians on prisoners during

- *Respect for persons:* Autonomy, self-determination, the right to deliberate about personal goals and act accordingly without interference.
- *Nonmaleficence:* The obligation to do no harm to others.
- *Beneficence:* The obligation to do good or promote the good of others.
- *Justice:* Fairness; equitable distribution of benefits and burdens.

FIGURE 6–2   Fundamental Principles of Biomedical Ethics

World War II received worldwide attention at the Nuremberg trials that attention was drawn to the need for society to define basic ethical principles (Figure 6–2) of research and not leave it solely to the researchers. As a result, the Nuremberg Code of 1947 defined the basic concepts that must be adhered to in research to uphold moral, ethical, and legal principles. It was not until the 1960s that the United States developed regulations addressing the protection of human subjects in clinical research. Despite this developing effort to ensure the protection of human subjects, in 1972 there was disclosure of the Tuskegee syphilis study in which hundreds of African-American males were intentionally not treated even after the therapy being tested was known to be effective. Since that time, numerous federal regulations and reports of national panels, including the Belmont Report, have resulted in the development of national ethical standards that govern the conduct of clinical research. The standards set by these groups include the major requirements that must be met in order for the clinical research to be conducted ethically: The selection of subjects must be just, the research must be designed to obtain useful knowledge, the subjects must give informed consent, and the privacy and confidentially of the subjects must be protected.

Currently, patient confidentially is a serious issue because of the progress in genetic testing and the ability to determine those at risk of cancer. There are groups, such as insurance companies, that would like access to this information to make decisions to deny benefits to individuals when they are known to be at risk. It is also an enormous issue because of the explosion of electronic communication. Patient databases are no longer on paper at the institution; they are part of integrated informatics systems that are difficult to protect. National panels have been formed by government and private groups for public discussion of these issues in order to ensure the development of careful guidelines that give proper consideration to the rights of patients. Such public forums are the proper approach to ensuring that ethical guidelines are developed for dealing with sensitive issues.

Assessment of Risks and Benefits

The federal regulations require that "risks to subjects are reasonable in relation to the anticipated benefits to the subjects, and the importance that the knowledge that may reasonably be expected to result." Because clinical trials by their very nature involve a certain degree of uncertainty, it is not possible to completely document all the risks of the research. In cancer clinical trials, this means balancing the risks and benefits of the study and continuing to monitor this balance throughout the study. In doing so, the principle stated by the Declaration of Helsinki must be employed: "Concern for the interest of the subject must always prevail over the interests of science and society." It is the anticipated risks and benefits that must be documented. Coupled with this consideration of risk are the design and conduct issues that ensure careful research and good care during the trial. It is not enough that the initial intent of the study is an ethical one. The responsibility continues throughout the duration of the study and the follow-up period.

Informed Consent

The process of informed consent is an essential component of clinical trials and is supported by federal regulation and international reports. The patient (human subject), as an autonomous individual, must voluntarily agree to participate after information has been provided. Then the individual, or an authorized representative, must sign a written consent form that has been approved by an Institutional Review Board. (The purpose of this local review process is to assure the institution and the potential research participants that the research is medically and ethically sound.) The key components of this consent are that it is completely voluntary and that there is comprehension of the research by the individual or the individual's authorized representative. To successfully address these components, adequate and accurate information must be presented in a way that is understandable and is consistent with the educational and cultural needs of the individual.

Since informed consent is an ongoing process and not a limited act, the nurse plays an important role in providing information to the individual considering participation in a clinical trial and during the trial once the patient has agreed to participate. It is therefore a responsibility of the nurse, as part of the health care team caring for individuals on a clinical trial, to ensure that fully voluntary and informed choice occurs. The nurse also has the responsibility to observe that the trial is being conducted with ethical integrity and that the subjects in the trial are aware that consent for participation can be withdrawn at any time with no penalty.

ISSUES AND CHALLENGES

Cancer clinical trials are an important part of cancer treatment and care. It is only through such research efforts that we will be able to prevent and successfully treat the various forms of cancer. Since nurses have historically had an integral professional role in clinical trials, it is important that they understand the nature and elements of these trials. This ongoing search for improved therapeutic interventions must be balanced with the responsibility to provide the highest standard of care to each individual.

There are multiple challenges ahead in cancer research due to the changing health care system and the explosion of biomedical knowledge. These challenges include the development of new, streamlined ways of conducting trials in the managed care environment, assurance of patient confidentiality in an electronic age, and the need for counseling of individuals involved in genetic testing studies. However, maintaining a balance among efficiency, quality, and ethical integrity in cancer clinical trials will be the most important challenge of all.

BIBLIOGRAPHY

Beauchamp, T., & Childress, J. (1994). *Principles of biomedical ethics* (4th ed.). New York: Oxford University Press.

Grant, M., & Padilla, G. (Eds.). (1990). *Cancer nursing research*. Norwalk, CT: Appleton & Lange.

Kreuger, J. (1980). Safeguarding the rights of human subjects. In A. Davis & J. Kreuger (Eds.), *Patients, nurses, and ethics* (pp. 35–49). New York: AJN Company.

McKenna, R. (1990). Reimbursement issues in cancer clinical trials. *Cancer, 65,* 2405–2410. (Suppl).

Miaskowski, C. (1990). The future of oncology nursing: A historical perspective. *Nursing Clinics of North America, 25,* 461–473.

The National Commission for the Protection of Human Subjects of Biomedical and Behavioral Research. (1979). *The Belmont report: Ethical principles and guidelines for the protection of human subjects of research.* Washington, DC: US Government Printing Office.

Newcomer, L. (1990). Defining experimental therapy—A third party payer's dilemma. *New England Journal of Medicine, 323,* 1702–1703.

7

Surgical Oncology

Cindy Stahl

Surgery as a treatment for cancer was recorded in Egyptian records as early as 160 BC. Throughout history techniques for excision of cancer have correlated with our understanding of tumor biology. In the Hippocratic era, one of the four humors of the body (black bile) was thought to be the cause of cancer. Surgical treatment was in the form of lancing or bloodletting to release the collection of cancer-causing humor. In the early 1800s, a better understanding of human anatomy and physiology replaced the humoral theories with the concept that cancer was a local disease. Until the 1960s, it was believed that cancer spread from the primary site to the lymphatic system and then to the circulatory system. This belief explains the reasoning behind the Halstead radical mastectomy and other en bloc tumor resections that left patients with drastic disfigurement and loss of function. Despite improved surgical techniques and better control of infection, morbidity was high. Currently, it is believed that cancer cells can spread into the circulatory system independent of lymphatic spread, and that cancer can spread to local lymph nodes in an unorderly fashion. The surgical trend has changed to more conservative surgery, sparing lymph nodes and tissue whenever possible.

Although surgery is still used as the primary treatment for localized disease, it is more common for cancer patients to receive a combination of treatment modalities. For example, a patient with early stage breast cancer may have a lumpectomy followed by radiation therapy and/or chemotherapy. This treatment modality leads to decreased length of stay in the hospital and increased use of outpatient services, and it minimizes the risk of decreased function in the adjacent arm.

PRINCIPLES OF CANCER SURGERY

There are several principles that guide the surgical oncologist in the decision to perform surgery for the treatment of cancer:

80

1. Slow-growing and locally confined tumors are most amenable to surgical treatment.

2. A margin of normal tissue is removed with the tumor while functional and physical outcome are also considered.

3. Adequate staging should be done prior to definitive surgery, to determine the best therapeutic approach.

4. Techniques are utilized that should decrease the local and systemic spread of cancer during surgery.

5. The possible extent of dysfunction related to the surgery must be explained and be acceptable to the patient.

6. The initial surgery for removal of a primary cancer has a better chance for success than a second surgery for recurrent disease.

ROLE OF SURGICAL ONCOLOGY

Surgery may be used for several different purposes in oncology. Those purposes include diagnosis, staging, prevention, treatment, reconstruction, insertion of therapeutic or supportive devices, and treatment of oncologic emergencies.

Diagnosis

A tumor sample is obtained surgically to confirm the **diagnosis** and determine the specific type of cancer **histology.** The tumor histology is important because each type of cancer responds differently to treatment. Treatment decisions are based on diagnosis and histology.

There are many surgical techniques used to obtain a tissue biopsy (see Table 7–1). Criteria for choosing a technique depend on the type, size, location, and growth characteristics of the suspected tumor. Guidelines for performing a biopsy follow:

1. The biopsy site should be in an area that will be removed at the time of surgery, or the biopsied specimen should contain the entire tumor with clean margins, to reduce the possibility of seeding cancer cells along the incision site.

2. The incision line, when possible, should be cosmetically acceptable and in skin folds.

3. The tissue sample must be intact and contain normal tissue for comparison.

Nurses can help ease patient anxiety by informing patients and their families about the procedure and the time required to obtain results. It is not unusual to have a 2-week waiting period between the time of biopsy and the definitive surgery. The waiting period may help patients and their families adjust to the diagnosis of cancer and allow them the time needed to make decisions about treatment options. Patient/family instruction should include caring for the

TABLE 7-1 Surgical Techniques for the Diagnosis of Cancer

Technique	Method	Benefits/Risks
Needle aspiration/biopsy Use: diagnosis	Needle inserted into tumor Percutaneous or during surgery Sample may be fluid or tissue Fine-needle (21-22 gauge) or core-needle (cutting needle)	Simple to perform Less tissue trauma Needle may miss the tumor or malignant cells Possible to seed tumor cells along the needle tract, causing recurrence
Excisional biopsy Use: diagnosis, treatment	Removal of the whole tumor with an effort to obtain clean margins Most commonly used biopsy method Tumor usually ≤ 3cm and accessible	Can be definitive therapy Outcome should be cosmetically acceptable Possible to seed tumor cells into tissue and incision, causing recurrence
Incisional biopsy Use: diagnosis	Removal of a piece of the tumor Tumors usually > 3cm	Additional surgery required to remove tumor Risk of profuse bleeding Specimen may be too small to make a diagnosis Margins not defined

Needle localization biopsy *Use*: diagnosis, treatment	Needle placed by stereotactic guidance to mark the tumor, then tumor excised Tumor usually nonpalpable, but seen as mammographic abnormality	Radiograph of specimen is necessary to ensure correct tissue was excised Done in outpatient radiology clinic
Endoscopy *Use*: diagnosis, treatment	Tumor visualized through endoscope and a piece of tumor removed with forceps Commonly used for tumors of GI tract, GU tract, and respiratory tract Can be incisional or excisional	Risk of perforation, hemorrhage Increases accessibility of tumors Avoids surgical trauma
Laparoscopy *Use*: diagnosis, staging, treatment	Tumor visualized through endoscope and a specimen can be taken using one or more techniques (incisional, excisional, scraping, or peritoneal washing)	Can detect metastatic disease not seen on imaging scans Risk of perforation, hemorrhage Increases accessibility of tumors Avoids surgical trauma
Laparotomy *Use*: diagnosis, staging, treatment	Exploratory surgery used to rule out metastases to other organs All types of biopsies can be done (needle biopsy, incisional, excisional, scraping, or peritoneal washing)	Useful when tumors are incorrectly staged by other techniques (e.g., CT scan), inaccessible, or difficult to evaluate

biopsy site, identifying and reporting signs of infection and continued bleeding, and accessing the health care system to ask questions and report untoward symptoms during and after office hours.

Staging

Surgical **staging** can be done at the time of diagnosis and will provide information regarding tumor location, extent of disease, and prognosis. The surgical oncologist uses staging information to determine the best surgical approach and the need for other treatment following surgery. Two procedures for surgical staging (laparoscopy and laparotomy) are identified and described in Table 7–1.

Prevention

There are some conditions that are considered high risk for cancer. Surgery may be performed on individuals with these conditions to prevent the occurrence of cancer. For example, benign polyps of the colon and ulcerative colitis are associated with colon cancer. The preventive *(prophylactic)* surgery that might be performed would be a colectomy to remove the affected part of the colon. The surgical oncologist considers the following factors when identifying the need for prophylactic surgery:

- The presence or absence of symptoms (e.g., intestinal symptoms with colon polyps).
- Potential risks related to the patient's age.
- Risk for cancer based on medical and family background.
- The ability to detect cancer at an early stage if prophylactic surgery is not done.
- Postoperative outcome (is it acceptable to the patient?).

Surgeries for precancerous and in-situ lesions are considered preventive because they prevent histologic progression to cancer. For precancerous and in-situ lesions of epithelial surfaces (e.g., skin and cervix), surgery is the treatment of choice and is usually curative.

Treatment

Surgical treatment for cancer is applied throughout the cancer trajectory and has the following specific goals.

Primary Treatment   Surgery as a primary treatment involves removal of the entire tumor with a margin of normal tissue. The goal is to cure the patient of cancer by removing the total tumor burden. The technique for removal of the tumor can be local excision or wide excision (en bloc dissection). Local excision involves cutting out the tumor with a narrow margin of normal tissue. It is commonly used for cancers of the skin, nose, lip, and ear. Wide excision is the removal of tumor, regional lymph nodes, lymphatic channels, and involved adjacent structures. Examples of surgical procedures using wide excision are radical mastectomy for breast cancer, pancreaticduodenectomy for pancreatic cancer, and subtotal gastrectomy with radical lymphadenectomy for gastric cancer. There are a variety of surgical techniques (e.g., laser surgery, cryosurgery, and electrosurgery) used for curative treatment of cancer in situ that cause little or no damage to healthy tissue.

There are some unique surgical techniques used in cancer treatment (e.g., laser surgery, electrosurgery, and cryosurgery). Laser surgery kills cancer cells by using intensive thermal energy and is used for local excision of gynecological and skin cancers. Electrosurgery kills cancer cells by using electrical current and is used to treat skin, oral cavity, and rectal cancers. Cryosurgery kills precancerous lesions and cancers in situ by deep freezing the tumor with liquid nitrogen or freon (common freezing agents), to treat skin and gynecological cancers.

Adjuvant Treatment   Surgery as an adjuvant treatment involves the removal of tumor to decrease the risk of cancer incidence (prophylactic surgery), progression, or recurrence. One form of surgical adjuvant therapy is **cytoreductive (debulking)** therapy. The goal is to remove as much of the tumor burden as possible. By removing the bulk of the tumor cells, other therapies (e.g., chemotherapy, radiation therapy, and/or biotherapy) can be used to kill the remaining tumor cells.

Salvage Treatment   Surgery as a salvage treatment involves removal of a recurrent tumor after a more conservative primary treatment has failed (e.g., a radical prostatectomy after primary radiation therapy or a mastectomy after primary lumpectomy and radiation therapy). Surgeries for recurrence of cancer are more radical because more tissue is removed in an attempt to excise all of the cancer. The goal is still to cure, but as stated earlier, secondary surgery for recurrence has less chance for success.

Palliative Treatment   Surgery as a palliative treatment is used to enhance patient comfort and decrease the disease or its related symptoms. Palliative treatment is not curative. The decision to use surgery for palliation depends on the patient's projected life expectancy, tumor growth rate, expected outcome, and expected benefit to the patient. Examples of palliative treatments include surgical procedures that help manage cancer pain (e.g., nerve blocks, neurectomy, or cordotomy), treatment of complications caused by other therapies (e.g., skin breakdown or radiation proctitis), and relief of life-threatening obstruction or bleeding.

Combination Treatment   It is common to see surgery combined with other modalities such as chemotherapy, radiation therapy, and/or biotherapy. Surgery is used in combination with other modalities to improve treatment outcomes by limiting changes in function and appearance, improving tumor resectability, and decreasing the amount of tumor that has to be removed. For example, any of the three methods mentioned (chemotherapy, radiation therapy, or biotherapy), can be used preoperatively to shrink the tumor and improve its resectability. When the same therapies are used intraoperatively or postoperatively, the goal is to kill any remaining tumor cells. Research in this area focuses on the timing and sequence of the therapies as well as identifying which combinations are most effective at controlling cancer while minimizing side effects.

Reconstruction

Cancer surgery may result in anatomic defects and loss of function. Reconstructive surgery is used to improve function and cosmetic appearance after extensive cancer surgery. The options for reconstructive surgery should be discussed with the patient prior to the primary surgery. Some reconstructive surgeries are performed during the primary surgery (e.g., postmastectomy breast reconstruction), and some require multiple surgeries (e.g., facial reconstruction and tissue grafts).

Insertion of Therapeutic Devices

Many patients require surgically implanted therapeutic and/or supportive devices to facilitate the delivery of treatment and increase patient comfort. Examples include catheters, tubes, implanted ports, and implanted reservoirs. Catheters and implanted ports can provide vascular, intraperitoneal, and epidural access for the delivery of cytotoxic therapy, nutritional therapy, and pain management, and they may also be used to monitor a patient's condition (e.g., blood draws). Implanted reservoirs can provide intraventricular and epidural access for the delivery of cytotoxic therapy, patient monitoring, and pain management. (See Chapter 15 for additional information on vascular access devices.)

Surgery for Oncologic Emergencies

Surgery is frequently used in the management of oncologic emergencies. The emergency can be caused by the primary tumor or as a result of treatment. For example, a patient who presents with an intestinal obstruction or perforation caused by a tumor in the colon may require a primary resection to correct the emergency, or a patient with constrictive pericarditis caused by radiation to the chest may need placement of pericardial windows or a pericardiectomy to manage the emergency. (See Chapter 17 for additional information on oncologic emergencies.)

NURSING CONSIDERATIONS

Care of the surgical cancer patient must incorporate the principles of nursing care for the general surgical patient *and* for the cancer patient. For specific nursing care related to the operative site (tissue, organ, or system) and surgical procedure, the reader is referred to a general surgical nursing textbook. Nursing management is critical to provide a comprehensive plan of care and improve patient outcomes. Preoperative assessment should include the patient's age and developmental stage; the purpose and type of surgery; and the patient's and family's or caregiver's understanding of the surgery, diagnosis, and the possibility for additional therapies and expected outcomes. The answers to these questions can help the nurse identify present and future physical and psychosocial needs of the patient and family.

Reducing anxiety can be very challenging. Anxiety affects mood and the ability to learn, and, if uncontrolled, it can manifest as physical symptoms such as respiratory distress. Nurses can help reduce anxiety by addressing the patient's and family's misconceptions and fears about the surgery, diagnosis, and what to expect throughout treatment. Age-specific instruction on pain management throughout the patient's treatment is very important in reducing anxiety. All patient and family education should be repeated several times verbally and in writing, beginning preoperatively and continuing throughout treatment. Validation of the patient's/family's or caregiver's understanding of the content should be assessed and documented. Many patients state that they do not remember anything that is said after the word *cancer* or *surgery* is mentioned. Referrals to institutional and community resources (e.g., support groups) and plans for rehabilitation should begin preoperatively. There are several organizations that offer preoperative counseling and support to help reduce patient anxiety (Reach to Recovery, Ostomate, and Y-Me National Breast Cancer Organization). Considerations specific to oncology are addressed in the following paragraphs.

Nutrition

Cancer patients are at risk for malnutrition due to decreased food intake and increased energy expenditure resulting from the cancer and treatment regimens. Surgery and wound healing further increase metabolic demands and make the risk for malnutrition even greater. As a result, the cancer patient has an increased potential for complications of anemia, infection, sepsis, pneumonia, compromised wound healing, and increased morbidity. Management involves preventing or minimizing weight loss before surgery and aggressive nutritional management after surgery. (Specific nursing management to improve nutrition is discussed in Chapter 16.)

Blood Disorders

Cancer patients are at risk for anemia, thrombocytopenia, leukopenia, and alterations in hemostasis due to tumor burden and/or side effects of treatment regimens. Assessment and management of thrombocytopenia and leukopenia must be addressed preoperatively to prevent intraoperative and postoperative hemorrhage or infection. Assessment for shortened prothrombin, partial thromblastin time, and prolonged coagulation times are essential because cancer patients are at risk for hypercoagulation and thrombosis. Nursing management includes early postoperative ambulation to prevent deep vein thrombosis. (For additional information on bone marrow suppression, see Chapter 13.)

Combination Therapy

The cancer patient who has received radiation or chemotherapy is a high surgical risk. Short- and long-term side effects from radiation or chemotherapy can increase the incidence of postoperative complications. Tissue damage from radiation therapy (past or concurrent) can compromise wound healing in the radiated area. Some cytotoxic drugs (Doxorubicin, 5-fluorouracil, and cyclophosphamide), when given within the first few postoperative days, can compromise wound healing and increase the risk of dehiscence. Concurrent cytotoxic drug therapy will increase the risk of infection and bleeding due to the drugs' effect on the hematopoietic system. (See Chapter 9 for side effects of chemotherapy.) Specific organ systems can be affected by cytotoxic drugs and require special attention. Bleomycin can cause interstitial fibrosis and predispose the patient to postoperative adult respiratory distress syndrome. Cisplatin can cause a decrease in glomerularfiltration rate, resulting in renal failure.

Due to current changes in health care delivery and an attempt to reduce costs, patients are being discharged earlier. This presents a challenge for the health care provider, patient, and family. Nurses are responsible for instructing the patient's caregiver about the patient's needs. Good communication among the inpatient staff, home health care staff, patient, and family caregiver are essential to decreasing the anxiety of the patient and family caregiver and improving patient outcome.

LATE EFFECTS

The increased number of cancer survivors has challenged health care professionals to focus on late treatment effects and quality of life. Late effects research is valuable to understand the long-term effects of treatment on the patient and family as well as to identify how health care professionals can help to improve or maintain quality of life for cancer survivors. Health care professionals are obligated to identify potential late treatment effects for patients and families. Patients and families need to be informed of possible late effects in order to make informed treatment choices. The health care provider can use this information to teach the importance of rehabilitation and be sensitive and proactive toward psychological stressors. The extent and possibility of late effects from oncologic surgery depend on the type of surgery, amount of tissue and/or organ removed, age of the patient, and meaning the patient places on the treatment outcome. Some possible late effects as a result of surgery follow.

Physical Asymmetry

Surgeries that involve removal of bone (e.g., long bone) can affect growth of the bone and result in asymmetry. For example, surgery and irradiation to the head and neck can alter growth of facial bones in pediatric patients and require reconstructive surgery. The health care professional should give anticipatory guidance to assist the patient and family in dealing with the visible deformity.

Renal Effect

A nephrectomy for treatment of Wilms' tumor predisposes a patient to urinary tract infections and requires lifelong monitoring of renal function. Abdominal-perineal surgeries for prostate cancer and gynecological cancers can predispose the patient to urinary tract infections, stress incontinence, and urgency.

Lymphedema

Patients who have a radical mastectomy and/or radiation therapy for breast cancer are at greatest risk for lymphedema. Lymphedema usually occurs on the affected side. Symptoms include loss of strength and function in the affected arm, pain and altered sensation due to swelling in the arm, skin breakdown, and joint complications. Procedures (e.g., venipuncture, measuring blood pressure) should not be done on the arm with lymphedema because there is a greater risk for infection and compromised wound healing in the limb. Treatment for lymphedema includes elevation, limb exercises, and compression bandage therapy to the affected arm. (For additional information on lymphedema, see Chapter 24.)

Sexual

There may be psychological and physical late effects of surgery on sexuality. Pelvic surgeries for prostate cancer are associated with erectile and ejaculatory impairments from nerve and vascular damage. Possible late effects of pelvic surgery for gynecologic cancers include vascular damage, fistula formation, adhesions, and coital discomfort. While current surgical techniques are decreasing the incidence of this late effect, patients need to be prepared for possible changes. Other oncologic surgeries (e.g., mastectomy, colostomy, tracheostomy) can affect body image. Alteration in body image can occur in patients with cancer regardless of the actual physical, functional, or cosmetic outcomes. For many patients, support from others who have experienced the same surgery can be helpful. Thus, nurses need to be aware of hospital and community resources to help patients and families cope with this difficult issue. (See the Appendix for the sources and Chapter 18 for additional information on sexuality.)

CONCLUSION

The trends in cancer treatment follow advances in biology, technology, and the dynamic changes in our health care system. Surgical treatment of cancer, in many cases, is less radical than before (e.g., lumpectomies). Minimal-access surgical techniques have decreased the length of hospital stay. Use of surgery in multimodal therapies (e.g., surgery and radiation and surgery and chemotherapy), can lengthen survival time and improve quality of life. Nurses caring for the surgical oncology patient are challenged to be experts in the art of pain management, patient/family education, side effects management, and psychosocial support.

BIBLIOGRAPHY

Greene, F. L., & Rosin, R. D. (Eds.). (1995). *Minimal access surgical oncology*. New York: Radcliffe Medical Press.

Havard, C. P., & Topping, A. E. (1991). Surgical oncology. In S. B. Baird, R. McCorkle, & M. Grant (Eds.), *Cancer nursing: A comprehensive textbook* (pp. 235–245). Philadelphia: W. B. Saunders.

Harvey, J. C., & Beattie, E. J. (Eds.). (1996). *Cancer surgery.* Philadelphia: W. B. Saunders.

Pfeifer, K. A. (1994). Surgery. In S. E. Otto (Ed.), *Oncology nursing* (pp. 443–466). St. Louis: Mosby.

Szopa, T. J. (1992). Implications of surgical treatment for nursing. In J. C. Clark & R. F. McGee (Eds.), *Oncology nursing society core curriculum for oncology nursing* (pp. 309–318). Philadelphia: W. B. Saunders.

8

Radiation Therapy

Ryan R. Iwamoto

Radiation therapy is one of the major treatment modalities for cancer. Approximately 60% of all people with cancer will be treated with radiation therapy sometime during the course of their disease. Its effectiveness as a treatment for cancer was first reported in the late 1800s. Advances in equipment technology, combined with the science of radiobiology, have led to today's highly sophisticated treatment centers. Radiation therapy can now be delivered with maximum therapeutic benefits, minimizing toxicity and sparing healthy tissues.

BIOLOGIC EFFECTS OF RADIATION

Radiation therapy uses high-energy ionizing radiation to kill cancer cells. It is considered a local therapy because cancer cells are destroyed only in the anatomic area being treated. The radiation causes the breakage of one or both strands of the DNA molecule inside the cells, thereby preventing their ability to grow and divide. While cells in all phases of the cell cycle can be damaged by radiation, the lethal effect of radiation may not be apparent until after one or more cell divisions have occurred. Although normal cells can also be affected by ionizing radiation, they are usually better able to repair the DNA damage.

PRINCIPLES OF TREATMENT

The dose of radiation administered is determined by a number of factors, including the radiosensitivity of the tumor, the normal tissue tolerance, and the volume of tissue to be irradiated. The **Gray,** the Systeme Internationale unit, has now replaced the *rad* (radiation absorbed dose) as the accepted term for radiation dosage. One Gray (Gy) = 100 rads; therefore, 1 cGy = 1 rad.

A radiosensitive tumor is one that can be eradicated by a dose of radiation that is well tolerated by the surrounding normal tissues (see Table 8–1). The sensitivity of tumor cells to the effects of radiation is also dependent on the presence of oxygen. Killing hypoxic cells requires two to three times the dose of radiation required to achieve the same therapeutic effect in well-oxygenated cells. Hypoxic cells occur when tumor growth exceeds the blood supply and the central core of the tumor becomes necrotic. New strategies are being developed to increase the radiosensitivity of these hypoxic, resistant cells with chemicals that mimic the presence of oxygen or with hyperthermia (the use of heat).

The dose of radiation that can be delivered to a tumor is also limited by the radiation tolerance of the adjacent normal tissues. This limit is the point at which normal tissues are irreparably damaged. The maximum dose of radiation that can be administered to parts of the body varies with the tissue involved.

Because administration of the tumor-lethal dose of radiation in a single treatment would result in unacceptable toxicity or even death, the total prescribed dose of radiation is usually divided into several smaller doses, or **fractions.** Treatments are usually given on a daily basis, 5 days per week for an average of 25 to 30 treatments. With fractionation, a **tumoricidal** dose can be delivered while minimizing the damage to normal tissues. In addition, gradual shrinkage of the tumor during treatment brings hypoxic cells closer to the vascular supply, where they become oxygenated and more susceptible to the effects of radiation.

For some tumors, a "boost" or "reduced field" of radiation is administered to complete the course of therapy. These treatments are delivered to limited areas within the treatment field that are at greatest risk for recurrence. In this way, the tumor can be treated with a higher dose than the normal surrounding tissues would tolerate or need. The boost may be administered externally or internally.

USES OF RADIATION THERAPY FOR THE TREATMENT OF CANCER

Primary Therapy

Radiation therapy is a primary therapy for basal cell carcinomas of the skin, early stage Hodgkin's disease, non-Hodgkin's lymphomas, early stage breast cancer following lumpectomy, certain lung cancers, seminomas, carcinomas of the cervix, prostate cancers, bladder cancers, thyroid cancers, certain pediatric tumors, and certain brain tumors.

Radiation and surgery, both of which are local therapies, may achieve comparable responses and cure rates in some diseases; however, radiation may offer some treatment advantages to certain patients. In some cases, the functional and cosmetic outcomes of radiation therapy are superior to the results that can be achieved surgically. Also, some individuals may be unable to undergo surgery due to preexisting medical conditions, thus making radiation therapy the better treatment choice.

TABLE 8–1 Relative Radiosensitivity of Various Tumors and Tissues

Tumors or Tissues	Relative Radiosensitivity
Lymphoma, leukemia, seminoma, dysgerminoma	High
Squamous cell cancer of the oropharyngeal, glottis, bladder, skin, and cervical epithelia; adenocarcinomas of the alimentary tract	Fairly high
Vascular and connective tissue elements of all tumors; secondary neurovascularization, astrocytomas	Medium
Salivary gland tumors, hepatoma, renal cancer, pancreatic cancer, chondrosarcoma, osteogenic sarcoma	Fairly low
Rhabdomyosarcoma, leiomyosarcoma, and ganglioneuro-fibrosarcoma	Low

Source: P. Rubin. (1983). Principles of radiation oncology and cancer radiotherapy. In P. Rubin, (Ed.), *Clinical oncology for medical students and physicians* (p. 60). Atlanta: American Cancer Society. Reprinted with permission of the publisher.

Combined Modality Therapy

Radiation therapy may be used in addition to other primary treatment modalities. Postoperative radiation therapy is frequently used to decrease the risk of local recurrence following surgery for breast cancer, lung cancer, high-risk rectal cancers, and brain tumors. Preoperative radiation is used to shrink the size of a tumor so that a less radical or disfiguring surgical procedure is possible.

Radiation therapy and chemotherapy are frequently combined to increase tumor destruction. Certain chemotherapeutic agents increase the radiosensitivity of cancer cells. However, combination approaches may exacerbate known side effects of these therapies. For example, when cyclophosphamide, which damages bladder mucosa, is administered to someone receiving pelvic radiation, an increase in cystitis is noted. Tumor cells appear to be especially sensitive to heat. Hyperthermia is used in some treatment centers in conjunction with radiation therapy to potentiate the effects of radiation.

Prophylaxis

Radiation therapy may also be used to prophylactically treat tissues or organs before disease is clinically evident. The central nervous system is frequently treated with radiation to prevent relapse of certain forms of leukemia in the brain.

Palliative Therapy

Radiation therapy may be used to palliate the symptoms of metastases in patients with widespread disease. Pain, bleeding, compression of vital structures such as

1. Flush toilet twice after each use.
2. Wipe up spilled urine with a tissue and flush in the toilet.
3. Wash hands after using the toilet.
4. Immediately wash clothing or linen that becomes stained with urine or blood. Wash these items separately from other clothes and rinse thoroughly.
5. If you should cut yourself, wash away any spilled blood.

FIGURE 8–1   Precautions for Patients Treated with Strontium-89

the brain, ulcerating skin lesions, and metastases in weight-bearing bones that are susceptible to fracture can be managed with palliative radiation therapy.

Although external radiation therapy is commonly used to treat areas of painful bony metastases, in some instances internal radiation with strontium-89 is utilized. Strontium-89 is used to treat cancer pain from multiple bone metastases. This intravenous radioactive medication provides systemic radiation to the sites of bone metastases. Because the isotope will be present in blood and urine during the first week after the injection of the isotope, the patient is instructed on the precautions listed in Figure 8–1. Occasionally, some patients note an increase in pain in 2 or 3 days after the injection is given. This "flare" reaction usually lasts for about 3 days. Instruct the patient to continue or even increase the use of pain medications if this flare reaction occurs. Blood counts are monitored for the mild bone marrow suppression that may occur.

Oncologic Emergencies

Radiation therapy is also used in the management of **spinal cord compression, superior vena cava syndrome,** and symptomatic brain metastases. Refer to Chapter 17 for a discussion of these complications.

ADMINISTRATION OF RADIATION THERAPY

Radiation treatments can be administered externally or internally, depending on the type and extent of the tumor. X-rays, radioactive elements, and radioactive isotopes are most often used.

External Beam Radiation

External radiation treatments are administered with machines that deliver high-energy radiation (see Figure 8–2). These machines vary according to the amount and type of energy (electromagnetic or particulate) produced. The kind of machine used will differ depending on the type and extent of the tumor. The cobalt-60 was the first megavoltage machine, and it is still used in many institutions. Linear accelerators, which use high-energy x-ray beams, are now the most commonly used machines. Technological advances have permitted development

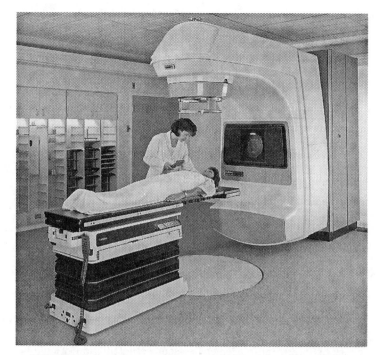

FIGURE 8–2   A linear accelerator is used to deliver external beam
radiation therapy.

Photo courtesy of Varian Associates, Palo Alto, CA.

of machines with increased energy, which allows for more precise treatments of
deeply seated tumors with less damage to superficial tissues.

Further technical refinement has enabled radiation oncologists to deliver a
large dose of radiation to a very limited and defined area. This treatment
method, known as *stereotactic radiosurgery* is delivered using a gamma knife, or a
modified linear accelerator. This technology was developed for the treatment of
arteriovenous malformations of the brain, a nonmalignant blood vessel condition. Commonly, persons with recurrent brain tumors or metastatic brain lesions
who have previously received whole-brain irradiation are treated with stereotactic radiosurgery. With this technique, the radiation beam can be directed to the
area of recurrence or metastasis while minimizing the dose to the immediate surrounding tissue.

Intraoperative Radiation Therapy

Intraoperative radiation therapy (IORT) is the technique used to deliver radiation directly to the tumor or tumor bed during the course of surgery. Locally
advanced nonmetastatic tumors of the gastrointestinal tract and peritoneum are
treated with IORT. While the patient is under anesthesia the surgeon locates the

tumor, and either before or after excision of the tumor, the patient is transported to the radiation treatment room and external beam radiation therapy is delivered from a linear accelerator. Normal tissues surrounding the tumor are shielded from the radiation with the use of special cones and devices. Once treatment
is delivered, the patient returns to the operating suite for surgical closure.

Simulation and Treatment Planning

The purpose of treatment planning is to determine the best way to deliver the
radiation treatment and to limit the radiation dose to normal tissues. An x-ray
machine called a *simulator* is used to visualize and define the exact treatment
area. Customized shielding devices (blocks) may be created to protect healthy
tissue from the radiation beam. Temporary dye or permanent tattoos about the
size of a small freckle may be used to mark reference points on the skin so that
exactly the same area is treated each day. In order to deliver treatments precisely, immobilization devices may be used to support and assist the patient in maintaining an exact position during treatment.

Internal Radiation

Internal radiation, or **brachytherapy,** is the use of radioactive isotopes for either
temporary or permanent implants. Methods of delivering brachytherapy include
intracavitary or interstitial placement of sources, instillation of colloidal solutions, and parenteral or oral administration. Sealed radioactive sources are those
encapsulated in a metal seed, wire, tube, or needle. Unsealed radioactive sources
are prepared in suspension or solution.

Encapsulated radioactive elements are placed in body cavities or inserted
directly into tissues with suitable applicators. The applicator is usually placed
into the body cavity or tissue surgically or using fluoroscopy. The applicators,
usually plastic or metal tubes, may be sutured into or near the tumor. Later, when
the patient returns to the hospital room, the radioactive isotope is placed into
the applicator. This "afterloading" technique is used to reduce the radiation
exposure to hospital personnel. These implants provide radiation to a limited
area while minimizing normal tissue exposure. Radioactive implants are used in
the treatment of cancers of the tongue, lip, breast, vagina, cervix, endometrium,
rectum, bladder, and brain.

Encapsulated sources may also be left within the patient as permanent
implants. "Seeding" with small beads of radioactive material is an approach that
can be used for the treatment of localized prostate cancers and localized but inoperable lung cancers. The patient's body attenuates, or blocks, most of the radiation, so radiation precautions are usually not required.

Radioactive isotopes can also be given orally or parenterally or instilled into
intrapleural or peritoneal spaces. Thyroid cancer, for example, is frequently treated with oral administration of radioactive iodine (^{131}I). The period of greatest
radioactivity for ^{131}I is 8 days.

NURSING CONSIDERATIONS

Many patients are frightened by the concept of radiation, making assessment of the patient's and family's knowledge and coping ability all the more important. Nurses can provide information about the use of radiation therapy in the treatment of cancer, the process of treatment planning, the treatment schedule, and the self-care activities the patient can perform to control treatment side effects. Inquiring about past experiences and coping abilities will help identify measures that have been effective for the individual. Giving time to the patient and family to talk about concerns related to illness and treatment is also beneficial.

With internal irradiation, patients may require special radiation precautions based on the principle of time, distance, and shielding. Health care personnel should limit the amount of time spent in close proximity to the patient, minimize the time spent in the room, and use lead shielding as appropriate.

Patients receiving internal irradiation via either sealed or unsealed sources are generally physically isolated from other patients and staff members in a private room. People under 18 years old and pregnant women are not permitted in the room. With sealed sources, body fluids and materials used by the patient are not radioactive and do not require handling special precautions. Bed rest may be required to prevent dislodging the radioactive source. Once the implant is removed and returned to the lead-lined container, the patient is no longer radioactive.

In patients treated with unsealed radioactive isotopes, secretions may be contaminated with radioactive material. Health care personnel should wear gloves when handling these secretions, and when possible, disposable items (e.g., eating utensils, urinals) should be used. Nondisposable items (equipment, linens, etc.) should be placed in plastic bags and left in the patient's room to be checked for radioactivity and removed when permissible. These patients may be discharged from the hospital when it is determined that the total body retention of the isotope is at a safe level.

Side effects occur as normal tissues within the treatment area are damaged by the radiation. Skin toxicity, fatigue, and anorexia can occur with treatment to any site, while other toxicities are seen when specific areas of the body are treated (Table 8–2). The severity of side effects depends on many factors, including volume of tissue treated, total dose, daily dose (fractionation) of therapy, method of treatment, and certain individual factors. Acute radiation reactions, such as skin reactions, occur during the course of therapy and generally resolve 2 to 4 weeks following the completion of therapy. However, delayed side effects may occur many months or years after treatment and may persist on a long-term basis.

Nursing care for side effects involves assessment and intervention to prevent or minimize the occurrence of the side effects and to provide relief of symptoms that do occur. Figure 8–3 lists nursing measures to manage side effects associated with radiation therapy.

TABLE 8–2 The Immediate and Delayed Response of Tissues to Radiation Exposure

Site of Radiation Exposure	Acute Response to Radiation	Subacute Response to Radiation	Late Response to Radiation
Skin	Denuding of the epidermal layer; redness, edema, itching, dryness, and weeping may occur; begins in 1–6 weeks and recovers 2–3 weeks after the exposure to radiation ends	Fibrosis, atrophy, telangiectasis, and a tan appearance ⟶	
Epithelial lining of the gastrointestinal tract:			
Oral cavity	Dryness, redness, edema, denuding, ulceration, pain, necrosis, taste alterations, anorexia	Fibrosis, telangiectasis, taste alterations ⟶	
Esophagus	Denuding and sloughing of epithelial cells, necrosis, ulceration, pain, anorexia	Fibrosis ⟶	
Stomach	Sloughing of epithelial cells, nausea, vomiting	Infarction, fibrosis, necrosis	Ulceration, obstruction
Intestines	Sloughing of intestinal villi, diarrhea	Infarction, fibrosis, necrosis	Ulceration, obstruction
Epithelial lining of the genitourinary tract:			
Kidneys		Vascular occlusion leading to radiation nephritis, renal shutdown ⟶	
Bladder	Cystitis, ulceration	Fibrosis, contracted bladder ⟶	
Bone marrow	Depression of the white blood cells (neutrophils), platelets, and red blood cells; complete recovery of the neutrophils and platelets in 2–6 weeks	Anemia ⟶	
Hair follicle	Hair loss	Permanent hair loss ⟶	
Respiratory system	Pneumonitis; significant if 25% of the lung tissue is involved, fatal if 75% of the lung tissue is involved	Fibrosis ⟶	

System	Response	
Cardiovascular system	Rare myocarditis or pericarditis	Fibrosis ⟶
Central nervous system:		
Brain and spinal cord	Inflammation and edema	Vascular obliteration leading to infarction and occlusion ⟶
Peripheral nerves	Inflammation and edema	
Eyes	Lenticular opacities	Cataracts ⟶
Bones and cartilage:		
Child	No response	Arrest of growth, shortening of bone ⟶
Adult		⟶
Gonads:		
Sperm	Radioresistant, will remain for 90–120 days	
Mature sperm	Some possibility of mutation	
Spermatogonia	100–300 cGy, temporary sterility with possible mutations	Normal levels with 100–300 cGy
	300–600 cGy, permanent sterility ⟶	⟶
Ovary	All oocytes are present; 600–1000 cGy permanent sterility	⟶

Special Note: The fetus is very sensitive to radiation. Pregnant women or those women who suspect they may be pregnant must avoid all possible exposure to sources of radiation. The most radiosensitive period for the fetus is during the period of organ development, which is 2–12 weeks post-conception. Congenital abnormalities have been detected at doses of 5 cGy with radiation-induced abortion occurring at 500 cGy. The development of cancer, especially leukemia and thyroid cancer, as well as the central nervous system disorders of microencephaly and mental retardation, are the defects most often reported when the fetus is exposed to a source of radiation.

Source: From *Care of the Client Receiving External Radiation Therapy.* (pp. 53–54) by J. M. Yasko, 1982. Reston, VA: Reston Publishing Co. Inc. Reprinted with permission of Appleton Lange, Norwalk, CT.

Skin Reaction

1. Assess skin within the treatment area for erythema, pain, and dry or moist desquamation (peeling of skin).
2. Markings on skin for treatment purposes must not be removed unless otherwise instructed.
3. Wash the treated area only with tepid water and a soft wash cloth.
4. Within the treatment area, avoid use of soaps, deodorants, powders, perfumes, cosmetics, heavily scented lotions, and skin preparations.
5. Avoid wearing tight-fitting clothing over treatment area.
6. Wear cotton clothing close to the skin.
7. Items that produce extreme temperatures, such as hot water bottles, electric heating pads, and hot and cold packs, must not be applied to the treatment area.
8. Protect the treatment area from the sun, wind, and cold. Utilize protective clothing. Following treatment, if sun exposure to the treatment area is unavoidable, use an SPF 15 sunscreening agent. Increased skin sensitivity within the treatment area may be a permanent outcome of irradiation.
9. If dry desquamation occurs, a moisturizing lotion may be prescribed.

Fatigue

1. Assess level of fatigue.
2. Determine activities that increase fatigue.
3. Identify activities that reserve energy; plan rest periods throughout the day.
4. Assist patient and family in obtaining resources for transportation, chores, and meal preparation.
5. Assure optimal nutritional status.

Anorexia

1. Assess nutritional status, food intake, weight.
2. Suggest small, frequent meals, high-protein and high-calorie foods and snacks.
3. Utilize nutritional supplements.

Oral Stomatitis

1. Assess oral cavity at least daily.
2. Review mouth care: Brush teeth after each meal, floss teeth once a day (if tolerated).
3. Rinse mouth with warm saline every 2 hours or as needed.
4. When mouth is tender, select soft, nonirritating foods and fluids to consume.
5. Utilize topical anesthetics or analgesics as ordered before meals to improve comfort with eating.

Taste Changes

1. Assess for taste changes.
2. Recommend experimenting with a variety of foods to find foods that provide some satisfying taste.
3. Perform mouth care before meals.

FIGURE 8–3   Nursing Measures to Manage Side Effects
Associated with Radiation Therapy

Xerostomia

1. Assess for xerostomia.
2. Inspect oral cavity for signs of infection.
3. Provide soft and moistened foods.
4. Provide fluids with meals and snacks.
5. Use saliva substitutes.

Pharyngitis and Esophagitis

1. Assess for sore throat, esophagus.
2. Provide soft, nonirritating foods.
3. Utilize topical anesthetics or analgesics prior to meals as ordered.

Cough

1. Assess for cough, fever, chills, or sweats.
2. Provide cough medications, antibiotics as ordered.
3. Encourage fluid intake as tolerated.
4. Encourage warm saline gargles as needed.

Nausea and Vomiting

1. Assess for nausea and vomiting.
2. Prophylactically use antiemetic for treatments that are emetogenic.
3. Utilize antiemetic as needed.
4. Monitor hydration status and encourage fluids.
5. Encourage small, frequent meals.
6. Encourage resting after meals.

Diarrhea

1. Assess for diarrhea.
2. Utilize low-residue diet when diarrhea occurs.
3. Utilize antidiarrheal medications as needed.
4. Monitor hydration status.
5. Assess perianal tissues for excoriation.

Cystitis

1. Assess for cystitis, dysuria, frequency.
2. Assess for bladder infection.
3. Encourage fluid intake.
4. Utilize medications as ordered.

FIGURE 8–3 (Continued)

CONCLUSION

Nursing care of the person receiving radiation therapy involves provision of symptom management and patient and family education. An additional role of the nurse is the identification of resources for the patient and family in the community. Receiving radiation therapy impacts the family's financial, time, energy, and emotional resources. By providing care that is attentive to psychosocial as well as physical needs, the nurse will assist the patient and family in adapting to the illness and treatment.

BIBLIOGRAPHY

Bruner, D. W., Iwamoto, R., Keane, K., & Strohl, R. (Eds.). (1992). *Manual for radiation oncology nursing practice and education*. Pittsburgh: Oncology Nursing Society.

Dow, K. H., & Hilderley, L. J. (Eds.). (1992). *Nursing care in radiation oncology*. Philadelphia: W. B. Saunders.

Fleming, I. D., Brady, L. W., Mieszkalski, G. B., Cooper, M. R., & Cooper, Michael R. (1995). Basis for major current therapies for cancer. In G. P. Murphy, W. Lawrence Jr., & R. E. Lenhard Jr. (Eds.), *Clinical oncology* (2nd ed.) (pp. 96–134). Atlanta: American Cancer Society.

Hilderley, L. J., & Dow, K. H. (1996). Radiation oncology. In S. B. Baird, R. McCorkle, M. Grant, & M. Frank-Stromborg, (Eds.), *Cancer nursing: A comprehensive textbook* (2nd ed.). Philadelphia: W. B. Saunders.

Sitton, E. (1992). Early and late radiation-induced skin alterations: Mechanisms of skin changes. Part 1. *Oncology Nursing Forum, 19*, 801–807.

Sitton, E. (1992). Early and late radiation-induced skin alterations: Nursing care of irradiated skin. Part 2. *Oncology Nursing Forum, 19*, 907–912.

9

Chemotherapy

Margaret Barton Burke

Chemotherapy is the primary treatment of choice for many cancers. It differs from surgery and radiation therapy in that chemotherapy is a systemic treatment that can reach metastatic and sanctuary sites not always amenable to other therapies.

The modern era of chemotherapy was initiated by the discovery of the effective use of estrogens in prostate and breast cancer. Alkylating agents were discovered as a result of a wartime investigation in which sailors exposed to poisonous mustard gas developed marrow and lymphoid hypoplasia. The eventual result was the treatment modality of chemotherapy. The first chemotherapeutic agent, nitrogen mustard, is still a prominent agent in many treatment protocols. There are over 50 chemotherapeutic agents in current use (Figure 9–1), with many more compounds in the drug development pipeline.

New drugs are analyzed regularly for anticancer effects through investigational protocols. These protocols have four phases of clinical investigation. The purpose of a Phase I **clinical trial** is to determine the associated toxicity, maximum tolerated dose, and optimal schedule or mode of delivery of a new drug. Phase II trials test the new drug's efficacy in patients with a variety of tumors. In Phase III trials, the efficacious new drug is compared to the standard or best available therapy for each type of tumor tested. In Phase IV, postmarketing studies are conducted to define new uses, dosing schedules, and additional information about the drug.

RATIONALE FOR USE OF CHEMOTHERAPY

To understand the use of chemotherapy as a rationale for treatment, one must understand normal cell cycle kinetics, the changes occurring once a cell becomes

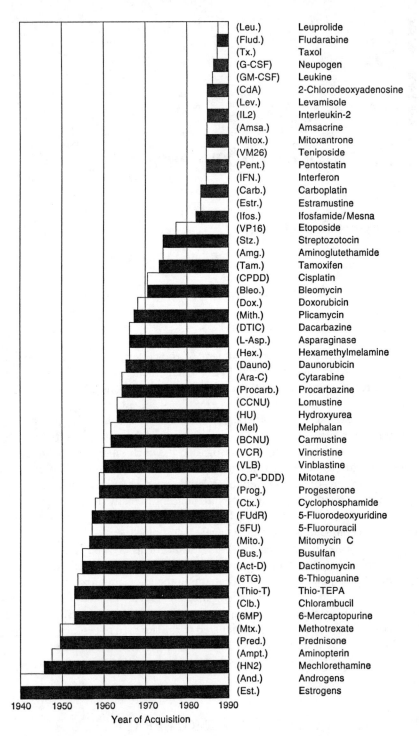

FIGURE 9–1 Acquisition of New Anticancer Drugs, 1940 to 1990

Source: Reprinted with permission from Krakoff, I. (1991). Cancer chemotherapeutic and biologic agents. *CA—A Cancer Journal for Clinicians, 41*(5), 264–278.

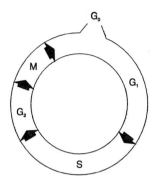

M	Period of cell division
G_1	Postmitotic period in proliferative cycle (RNA and protein synthesis)
G_0	Postmitotic period, temporarily out of proliferative cycle, "resting cells" - when stimulated, cells move into G_1, and begin to multiply again
S	Period of DNA synthesis
G_2	Premitotic period (RNA and protein synthesis)

FIGURE 9-2   The Cell Cycle

malignant (see Chapter 2), the goals of chemotherapy treatment, and the mechanisms of action of these agents.

The **cell cycle** is a sequence of steps through which both normal and neoplastic cells grow and replicate. This process of cell growth and replication involves five phases that are designated by the letters and subscripts G_0, G_1, S, G_2, and M (Figure 9-2).

Most antineoplastic agents are classified according to both their cell cycle activity and cellular function. If classified by cellular activity, chemotherapeutic agents are considered either cell cycle [phase] specific or cell cycle [phase] nonspecific. Functional classifications specify agents as alkylators, antimetabolites, antitumor antibiotics, plant alkaloids and natural products, and hormones.

Cell cycle [phase] specific agents kill proliferating cells only in a specific phase of the cell cycle (i.e., phases G_1 through M). Theoretically, when chemotherapy is given to frequently cycling cells there is more cell kill. **Cell cycle [phase] nonspecific** agents do not depend on the phase of the cell cycle to be active. Instead, these agents affect cells in all phases of the cell cycle. Resting cells are as vulnerable as dividing cells to the cytotoxic effects of these agents. A list of common chemotherapeutic agents classified by cell cycle activity as well as function can be found in Table 9-1.

The goals of chemotherapy are cure, control, or palliation. Additionally when there is high probability of residual microscopic disease and increased risk of systemic recurrence, agents may be given as **neo-adjuvant therapy** or as **adjuvant therapy,** that is as a treatment prior to either surgery, radiation, or biotherapy or in addition to these therapies. In theory, combining local and systemic therapies will achieve a greater response to treatment.

Understanding the mechanism of action and the purpose of treatment are paramount to understanding the logic behind combination therapy, the usual way chemotherapy is given. In combination therapy, agents that differ in both cell cycle specificity and toxicities are combined to achieve maximum cell kill with minimum side effects. Examples of standard combination therapy are the CMF (cyclophosphamide, methotrexate, 5-fluorouracil) protocol for breast

TABLE 9–1   Cell Cycle Activity of Selected Chemotherapeutic Agents

| | *Cell Cycle Phase-Specific Agents* | | |
G₁ Phase	*G₂ Phase*	*S Phase*	*M Phase*
L-asparaginase	Bleomycin	Cytarabine	Vinblastine
Hormones	Etoposide	5-flourouracil	Vincristine
Corticosteroids		Hydroxyurea	Vindesine
Bleomycin		Methotrexate	Pacitaxel
		Thioguanine	Bleomycin

| | *Cell Cycle Phase-Nonspecific Agents* | | |
Alkylating Agents	*Nitrosoureas*	*Antibiotics*	*Miscellaneous*
Busulfan	Carmustine (BCNU)	Dactinomycin	Dacarbazine
Chlorambucil	Lomustine (CCNU)	Daunorubicin	Procarbazine
Cisplatin	Semustine (MeCCNU)	Doxorubicin	CPT-11
Cyclophosphamide	Streptozocin	Mitomycin	Suramin
Ifosfamide		Plicamycin	Topotecan
Mechlorethamine			Asparaginase
Melphalan			

Source: Adapted from Barton Burke, M., Wilkes, G., & Ingwersen, K. (1996). *Cancer chemotherapy: A nursing process approach* (2nd ed.). Sudbury, MA: Jones and Bartlett.

cancer and a MOPP (methotrexate, Oncovin®, prednisone, procarbazine) protocol for Hodgkin's disease.

CHEMOTHERAPEUTIC AGENTS

The mechanisms of action for these drugs are based on the functional classifications mentioned earlier.

Alkylating agents are drugs that work by interacting chemically with the cellular deoxyribonucleic acid (DNA) to prevent replication of the cell. As a class, these chemotherapy agents are considered cell cycle [phase] nonspecific. Alkylating agents have been proven to be cytotoxically active against chronic leukemias; lymphomas; Hodgkin's disease; and certain carcinomas of the breast, lung, prostate, and ovary. Nitrosoureas act similarly to alkylating agents by inhibiting enzymatic changes necessary for DNA repair. These agents cross the blood-brain barrier and are used to treat brain tumors, lymphomas, multiple myeloma, and malignant melanoma.

Antimetabolites are a group of agents that interfere with DNA and ribonucleic acid (RNA) synthesis by mimicking the chemical structure of essential metabolites. They prohibit cell replication in one of two ways: (1) by deceiving cells into incorporating the agent into certain metabolic pathways essential for the synthesis of RNA or DNA so that a false genetic message is transmitted, or (2) by blocking the enzymes necessary for the synthesis of essential compounds. The end result is that DNA synthesis is prevented. These drugs are cell cycle [phase] specific and are used in the treatment of acute and chronic leukemias and tumors of the gastrointestinal tract, breast, and ovary.

Antitumor antibiotics are cytotoxic agents derived from microorganisms and have both antimicrobial and cytotoxic activity. Several of these drugs interfere with DNA through an interaction called intercalation: The drug is able to be inserted between DNA base pairs. Others are chemically able to inhibit cellular enzymes and mitosis or alter cellular membranes. These agents are considered cell cycle [phase] nonspecific and are widely used in the treatment of a variety of malignancies.

Plant alkaloids and natural products fall into three categories: mitotic inhibitors, enzymes, and enzyme inhibitors. Mitotic inhibitors work in two ways. The first mechanism of action is to cause crystallization of the microtubules during mitosis, causing mitotic arrest and cell death. The second mechanism of action is to enhance microtubular formation, resulting in a stable, albeit nonfunctional microtubule capable of causing cellular death. Enzymes act by inhibiting protein synthesis, thereby depriving tumor cells of the amino acids necessary for cell replication. Enzyme inhibitors, such as topoisomerase inhibitors, have been found to inhibit enzymes that break and reseal DNA strands. These drugs form a stable complex by binding to DNA and topoisomerase enzymes, resulting in DNA damage that interferes with replication and transcription.

Hormones are useful in treating some types of tumors by changing the environment in which the tumor originates and grows. Once the environment is changed, tumor growth is impaired or arrested; however, the specific mechanism of action is not clear. This group of agents is effective against hormone-dependent tumors such as breast, prostate, or testicular cancer.

Mechanisms of action of several of these drugs are illustrated in Figure 9–3.

ADMINISTRATION ISSUES

The administration of cancer chemotherapeutic agents differs from other medication administration in that it requires specialized education including both didactic theory and supervised clinical experience. Nurses should be familiar with the agent(s) to be administered by knowing the dosage, route of administration, and toxicity. Chemotherapy doses are usually based on body surface area (m^2) and are calculated from an individual's height and weight. The sequence of drug administration may be crucial to effectiveness; therefore, familiarity with the chemotherapy protocol is critical. Careful adherence to written chemotherapy orders prevents errors in scheduling or method of administration.

Chemotherapeutic agents are administered via the following routes: oral, intravenous, intramuscular, intracavitary, intraperitoneal, intrathecal, intrapleural, intravesicular, topical, and intra-arterial. Several chemotherapeutic

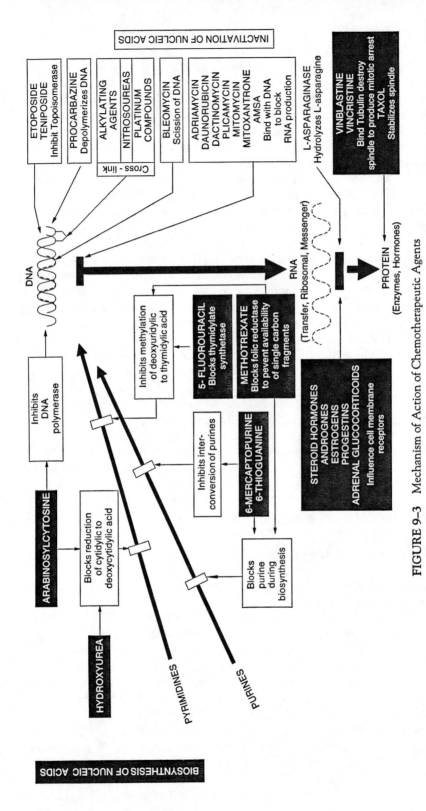

FIGURE 9-3   Mechanism of Action of Chemotherapeutic Agents

Source: Reprinted with permission from Krakoff, I. (1991). Cancer chemotherapeutic and biologic agents. *CA—A Cancer Journal for Clinicians, 41*(5), 266.

agents are considered irritants and vesicants and when given intravenously can cause either irritation to the vein or, if improper technique is used, **extravasation** and subsequent tissue damage. Such damage might include hyperpigmentation, burning, erythema, inflammation, ulceration, necrosis, prolonged pain, tissue sloughing, infection, and loss of mobility. A careful intravenous technique or the use of an implantable device (see Chapter 15) minimizes the possibility of extravasation.

A comprehensive chemotherapy checklist may be found in Figure 9–4.

Some chemotherapeutic agents are known to cause allergic or hypersensitive reactions that vary from mild to life threatening. Although it is impossible for a nurse to recall all the side effects for every drug, it is the nurse's responsibility to be aware of potential allergic or hypersensitive reactions to specific drugs. These drugs must be given with caution, and emergency medications should be readily available in case of anaphylactic reaction.

NURSING CARE

Chemotherapeutic agents damage proliferating and resting cells, healthy and cancerous cells alike. The most vulnerable cells are those with rapid doubling times in the hematopoietic, integumentary, gastrointestinal, respiratory, cardiovascular, genitourinary, nervous, and reproductive systems. Table 9–2 highlights the potential problems or nursing diagnoses and the assessment parameters, as well as the drug- and dose-limiting side effects for chemotherapeutic agents. This information foms the foundation for care given to patients receiving chemotherapy.

SAFE HANDLING OF CANCER CHEMOTHERAPEUTIC AGENTS

Controversy regarding the potential health hazards of exposure to **cytotoxic agents** has been debated since the late 1970s, when research revealed possible genotoxic (DNA-damaging), carcinogenic (cancer-causing), teratogenic (causing abnormal structures in the embryo or fetus), and fetotoxic (capable of causing fetal death) characteristics of cytotoxic agents. Research findings are inconclusive; however, these findings sparked the development of Occupational Safety and Health Administration (OSHA) guidelines for safe handling of chemotherapeutic agents to guide practice and minimize health care workers' exposure.

The main routes of cytotoxic drug exposure are inhalation, absorption, and ingestion. At risk are health care personnel who come in contact with these drugs, including nurses, pharmacists, physicians, nursing assistants, and housekeeping staff. Additionally, patients and family members who handle either the chemotherapeutic agent(s) or the human excreta are at risk of exposure. Figure 9–5 offers guidelines for handling cytotoxic drugs safely.

It is the responsibility of nurses to incorporate such guidelines into their practice in order to minimize exposure both to themselves and to their patients.

1. Verify informed consent. May be written or oral depending on institution policy, but it is required before chemotherapy administration.
2. Know the drug phamacology: mechanism of action, usual dosage, route of administration, acute and long-term side effects, and route of excretion.
3. Review laboratory data, keeping in mind acceptable parameters. Report abnormalities to the physician.
4. Complete prechemotherapy assessment of patient, medical history, and prior chemotherapy.
5. Check physician order for name of drug(s), dosage, route, rate, and timing of drug(s) administration. (Question anything that seems out of the ordinary.)
6. Recalculate dosage. Check height and weight; calculate body surface area (BSA).
7. Verify physician orders and dosage calculations with another nurse.
8. Premedication: Administer most premedications at least 20–30 minutes before chemotherapy starts. In some cases, may want to start the patient on antiemetic therapy the night before or the morning of therapy.
9. Patient education: Teach and review with the patient and family details of the chemotherapy schedule, expected side effects, and self-care preventive management suggestions to minimize untoward side effects. Provide written explanations the patient can refer to later since this information may be overwhelming. Refer questions to physician as necessary.
10. Provide patient with telephone numbers for physician and clinic, as appropriate.
11. Reconstitute drug(s) according to manufacturer suggestions, OSHA guidelines, and institution procedures. May be the responsibility of the nursing or the pharmacy department depending on the institution's policy.
12. Gather appropriate equipment. D_5W or normal saline (NS) are commonly used to infuse chemotherapy, but not exclusively. Use the correct solution and volume. Protect from direct sunlight if applicable.
13. Administer chemotherapy agents according to written policies and procedures using proficient intravenous therapy skills and techniques.
    a. Administer all medications using the five rights:
       (1) Right patient
       (2) Right drug
       (3) Right dose
       (4) Right route
       (5) Right time
    b. If no information is available, assume the drug you are giving is a vesicant and administer it with caution, according to institutional policy and procedure.
    c. Avoid drug infiltration. If unsure whether the IV is infiltrated, discontinue it and restart another IV rather than risk extravasation. *When in doubt, pull it out.*
    d. Do not mix drugs together when administering combination therapy. Use syringe or intravenous of NS to flush before first drug, in between drugs, and upon completion of all drugs.
    e. It is not optimal to administer vesicant drugs through an indwelling peripheral IV (one that has been in place 4–6 hours or more). It is important to preserve veins, but it is more important to prevent potential extravasation.
    f. Nonvesicant chemotherapy drugs may be administered through an existing IV, once the site has been fully assessed for patency and lack of infiltration.
    g. If unable to start an IV after two attempts, consult a colleague for assistance.

FIGURE 9–4   Chemotherapy Checklist

14. Do not allow anyone to interrupt you during the preparation or administration of chemotherapy.
15. Do not foster a patient's dependency on one nurse.
16. Always have emergency drugs and an extravasation kit readily available should an adverse reaction occur.
17. Always listen to the patient. The patient's knowledge and preference should be utilized as frequently as possible. As the patient becomes more knowledgeable regarding IV techniques, his or her personal experience with successful IV sites, methods, and sensations can be a great aid to the nurse. There are times when the patient's preference may not be the best choice, but his or her participation should always be encouraged.
18. Dispose of intravenous supplies according to OSHA guidelines and institution policy and procedure.
19. Document drug administration according to institution policy and procedures. Use time savers in documentation. For example, instead of writing step-by-step how a vesicant was given, write "(Name of drug) administered according to institution policy and procedure for vesicants."
20. Observe for adverse reactions.
21. Use the opportunity to teach and counsel the patient and the family while administering the chemotherapy.

FIGURE 9–4 Continued

Source: Barton Burke, M., Wilkes, G., & Ingwersen, K. (1996). *Cancer chemotherapy: A nursing process approach* (2nd ed., pp. 536–537). Sudbury, MA: Jones and Bartlett.

CONCLUSION

Nurses who treat patients with cancer chemotherapy realize that their practice is both an art and a science. Knowing that these drugs are cellular poisons compels the nurse to have a healthy respect for, as well as an indepth scientific understanding of, their therapeutic use. The actual administration of these agents requires skilled techniques and a thorough understanding of the tasks involved in specific administration procedures.

The Oncology Nursing Society and the Association of Pediatric Oncology Nurses recommend that only registered nurses who have received both didactic theoretical training and supervised clinical experience administer cancer chemotherapy. This training ought to be authenticated in writing in the nurse's personnel record.

Additionally, patients should be educated about the chemotherapy regimen that they are going to receive and should give their informed consent to such treatment. This teaching should be documented in the patient's chart for ethical and legal reasons.

The days of "pushing poisons" are gone. The role of the chemotherapy nurse has expanded to include giving drugs, educating the patient about treatment expectations, and managing the side effects of that treatment.

TABLE 9–2 Prechemotherapy Nursing Assessment Guidelines

Potential Problems/Nursing Diagnoses	Physical Status: Assessment Parameters/Signs and Symptoms	Drug- and Dose-Limiting Factors
Hematopoietic system		
A. Impaired tissue perfusion related to chemotherapy-induced anemia	• Hgb g(norms 12–14; 14–16) • Hct% (norms 32–36; 36–40) • Vital signs (BP, pulse, respiration) • Pallor (face, palms, conjunctiva) • Fatigue or weakness • Vertigo	Hgb < 8g Hct < 20% Blood transfusions not initiated
B. Impaired immunocompetence and potential for infection related to chemotherapy-induced leukopenia	• WBC (norm 4,500–9000/mm^3) • Pyrexia/rigor, erythema, swelling, pain any site • Abnormal discharges, draining wounds, skin/mucous membrane lesions • Productive cough, SOB, rectal pain, urinary frequency	WBC < 3,000/mm^3 Fever > 101°F • Hold all myelosuppressive agents (exceptions may include leukemia, lymphoma, and/or situations in which there is neoplastic marrow infiltration)
C. Potential for injury (bleeding) related to chemotherapy-induced thrombocytopenia	• Platelet count (150,000–400,000/mm^3) • Spontaneous gingival bleeding or epistaxis • Presence of petechiae or easy bruisability • Hematuria, melena, hematemesis, hemoptysis • Hypermenorrhea • S/s of intracranial bleeding (irritability, sensory loss, unequal pupils, headache, ataxis)	Platelet count < 100,000/mm^3 • Hold all myelosuppressive agents (exceptions may include leukemia, lymphoma, and/or situations in which there is neoplastic marrow infiltration)

Integumentary system
Alteration in mucous membrane of mouth, nasopharynx, esophagus, rectum, anus, or ostomy stoma related to chemotherapy-induced tissue changes

Mucositis Scale
0 = pink, moist, intact mucosa; absence of pain or burning
+1 = generalized erythema with or without pain or burning
+2 = isolated small ulcerations and/or white patches
+3 = confluent ulcerations with white patches on 25% mucosa
+4 = hemorrhagic ulcerations

+2 mucositis
- Hold antimetabolites (esp. methotrexate, 5-FU)
- Hold antitumor antibiotics (esp. doxorubicin, dactinomycin)

Gastrointestinal system
Discomfort, nutritional deficiency, and/or fluid and electrolyte disturbances related to chemotherapy-induced:

A. Anorexia
- Lab values: albumin and total protein
- Normal weight/present weight and % of body weight loss
- Normal diet pattern/changes in diet pattern
- Alterations in taste sensation
- Early satiety

B. Nausea and vomiting
- Lab values: electrolytes
- Pattern of nausea/vomiting (incidence, duration, severity)
- Antiemetic plan
- Drug(s), dosage(s), schedule, efficacy
- Other (dietary adjustments, relaxation techniques, environmental manipulation)

Intractable nausea/vomiting × 24 hrs if IV hydration not initiated

C. Bowel disturbances
1. Diarrhea
- Normal pattern of bowel elimination
- Consistency (loose, watery/bloody stools)
- Frequency and duration (#/day and # of days)
- Antidiarrheal drug(s), dosage(s), efficacy

Diarrheal stools × 3 per 24 hrs
- Hold antimetabolites (esp. methotrexate, 5-FU)

Continued

113

TABLE 9–2 Continued

Potential Problems/Nursing Diagnoses	Physical Status: Assessment Parameters/Signs and Symptoms	Drug- and Dose-Limiting Factors
2. Constipation	• Normal pattern of bowel elimination • Consistency (hard, dry, small stools) • Frequency (hours or days beyond normal pattern) • Stool softener(s), laxative(s), efficacy	No BM × 48 hrs past normal bowel patterns • Hold vinca alkaloids (vinblastine, vincristine)
D. Hepatotoxicity	• Lab values: LDH, SGOT, alk phos, bilirubin • Pain/tenderness over liver, feeling of fullness • Increase in nausea/vomiting or anorexia • Changes in mental status • Jaundice • High-risk factors • Hepatic metastasis • Viral hepatitis • Abdominal XRT • Concurrent hepatotoxic drugs • Graft vs. host disease • Blood transfusions	Evidence of chemical hepatitis • Hold hepatotoxic agents (esp. methotrexate, 6-MP) until differential dx established
Respiratory system Imparied gas exchange or ineffective breathing pattern related to chemotherapy-induced pulmonary fibrosis	• Lab values: PFTs, CXR • Respiration (rate, rhythm, depth) • Chest pain • Nonproductive cough • Progressive dyspnea • Wheezing/stridor	Acute unexplained onset respiratory symptoms • Hold all antineoplastic agents until differential dx established

- High-risk factors
  - Total cumulative dose of bleomycin
  - Preexisting lung disease
  - Prior/concomitant XRT
  - Age > 60 yrs
  - Concomitant use of other pulmonary toxic drugs
  - Smoking hx

Cardiovascular system
Decreased cardiac output related to chemotherapy induced:
A. Cardiac arrhythmias
B. Cardiomyopathy

- Lab values: cardiac enzymes, electrolytes, EKG, ECHO, MUGA
- Vital Signs
- Presence of arrhythmia (irregular radial/apical)
- S/s of CHF (dyspnea, ankle edema, nonproductive cough, rales, cyanosis)
- Hold anthracyclines
- High-risk factors
  - Total cumulative dose anthracyclines
  - Preexisting cardiac disease
  - Prior/concurrent mediastinal XRT
  - Bolus administration higher drug doses

- Acute s/s of CHF and/or cardiac arrhythmia
  - Hold all antineoplastic agents until differential dx established
- Total dose doxorubicin or daunorubicin > 550 mg/m^2

Genitourinary system
A. Alteration in fluid volume (excess) related to chemotherapy-induced:
  1. Glomerular or renal tubule damage
  2. Hyperuricemic nephropathy
B. Alteration in comfort related to chemotherapy-induced hemorrhagic cystitis

- Lab values: BUN, creatinine clearance, serum creatinine, uric acid, electrolytes, urinalysis
- Color, odor, clarity of urine
- 24 hr fluid I&O (estimate/actual)
- Hematuria; proteinuria
- Development of oliguria or anuria

- Hematuria
  - Hold cyclophosphamide
- Serum creatinine > 2.0 and/or creatinine clearance < 70 ml/min
  - Hold Cis-platinum, streptozocin
- Anuria × 24 hrs
  - Hold all antineoplastic agents

Continued

TABLE 9-2 *Continued*

Potential Problems/Nursing Diagnoses	Physical Status: Assessment Parameters/Signs and Symptoms	Drug- and Dose-Limiting Factors
	• High-risk factors • Preexisting renal disease • Concurrent treatment with nephrotoxic drugs (esp. aminoglycoside antibiotics)	
Nervous system A. Impaired sensory/motor function related to chemotherapy-induced: 1. Peripheral neuropathy 2. Cranial nerve neuropathy	Paresthesias (numbness, tingling in feet, fingertips) • Trigeminal nerve toxicity (severe jaw pain) • Diminished or absent deep tendon reflexes (ankle and knee jerks) • Motor weakness, slapping gait, ataxia • Visual and auditory disturbances	Presence of any neurologic s/s • Hold vinca alkaloids, Cis-platinum, hexamethylmelamine, procarbazine until differential dx established
B. Impaired bowel and bladder elimination related to chemotherapy-induced autonomic nerve dysfunction	• Urinary retention • Constipation, abdominal cramping and distention • High-risk factors • Changes in diet or mobility • Frequent use of narcotic analgesics • Obstructive disease process	Presence of any neurologic s/s • Hold vinca alkaloids until differential dx established
Reproductive System A. Altered sexuality patterns related to body image changes and decreased level of sexual excitement	Side effects of chemotherapy • Alopecia • Weight loss related to nausea/vomiting • Diarrhea • Fatigue • Decreased libido	Most chemotherapeutic agents have the potential to cause this problem, although this is not a drug- or dose-limiting side effect.

B. Alterations in the ability to achieve sexual fulfillment

Side effects of chemotherapy
- Dryness of vaginal mucosa secondary to decreased estrogen levels
- Inflammation and ulceration of vaginal mucosa (mucositis) secondary to stem cell injury

Other possible factors
- Altered role function
- Fear
- Fatigue
- Anxiety
- Lack of privacy
- Anger
- Medications/alcohol/analgesics

Side effects of chemotherapy
- Temporary impotence possibly related to fatigue
- Pain

Some chemotherapeutic agents or the psychosexual sequelae of the disease may cause this potential problem, although this is not a drug- or dose-limiting side effect.

C. Sexual dysfunction

Side effects of chemotherapy
- Temporary or permanent sterility
  Ovarian fibrosis with decrease in estrogen levels, decrease in number of available ova, especially with higher-dose alkylating agents and age over 30
  Atrophy of endometrial lining of uterus
  Irregular menses or amenorrhea (may be reversible under 30 years of age)
- Potential for mutation of available ova (especially by alkylating agents)
  Spontaneous abortion, stillbirth, birth defects
  May have normal children who should be followed by a pedioncologist

Some chemotherapy causes sexual infertility:
chlorambucil
cyclophosphamide
doxorubicin
cytarabine
procarbazine
vinblastine

Continued

TABLE 9-2 *Continued*

Potential Problems/Nursing Diagnoses	Physical Status: Assessment Parameters/Signs and Symptoms	Drug- and Dose-Limiting Factors
	• Temporary or permanent sterility Damage and destruction of testicular germ cells and epthelium of seminiferous tubules Oligospermia or azoospermia 90–120 days after treatment begins; normal sperm levels may be achieved several years after therapy Testosterone levels not altered • Possible sperm mutation Spontaneous abortion, stillbirth, birth defects Normal children have been fathered; child should be closely followed by pedioncologist	
D. Alterations in fetal development	Possible side effects of chemotherapy • Drugs cross placental barrier • Antimetabolites (e.g., MTX) and alkylating agents most harmful • First trimester: Drugs can cause cellular damage and destruction leading to spontaneous abortion • Second, third trimester: Cellular destruction leads to low birth weight or premature infant, stillbirth, birth defects, great potential for development of malignancy; there may be mutation of ova of female child Access options regarding alternative methods of family planning • Foster parenthood • Adopting • Provide information on sperm banking	

Source: Adapted from Barton Burke, M., Wilkes, G. & Ingwersen, K. (1996). *Cancer chemotherapy: A nursing process approach* (2nd ed., pp. 541–543). Sudbury, MA: Jones and Bartlett.

Preparation
- Wash hands thoroughly.
- Put on protective disposable gown made of lint-free, low-permeability material with long sleeves and elastic or knit-closed cuffs.
- Put on nonpowdered surgical latex gloves (powdered gloves may cause exposure to drug through the powder residue).
- Double-gloving has been recommended if it does not interfere with technique; gloves should be changed hourly or if they have a tear.
- Surgical masks do not protect against the inhalation of aerosols.
- A biological safety cabinet is essential. It should conform to OSHA guidelines. It should be inspected and cleaned according to guidelines.
- A respirator with a high-efficiency filter (powered air-purifying respirator) should be used if a BSC is unavailable.
- Plastic face shields and splash goggles should be used with the respirator if a BSC is unavailable.
- Disposable, plastic-backed absorbent pads should be used to protect the preparation area.
- A Leur-lock system for syringes, needles, tubing, and connectors should be used.
- Use aseptic technique when reconstituting cytotoxic drugs. Avoid overfilling containers; slowly add diluent. Use sterile gauze around the neck of glass ampules when opening.
- IV tubing should be primed with the solution before the cytotoxic drug is added.
- All syringes and containers should be wiped, cleaned, and labeled as cytotoxic drug.
- All needles and syringes should be discarded in a puncture-proof container labeled as hazardous waste.
- Do not recap or clip needles.
- Discard protective clothing and other contaminated equipment in appropriately labeled containers that conform to OSHA guidelines.
- Wash hands thoroughly after removing gloves.

Administration
- Cytotoxic drugs should be labeled appropriately in clean, dry syringes or IV bags.
- Syringes should be kept in zip-closed plastic bags.
- Wash hands thoroughly.
- Wear nonpowdered surgical latex gloves.
- Wear a disposable gown of low-permeable or nonpermeable fabric with a closed front and long sleeves with elastic or knit-closed cuffs.
- Use a disposable plastic-backed pad on the administration area to absorb any drips.
- Use Leur-lock IV tubing, syringes, and connector sites during administration.
- If tubing is not primed, it should be primed into a gauze pad inside a zip-closed plastic bag or piggybacked into a plain IV fluid and primed by retrograde flow (back-primed).
- Tape all Leur-lock connections and Y-sites. Keep gauze available to wipe droplets off Y-sites and connectors.
- Watch infusion sets and pumps for signs of leakage.
- Do not expel air from syringes.

FIGURE 9–5   Guidelines for Handling Cytotoxic Drugs

- Do not use venting tubing with IV bottles.
- Do not clip or recap needles.
- Discard needles and syringes into an appropriately labeled puncture-proof container.
- Wash hands thoroughly after removal of gloves.

Disposing of Body Fluids
- Surgical latex gloves and disposable gowns should be worn when handling body fluids (blood, urine, stool, emesis) up to 48 hours after the patient has received a cytotoxic agent.
- Provide urinals with a tight-fitting lid for male patients.
- Avoid back-splashing when disposing of urine and stool by placing a waterproof pad over the top of the bedpan or toilet.
- Use gloves when handling linens contaminated with cytotoxic drugs and body fluids for up to 48 hours after drug administration. Place contaminated linens in appropriately labeled double bags that are designated for separate laundering.

Managing a Cytotoxic Drug Spill
- Know where the spill kit is located. Be knowledgeable about the proper procedure for managing a spill.
- For overt contamination of gloves or gowns, remove them immediately.
- For skin exposure, wash affected area with soap and water.
- For exposure to eyes, use water or an isotonic eyewash for at least 5 minutes. Obtain medical attention immediately.
- For small spills (less than 5 ml or 5 gm), personnel should wear gowns, double gloves, and facial protection. Care should be taken to remove any glass fragments and dispose of them in a properly labeled container. Spill pads should be used to absorb a liquid, and a dampened disposable gauze pad should be used to remove a powder. The area should then be rinsed with water and cleaned with a detergent. All the contaminated wastes should be disposed of properly.
- For large spills, a respirator should be worn in case of aerosols or airborne powder. The spread should be limited by covering the spill with absorbent sheets or spill-control pillows. Damp towels or cloths can control a powder spill. Caution should be taken not to generate aerosols. Restrict access to the spill area. The area should be washed thoroughly with detergent and then wiped with clean water. All contaminated equipment and wastes should be disposed of properly.
- For spills in the BSC hood, follow the procedures for any spill. If the HEPA filter is contaminated, the BSC should be labeled "Contaminated: Do not use." Changing and disposal of the filter must be done immediately by properly trained personnel.

FIGURE 9–5 Continued

Source: Barton Burke, M., Wilkes, G., & Ingwersen, K. (1996). *Cancer chemotherapy: A nursing process approach* (2nd ed.). Sudbury, MA: Jones and Bartlett. Adapted from Occupational Safety and Health Administration. (1995). *Work-practice guidelines for personnel dealing with cytotoxic (antineoplastic) drugs.* Washington, DC: OSHA; and Yodaiken, R. E., & Bennett, D. (1986). OSHA work-practice guidelines for personnel working with cytotoxic (antineoplastic) drugs. *American Journal of Hospital Pharmacy, 43*, 1193–1204.

BIBLIOGRAPHY

Barton Burke, M., Wilkes, G., & Ingwersen, K. (1996). *Cancer chemotherapy: A nursing process approach* (2nd. ed.). Sudbury, MA: Jones and Bartlett.

Barton Burke, M., Wilkes, G., & Ingwersen, K. (1992). *Chemotherapy care plans: Designs for nursing care.* Sudbury , MA: Jones and Bartlett.

Fischer, D. S., Knobf, M. T., & Durivage, H. J. (1993). *The cancer chemotherapy handbook* (4th ed.). St. Louis: Mosby.

Fleming, I. D., Brady, L. W., Mieszkalski, G. B., & Cooper, M. R. Basis for major current therapies for cancer. In G. P. Murphy, W. Lawrence, & R. E. Lenhard (Eds.), *American Cancer Society textbook of clinical oncology* (2nd ed.) Atlanta: American Cancer Society.

Krakoff, I. (1991). Cancer chemotherapeutic and biologic agents. *CA—A Cancer Journal for Clinicians, 41*(5), 264–278.

Occupational Safety and Health Administration. (1995). *Work-practice guidelines for personnel dealing with cytotoxic (antineoplastic) drugs.* Washington, DC: Office of Occupational Medicine, Directorate of Technical Support, Occupational Safety and Health Administration.

Oncology Nursing Society. (1996). *Cancer chemotherapy guidelines and recommendations for practice.* Pittsburgh: Oncology Nursing Press.

Wilkes, G., Ingwersen, K., & Barton Burke, M. (1994). *Oncology nursing drug reference.* Sudbury, MA: Jones and Bartlett.

Yodaiken, R. E., & Bennett, D. (1986). OSHA work-practice guidelines for personnel dealing with cytotoxic (antineoplastic) drugs. *American Journal of Hospital Pharmacy, 43,* 1193–1204.

10

Biotherapy

Elizabeth Abernathy

Biological response modifiers (BRMs) can be defined as agents or approaches that modify the host's biologic response to his or her own tumor in an attempt to treat the cancer by modulating one of the body's systems involved in the growth of the cancer. The scientific and medical communities have recently begun to recognize the use of BRMs as the fourth treatment modality for patients with cancer. The other three are surgery, chemotherapy, and radiation therapy. **Biotherapy** refers to the use of agents derived from biological sources or of agents or approaches that affect the body's biological responses. **Gene therapy** is included in this classification since it attempts to modify the body's biological response through genetic manipulation. BRMs can be divided into three categories:

1. Agents that augment, restore, or modify the host's immune response.
2. Agents with direct cytotoxic activity.
3. Agents that modify the tumor's biology or other biological activity.

HISTORICAL PERSPECTIVE

The idea of manipulating the body's biology, especially the immune system, to fight cancer is not a new idea. In the late 1800s a New York surgeon, Dr. William Coley, began a series of experiments whereby he injected cancer patients with live bacteria in an effort to induce an immune response to the bacteria and hopefully to the cancer. The therapeutic responses obtained were mixed.

A core group of scientists remained very interested in biotherapy throughout the 1900s. However, it was not until the refinement of DNA technology and the advent of sophisticated computers in the early 1980s, that researchers had the technology to isolate, understand, and produce the different components of the body's biological systems that are crucial in the development and growth of cancer. These developments, along with new information on genetics, have given researchers the ability to explore the genetic basis of cancer as well as to attempt to treat cancer through the alteration or manipulation of genes.

Currently there are 9 BRMs approved for use in patients with cancer and more than 25 additional BRMs in clinical trials (see Table 10–1).

OVERVIEW OF THE IMMUNE SYSTEM

The immune system remains key in the body's ability to prevent, control, and destroy cancerous growth. The purpose of the immune system is threefold: to recognize, destroy, and clear that which is foreign from the body. To do this the body must be able to determine what naturally belongs to it and is not harmful (*self*) from that which is foreign and potentially harmful (**antigen**). It is believed that the body has, or can have, the ability to recognize cancer as foreign and can elicit an immune response in an attempt to destroy it, the same as it does against a bacterium that has invaded the body.

The cells that carry out the functions of the immune system are primarily white blood cells (*leukocytes*). These cells are produced in the bone marrow and continuously circulate through the vascular and lymphatic systems, prepared to fight off any foreign invaders. The inflammatory response is the initial defense of the immune system to foreign invaders in the body. *Neutrophils*, a group of leukocytes, migrate to the area of the invasion and attempt to destroy the invaders. However, a more complicated response becomes activated once the inflammatory response is initiated. This is referred to as **specific immunity,** and it occurs when an antigen is recognized by a particular group of leukocytes, the **lymphocytes,** which in turn trigger a cascade of events to destroy the invader. One of the outcomes of this activation is that memory of the invader occurs for a group of lymphocytes, providing for a strong, rapid immune response if a reencounter with the same antigen occurs at some future time. This is the basis for immunization procedures such as those for measles, tetanus, and polio.

Specific immunity can be divided into humoral and cell-mediated immunity (Figure 10–1). **Humoral immunity** refers to immunity conferred by a subset of lymphocytes, B-cells. Upon activation, B-cells secrete plasma cells, which in turn produce antibodies. **Antibodies** (*immunogloblins*) have the ability to bind to surface receptors on antigens, either neutralizing the antigen or activating additional components of the immune system, such as **complement,** to destroy the antigen. The antigen/antibody interaction is highly specific, meaning that the antibody that binds to the antigen is capable of binding to that particular type of antigen only and no other.

One particular form of biotherapy, serotherapy, is modeled after the antigen antibody interaction. **Serotherapy** is the use of antibodies that have been created to recognize and bind with antigens expressed by a particular tumor.

The second type of specific immunity, **cell-mediated immunity,** refers to immunity conferred by T-lymphocytes. Upon activation, T-lymphocytes mature into cells with different functions, including the following:

TABLE 10–1 Approved Biologic Agents

Agent	Trade Name	Generic Name	Approved Indications	Date
CSFs				
G-CSF	Neupogen	Filgrastin	Chemotherapy-induced myelosuppression	1991
GM-CSF	Leukine	Sargramostim	Post-ABMT for lymphoid malignancy engraftment failure	1991
EPO	Epogen Procrit	Epoietin alfa	Anemia; chronic renal failure; AZT-treated HIV infection; chemotherapy-related	1989
Interferon				
Alpha			Hairy cell leukemia, condyloma, AIDS-related Kaposi's sarcoma, chronic hepatitis	1986
Beta			Multiple sclerosis	1992
Gamma			Chronic granulomatous disease	1992
Interleukin				
IL-2	Proleukin	Aldesleukin	Metastatic renal cell carcinoma	1992
Monoclonal antibodies				
Oncoscint		Oncoscint	Diagnostic testing for ovarian & colorectal cancer	1993
OKT-3		Orthoclone	Treatment of acute cell-mediated rejection in organ transplants	1986

Source: From Abernathy, E. A. (1996). Biotherapy. In McCorkle, R., Grant, M., Frank-Stromborg, M., & Baird, S. B. (Eds.), *Cancer nursing: A comprehensive textbook* (p. 436). Philadelphia: W. B. Saunders.

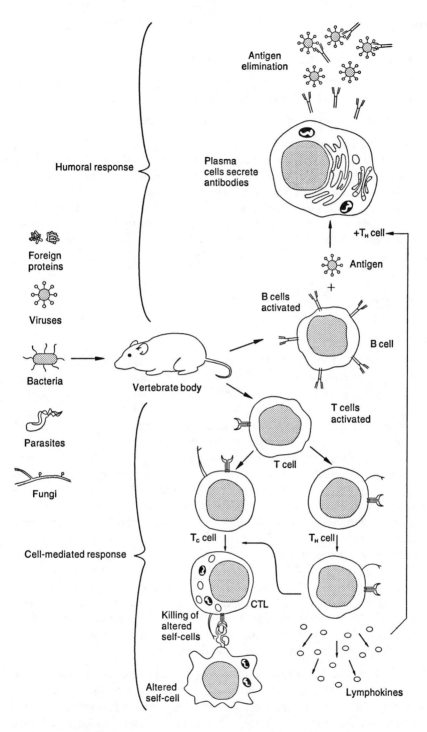

FIGURE 10–1 Humoral and Cell-Mediated Immunity

Source: IMMUNOLOGY 2/E by Kuby. Copyright © 1994 by W. H. Freeman and Company. Used with permission.

- Memory cells, which remember the antigen
- Killer cells, which destroy antigens
- Helper cells, which activate humoral immunity
- Suppressor cells, which inhibit the immune response

Activated T-lymphocytes secrete proteins, called **lymphokines,** that mediate the behavior of the immune system cells. Many of the BRMs in clinical use today are lymphokines. Lymphokines are a subgroup of **cytokines,** which refers to all proteins released by any activated cell that mediates the activity of the immune system. Other cells, such as **macrophages,** identify and clear invaders from the body. It is critical that all components of the immune system be functioning fully and correctly eliciting an immune response because of the interdependency of the reactions.

CYTOKINES

Interferon

In 1957 two British virologists identified a substance that had the ability to interfere with viral replication, and they named it *interferon*. Researchers over the next decade reported both antiproliferative and immunomodulatory effects of interferon that led to the discovery of its antitumor activity.

Interferons are a family of more than 20 different proteins produced by most human cells. There are three major types of interferon: alpha, beta, and gamma. Each type has distinct abilities as well as similar properties and toxicities. Alpha interferon, researched the most extensively with cancer patients, received FDA approval in 1986 for the treatment of **hairy cell leukemia.** Since then the following indications have been added: Kaposi's sarcoma, condyloma asuminatum, hepatitis C, chronic myelogenous leukemia, and melanoma. In addition, therapeutic activity has been documented in other hematologic malignancies and, to a lesser degree, in several solid tumors, such as renal and ovarian cancer.

Beta and gamma interferon have also shown antitumor activity in select cancers, and both have FDA approval, but for nonmalignant indications. Research continues in this area to determine additional indications for the use of interferons, as well as to determine the optimal mode and timing of delivery of the agents. Modes of delivery under research include use in combination with other BRMs or with chemotherapy or radiation therapy.

Administration and Toxicities   Interferon, like all cytokines, is a protein and cannot be administered orally because digestive enzymes would destroy it. Subcutaneous injection is the most common route, but it has been administered via intramuscular, intranasal, intralesional, intrathecal, and intracavity route, as well as intravenously or by bolus infusion. The route of administration has been shown to alter the pharmacokinetics and toxicities of the agent. Constitutional side effects are increased when interferon is administered intravenously.

The toxicities of the interferons are dose and route dependent and affect multiple systems. Low doses are well tolerated, whereas high doses cannot be maintained because cumulative toxicities cannot be tolerated. The most common side effect is the flu-like syndrome, which is associated with fever, chills, and muscle and joint aches. Fatigue may become so severe that a dose reduction of the agent is necessary.

Colony-Stimulating Factors

Colony-stimulating factors (CSFs) are cytokines that regulate the production, maturation, and function of blood cells. This process is referred to as **hematopoiesis,** and CSFs provide direction and regulation. Hematopoiesis occurs in the bone marrow, where pluripotent stem cells receive their direction by binding appropriate CSFs to their surface receptors. This binding activates the required cell line to enter into maturation. Because of the CSFs' role in stimulating maturation, the cell is released into circulation. CSFs are also referred to as *growth factors*.

CSFs are generally named after the lineage they influence. G-CSF is a growth factor affecting granulocyte, and GM-CSF is a growth factor affecting both granulocyte and macrophages. Three CSFs—G-CSF, GM-CSF, and erythropoietin— have received FDA approval, and several CSFs are in clinical trials, including interleukins, macrophage CSF (M-CSF), stem cell factor, and a CSF hoped to influence platelet recovery. CSFs have made a tremendous contribution to cancer care in preventing infection, which remains the leading cause of death for individuals with cancer. Often infection occurs during a time of **neutropenia** following chemotherapy, and CSFs have been able to speed the recovery of the granulocyte, thereby providing the patient better protection from infection. **Anemia** is also a significant problem in this population, requiring multiple transfusions for many individuals with cancer. Erythropoietin (EPO) provides valuable support in stimulating the production of erythrocytes and diminishing anemia (Table 10–2).

Administration and Toxicities   G-CSF, GM-CSF, and EPO have been given by a variety of routes, including subcutaneous injection and intravenously. Side effects appear to be influenced by the route of administration, with the intravenous route producing the most severe effects (Table 10–3).

In general, CSFs are well tolerated. At approved doses, patients report few side effects. Higher doses of the agents and combination therapy increase the toxicities experienced by patients.

Interleukins

Interleukins are a group of cytokines (lymphokines and **monokines**) named for their ability to "interlink" cells of the immune system and hematopoietic cells. By interlinking cells of the immune system, interleukins aid in the control of specific immune responses. Interleukins may directly influence hematopoiesis as CSFs, or they may indirectly aid in hematopoiesis by interacting with target

TABLE 10–2 Colony-Stimulating Factors

	Epoetin alfa (Epogen®)	Filgrastim (G-CSF, Neupogen®)	Sargramostim (GM-CSF, Leukine®)
What Is It?	A synthetic hormone produced by recombinant DNA technique	Hematopoietic growth factor, which promotes proliferation and maturation of neutrophil granulocytes	Hematopoietic growth factor, which stimulates production of monocytes, eosinophils, neutrophils, and megakaryocytes
Indications	Treatment of anemias associated with chronic renal failure and zidovudine therapy in patients with HIV infection; chemotherapy-induced anemia in patients with nonmyeloid malignancies receiving therapy with antineoplastic agents; autologous blood donation and presurgical blood loss; and other anemias of chronic disease	Prevent or reduce cytotoxic chemotherapy-induced neutropenia in cancer patients	Acceleration of myeloid recovery in patients with non-Hodgkin's lymphoma, acute lymphoblastic leukemia, and Hodgkin's disease undergoing autologous bone marrow transplant (ABMT), and persons with failed autologous BM engraftment
Dose	150 units/kg IV or SC 3 times/wk. Dose should be reduced when hematocrit reaches 30–33% or there is an increase of more than 4 points during any 2-wk period. Hematocrit should not rise above 36%	5 μg/kg/d administered SC or IV by short infusion of 20–30 min; continue daily for up to 2 wks or until absolute neutrophil count (ANC) has reached 10,000/mm³, after the expected nadir	250 μg/m²/d given SC or as a 1-h infustion. Begin 2–4 hrs after the ABMT infustion when ANC reaches 20,000 after the expected nadir

Onset of Activity	Approximately 7–10 days following 3 times/wk dosage	Rapid rise in neutrophil count within first 24 hrs following administration of IV filgrastim. Neutrophil counts continue to rise, reaching a plateau by day 3 of treatment, and remain continuously elevated during treatment	Similar to filgrastim
Labs	Hematocrit should be determined 2 times/wk. Dose should be reduced when HCT reaches 30–33% or if there is an increase of 4% in any 2-wk period. This sharp rise can bring on hypertension. HCT should not rise above 36%	CBC with platelets should be obtained prior to starting filgrastim and 2 times/wk during daily therapy	CBC with platelets should be obtained prior to therapy and 2 times/wk during therapy
Contraindications	Uncontrolled hypertension	Drug should be given not less than 24 hrs after last dose of chemotherapy and should be stopped at least 24 hrs before chemotherapy	Drug should be given not less than 24 hrs after chemotherapy and 12 hrs after last dose of radiation therapy
Adverse Reactions	Hypertension, functional iron deficiency	Mild to moderate bone pain	Fever, chills, rash, fatigue, myalgia, bone pain, dyspnea, peripheral edema; use caution in patients with preexisting edema or pericardial effusion

Source: Abernathy, E. A. (1994). Biotechnology: Exploring the fourth modality of cancer treatment. In L. P. Schwager & M. B. Whedon (Eds.), Quality of life: A nursing challenge. *Effects of Technology, 3*(2), 30–38.

TABLE 10–3 Side Effects of Biological Response Modifiers

Agent	Alteration in Hematologic Lab Value	Alteration in Mental Status	Anaphylaxis	Anorexia	Bone Pain	Bronchospasm	Capillary Leak Syndrome	Chills	Desquamation	Diarrhea	Edema, Peripheral	Edema, Pulmonary	Fatigue	Fever
Inteferon alpha and beta	+	O	R	+	O	R	R	+	R	O	R	R	+	+
Inteferon gamma	+	O	R	+	O	R	R	+	R	O	R	R	+	+
Granulocyte-macrophage colony-stimulating factor (GM-CSF)	+	R	R	O	O	R	R	O*	R	O	R	R	O	+
Granulocyte colony-stimulating factor (G-CSF)	+	R	R	R	O	R	R	R	R	R	R	R	R	R
Monoclonal antibodies	O	R	O	O	R	O	R	O	R	R	R	R	R	O
Tumor necrosis factor	+	O	R	+	R	R	R	+	R	O	R	R	+	+
Interleukin-2	+	O	R	+	R	R	+	+	O	+	+	O	+	+
Erythropoietin	+	R	R	R	R	R	R	R	R	R	R	R	R	R
Levamisole	O	O	R	R	R	R	R	R	R	O	R	R	O	R

+ = Common   O = Occasional   R = Rare
*Dose dependent; as dose increases, chills are more regularly seen preceding fever.
• Patients may exhibit 10–20 mm/Hg decrease in systolic blood pressure; however, symptomatic hypotension is generally seen at higher doses given intravenously.

Fluid Retention	Flushing	Headache	Hives	Hypotension	Liver Enzymes	Mucositis	Myalgias	Nausea	Pruritus	Rash	Tachycardia	Weight Loss	Weight Gain	Other Side Effects
R	O	+	R	O	+	R	+	O	O	O	O	+	R	Fever dissipates after first week
R	O	+	R	+	+	R	+	O	O	O	O	+	R	Fever higher and more persistant
O	O	O	R	+●	O	R	O	O	O	O	O	O	O	Erythema at injection site; fever generally low grade; first dose effect
R	R	R	R	R	O	R	R	R	R	R	R	R	R	Erythema at injection site
R	O	O	O	O	R	R	O	R	O	O	O	R	R	Side effects depend on what is attached
R	R	+	R	O	O	R	+	O	R	R	O	+	R	Severe rigors
+	+	+	R	+	+	O	+	+	+	+	+	+	+	Weight gain during treatment and weight loss over time due to decrease in appetite
R	R	O	R	R	R	R	R	R	R	R	R	R	R	Occasional increase in blood pressure if hematocrit rises rapidly
R	R	R	R	R	R	R	R	O	R	R	R	R	R	Rare occurrence of granulocytosis may provide a disulfiram-like reaction in combination with ethanol

Source: From *Biological response modifiers: A self-instruction manual for health professionals* (p. 65) by K. Rumsey and P. Rieger, 1992, Chicago: Precept Press. Copyright 1992 by Precept Press. Adapted with permission.

cells, thereby enabling their target cells to release CSFs. Over 15 interleukins have been identified; however, only one, Interleukin-2, has received FDA approval. Many of the other interleukins are being investigated in clinical trials to better determine their role in cancer therapy (Table 10–4).

Interleukin-2   **IL-2,** described originally in 1976 as T-cell growth factor, is a protein released by activated T-lymphocytes that directs T-lymphocytes to clone and perform a variety of activities, including killing cancer cells. The cytotoxic activity is thought to be due to IL-2's ability to activate antitumor cells, which attack the tumor. Cells activated by IL-2 include killer T-cells, **natural killer cells,** and very toxic killer cells, identified only after exposure to IL-2, called **lymphokine-activated killer (LAK) cells.** Another population of cells responsive to IL-2 are **tumor-infiltrating lymphocytes (TILs).** These highly cytotoxic cells are found infiltrating tumor cells. IL-2 also mediates the release of a spectrum of secondary cytokines, such as interferon gamma and **tumor necrosis factor.** These are thought to play a crucial role in the toxicities associated with IL-2.

IL-2 has documented activity in a variety of solid as well as hematologic malignancies. It currently has FDA approval for refractory renal cell cancer.

Administration and Toxicities   IL-2 can be administered as a subcutaneous injection or intravenously as a bolus injection or continuous infusion. Several very complicated protocols have been investigated in the administration of IL-2 with LAK or TIL cells, as well as in combination with other BRMs, chemotherapy, or radiation therapy.

Multisystem toxicities that can endanger life may occur with the administration of IL-2. These toxicities are dose and schedule dependent. Low-dose therapy (e.g., < 18IU given SubQ) is generally well tolerated; however, high-dose therapy (e.g., > 135IU given IV every 8 hours) is highly toxic and requires intense patient monitoring. The toxicities appear to be reversible once therapy is discontinued (Table 10–3).

SEROTHERAPY

Scientists have demonstrated that all cells, including tumor cells, have antigens on their surface that allow that cell to be identified by the immune system. As noted earlier, **serotherapy,** a biotherapy approach using the principles of humoral immunity, is the ability to deliver a treatment or label to tumor cells by binding with the surface antigens on tumor cells. Even though these surface antigens are specific for that type of tumor, they unfortunately can be found in lesser amounts on normal cells. Through the concept of antibody-antigen response, researchers have tailored an antibody to bind with the antigen associated with a specific tumor type.

In 1975, Kohler and Milstein developed the hybridoma technique for producing monoclonal antibodies. This is a complicated technique to produce antibodies from the same clone specific to an isolated antigen. All antibodies derived

TABLE 10-4 Names and Functions of ILs

IL	Name	Produced by	Functions
IL-1α, IL-1β	Endogenous pyrogen, lymphocyte-activating factor	Monocytes, macrophages, B- and T-cells and NK cells	IL-α: co-factor for hematopoiesis; stimulates B-, and NK cells, platelet and antibody proliferation. IL-1β: activates T- and NK cells, induces cytokines, acts in inflammation and disease mediation
IL-2	Killer helper factor, T-cell growth and activator	T-cells	Stimulates cytokine secretion, acts as growth factor and differentiation factor for T- and B-cells, enhances LAK, TIL, and NK cells
IL-3	Multi-CSF, eosinophil	T-cells	Stimulates pluripotent stem cells, pre-B (mast) cell growth, stimulates histamine
IL-4	B-cell growth factor	T-cells, mast cells, bone marrow	Growth factor for B-, mast, and resting T-cells; increases IgG and IgE secretion; enhances MHC Class II antigens on B cells; enhances phagocytic activity of macrophages and cytolytic activity of T-cells
IL-5	B-cell growth factor, eosinophil CSF	T- and mast cells	Stimulates growth and differentiation of B-cells and eosinophils, with IL-4 stimulates IgE
IL-6	B-cell stimulation factor	T-cells, monocytes, and macrophages	Increases secretion of immunoglobulins and antibodies, induces B-cell and myeloid stem cell differentiation, and stimulates T-cells
IL-7	preB-cell growth factor	Bone marrow	Growth of B-cell precursors and thymocytes, increases the expression of IL-2 by T-cells
IL-8	Neutrophil chemotactic factor	Monocytes, macrophages	Chemotactic attracts neutrophils, aids adherence and migration of neutrophils
IL-9	40 kD protein	T-helper cells	Increases IL-4 secretion for T-helper cell growth factor, assists in growth of mast cells
IL-10	Cytokine inhibitor	T- and B-cells, macrophages	Stimulates cytotoxic T-cells, suppresses cytokine secretion by T-helper cells
IL-11	None	Stromal fibroblasts	Stimulates T-cell dependent B-cells, with IL-3 participates in growth of early hematopoietic cells and platelets, suppresses lipase activity
IL-12	Cytotoxic maturer, NK activator	B-cells	Stimulates CD4 and CD8 cells, enhances NK and T-cell cytotoxicity
IL-13	P-600	T-cells	Increase B-cells
IL-14	B-cell growth factor	T-cells	B-cell proliferation

Source: From Dela Pena, L, Tomaszewski, J. Bernato, P., et al. (1996). Programmed Instruction: Biotherapy, Module IV. Interleukins. *Cancer Nursing,* 19(1), 62.

from a single clone are identical; hence the term **monoclonal antibodies (MoAbs).** This procedure involves injecting a specified antigen into a mouse to elicit the production of antibodies, then retrieving the desired antibody and fusing it with a myeloma cell to form a hybridoma, thereby allowing for the continued production of the desired antibody (Figure 10–2).

Therapeutic possibilities of MoAbs are endless, but their production process is very difficult, and many obstacles still impede their application. Potentially, MoAbs could be used to deliver toxic agents directly to tumor cells or for the identification of tumor cells. Oncoscint, an imaging monoclonal antibody, received FDA approval in 1993 for diagnostic imaging of colon and ovarian cancer. Many clinical trials have tested MoAbs alone or in combination *(conjugated)* with radioisotopes, toxins, chemotherapy, or biologic agents. In vitro, they have been used to remove tumor cells from the bone marrow prior to autologous transplant and to remove T-lymphocytes in order to lessen the incidence of graft-versus-host disease.

Administration and Toxicities   MoAbs are delivered intravenously to patients. Anaphylaxis, although rare, remains a potential risk associated with MoAb therapy, due to the delivery of a foreign serum (usually mouse) that contains the antibody into the body. Most associated toxicities are related to potential allergic responses or to that which is conjugated with the antibody, such as a toxin or radioisotopes.

GENE THERAPY

Gene therapy is defined as an attempt to alter patients' genetic material in order to fight or prevent disease. It is included in the biotherapy classification because of its ability to modify the body's biological response by genetic manipulation. Genes are biologic units of heredity contained in the DNA of every nucleated human cell that serve as a blueprint for a specific protein or enzyme. A flaw in any of the body's 100,000 genes or genetic order can result in disease. Gene therapy for cancer is complicated; cancer is generally not thought of as a single genetic deficit but as a combination of gene mutations.

A group of genes, termed **oncogenes,** have been identified which, on activation, can lead to the conversion of normal cells into cancer cells. Typically, oncogenes are involved in the growth and regulation of a cell. Another type of gene, the **tumor-suppressor gene,** is known to suppress cellular growth. Its absence aids tumor development and growth by allowing the oncogene to be activated. For example, mutations of p53, a tumor-suppressor gene, are common in a wide spectrum of tumors, including lung, colorectal, and breast; sarcomas; and cancer of the liver.

With the explosion of knowledge in genetics and cancer development, coupled with DNA technology, the exploration of gene therapy is clinically possible in select research settings. A variety of approaches are being tested in laboratories and in clinical research settings. Some of the approaches in cancer therapy

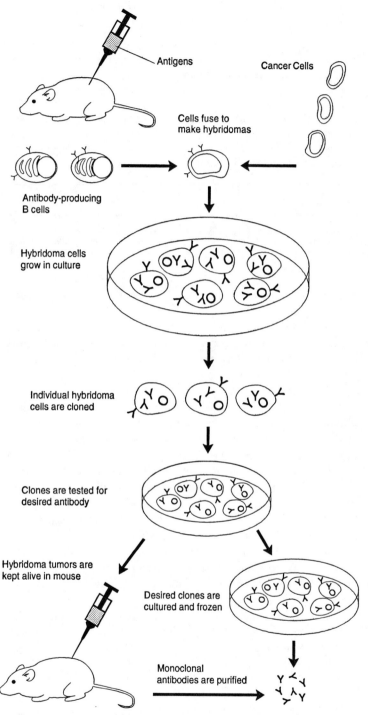

FIGURE 10–2 Use of Hybridoma Technique to Make Monoclonal Antibodies

Source: From Schindler, L. W. (1988). *Understanding the immune system* [NIH 88–529], p. 28. Bethesda, MD: U.S. Dept. of Health and Human Services.

- *Gene replacement:* Supply cells with healthy copies of missing or flawed genes.
- *Enhanced cytokine therapy:* Deliver cytokines by inserting their gene into either tumor cells or cells that infiltrate tumors.
- *Drug targeting therapy:* Inject a tumor with a gene that renders the tumor cell vulnerable to a drug.
- *Oncogene inhibition:* Deliver a synthetic agent capable of blocking the translation of an oncogene.
- *Gene marking:* Mark cells with a drug-resistant gene to determine whether transduced cells are sensitive to therapy.

FIGURE 10–3   Approaches of Gene Therapy in Cancer Treatment

Source: Abernathy, E. A. (1994). Biotechnology: Exploring the fourth modality of cancer treatment. In P. Schwager & M. B. Whedon (Eds.), Quality of life: A nursing challenge. *Effects of Technology,* 3(2), 31.

include gene replacement, enhanced cytokine delivery, and drug targeting therapy (Figure 10–3).

There are unknowns associated with any form of new therapy, and gene therapy is no exception. Possible associated risks include the chance of incorrectly inserting a gene that would trigger the development of cancer or other disease. With gene replacement therapy, transferred genes could be overexpressed, producing an excess of the missing protein. Other risks are more involved with the vector used to transfer the genetic information into the desired cells. In gene therapy for cancer, a deactivated retrovirus has been used most frequently as the vector, since it will only infect dividing cells such as cancer cells. By infecting the cancer cells, the deactivated retrovirus carrying the new genetic information is able to attach to the cancer cell and empty its new genetic content into the cell. As the cancer cell divides, each of its offspring will contain the new genetic code. Risks associated with this include the chance of infecting cells other than the targeted cells, as well as the chance that the retrovirus is not deactivated and might transfer its own genetic information (Figure 10–4).

The possible benefits of gene therapy in cancer treatment may not be immediate; however, as our knowledge and understanding of molecular biology increase, applications for therapeutic interventions could be realized. Social and ethical issues have arisen from the possibility that genetically altering human eggs and sperm could permanently alter human genetic inheritance. Gene therapy for cancer therapy does not yet involve alterations in somatic cells; however, this may become an issue as more is learned about the genetic influence on cancer development.

CONCLUSION

With the tremendous amount of information about biotherapy being generated, nurses face the challenge of keeping abreast of this complex area. Every week

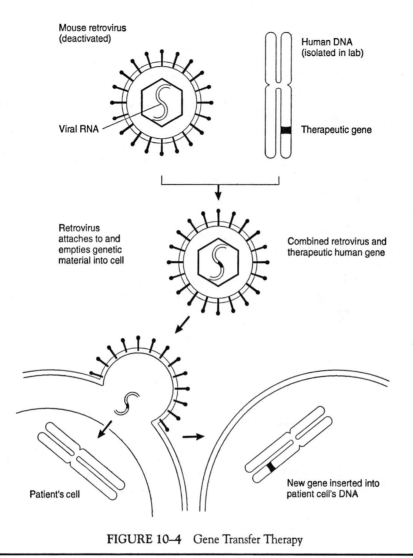

Mouse retrovirus
(deactivated)

Human DNA
(isolated in lab)

Viral RNA

Therapeutic gene

Retrovirus
attaches to and
empties genetic
material into cell

Combined retrovirus and
therapeutic human gene

Patient's cell

New gene inserted into
patient cell's DNA

FIGURE 10–4   Gene Transfer Therapy

Source: From Pizzo, P. A. (Ed.). (1993, Sept./Oct.) *NIH Observer*, p. 11.

new articles appear in the lay press regarding new developments in biotechnology. Patients and their families often turn to the nurse to explain or interpret new information about cancer and its therapy. This is a complex, difficult area to understand, involving immunology, physics, genetics, and molecular biology. Nurses must meet this challenge by obtaining the education they need to better understand this emerging technology, so that they can educate their patients, make astute observations of patients receiving biotherapy, and participate in research to ensure the advancement of nursing care for these patients.

BIBLIOGRAPHY

Abernathy, E. A. (1994). Biotechnology: Exploring the fourth modality of cancer treatment. In L. P. Schwager & M. B. Whedon (Eds.), Quality of life: A nursing challenge. *Effects of Technology, 3*(2), 30–38.

Applebaum, F. R. (1993). The application of hematopoietic colony stimulating factors in cancer management. In S. M. Hubbard, P. E. Greene, & M. T. Knobf (Eds.), *Current issues in cancer nursing practice updates* (pp. 1–13). Philadelphia: Lippincott.

Engelking, C. (1995). The human genome exposes: A glimpse of promise, predicament, and impact on practice. *Oncology Nursing Forum, 22*(2) (Suppl.), 3–9.

Goldenberg, D. M. (1995). New developments in monoclonal antibodies for cancer detection and treatment. *CA—A Cancer Journal for Clinicians, 44,* 43–64.

Hood, L. E., & Abernathy, E. A. (1996). Biologic response modifiers. In R. McCorkle, M. Grant, M. Frank-Stromborg & S. B. Baird (Eds.), *Cancer nursing: A comprehensive textbook* (pp.434–457). Philadelphia: W. B. Saunders.

Rieger, P. T. (1995). *Biotherapy: A comprehensive overview.* Sudbury, MA: Jones and Bartlett.

Sznol, M. (1994). Clinical applications of IL-2. *Oncology, 8*(6), 61–65.

Wheeler, V. (1995). Gene therapy: Current strategies and future applications. *Oncology Nursing Forum, 22*(2) (Suppl.), 20–26.

Wujcik, D. (1993). An odyssey into biologic therapy. *Oncology Nursing Forum, 20*(6), 879–887.

11

Hematopoietic Stem Cell Transplantation

Cynthia R. King

Much has changed in the field of hematopoietic **stem cell** transplantation (HSCT) since the first bone marrow transplant (BMT) was reported by Brown-Sequard in 1891. This first marrow was given orally, and the results were unclear. Throughout the 1950s and 1960s BMTs were performed with little success. This may have been due to the lack of knowledge regarding the importance of matching **human leukocytic antigens (HLAs).**

The first three successful **allogeneic bone marrow transplants** were performed in 1968 after years of research concerning the genetic factors involved in marrow grafting, **hematopoiesis,** blood component therapy, conditioning regimens, and supportive measures. In each of these three cases the donors and recipients were siblings and closely HLA matched. The first **peripheral blood stem cell transplants (PBCTs)** were performed in 1979 and involved infusing the cells over 8 to 14 days. In each case the patient failed to engraft. Successful PBCTs were finally performed between 1984 and 1986, and in each case the cells were infused over 1 to 2 days.

Much has changed since the early days of BMTs and PBCTs. In 1979 there were fewer than 400 BMTs performed worldwide. By the 1990s over 14,000 allogeneic transplants had been performed. Additionally, over 200 transplant centers have developed, and new transplant teams are joining the International Bone Marrow Registry at a rate of 20 to 25 per year. Most important, this field of marrow/stem cell transplantation, now called *hematopoietic stem cell transplantation, or HSCT,* has evolved from an experimental treatment modality of last resort to a recognized and effective modality for the treatment of various malignant and nonmalignant hematopoietic disorders.

RATIONALE FOR TRANSPLANTATION

There are two main reasons for performing marrow or stem cell transplantation. These are (1) to replace diseased stem cells that are causing an underlying disease with healthy stem cells and (2) to provide healthy stem cells to a patient whose marrow has been destroyed by high-dose chemotherapy and/or radiation.

TYPES OF TRANSPLANT

There are three types of HSCTs. They are named according to the source of the healthy donor cells. **Autologous** (self) transplants use cells obtained from the patient prior to transplantation. In this case the marrow must be healthy and free from disease. **Allogeneic** (donor) transplants use cells obtained from another donor (related or unrelated). Matching the donor and the patient according to human leukocyte antigen (HLA) typing is important. Some patients receive cells from HLA-matched or partially matched relatives. Other individuals must receive matched or partially matched cells from an unrelated donor. **Syngeneic** transplants use cells obtained from an identical twin. In each of these types of HSCTs the stem cells may be obtained from the bone marrow (BMT) or from the peripheral blood (PBCT).

Autologous

Autologous transplants are frequently used in the treatment of some hematologic malignancies, Hodgkin's disease, and non-Hodgkin's lymphoma, and in solid tumors such as neuroblastoma, germ cell tumors, breast cancer, and ovarian cancer. In recent years there has been a rapid increase in the use of autologous transplants because they allow intensive doses of chemotherapy and radiation that without transplantation would be too toxic. Moreover, this type of transplant does not require a genetically (HLA) matched donor, and thus there is minimal risk of **graft-versus-host disease (GVHD)**. GVHD is a life-threatening complication that occurs when the donor T-lymphocytes recognize the host antigens as foreign and mount an attack that results in damage to host tissues.

Allogeneic

Currently, allogeneic transplants are most often used in the treatment of acute or chronic leukemias, aplastic anemia, and some genetic diseases. When stem cells from a source other than the patient are used, the cells that are causing the underlying disease may be replaced by healthy cells. Some patients receive stem cells from an HLA-matched or partially matched relative, while others must obtain cells from an unrelated donor through a marrow registry (e.g., National Marrow Donor Program Registry). Although this type of transplant may be curative, it may be associated with substantial morbidity and mortality if the recipient develops GVHD.

HLA Typing   For allogeneic transplants, patients and donors are matched based on a histocompatibility system called the **human-leukocyte antigen (HLA)** system. This system contains antigens capable of mounting immune reactions. The HLA system is made up of multiple loci located on chromosome 6, which includes six antigen groups: HLA-A, B, C, DR, DQ, and DP. These antigen groups are typed by a variety of methods. The most frequent method is serological typing, which involves mixing viable lymphocytes with the appropriate antiserum and incubating the mixture. A positive reaction is determined by the bonding of antibody molecules to the HLA antigen on the cell surfaces. This will determine the A, B, C, and DR series of loci. In allogeneic transplantation, if HLA matching is incomplete between the recipient and donor, then the T-cells of the donor may attack the host cells and result in GVHD, which may be fatal.

Syngeneic

With syngeneic transplants, the stem cells of the donor are perfectly HLA matched to the recipient. This is the ideal type of transplant, but few patients are fortunate enough to have an identical twin. A higher incidence of leukemic relapse has been reported in syngeneic transplant patients than in allogeneic or autologous transplant patients. This may be due to the antileukemic effect provided by the GVHD associated with allogeneic transplants.

Peripheral Blood Stem Cell Transplants

Peripheral blood stem cell transplantation (PBCT) has been used with increasing frequency instead of or in addition to autologous bone marrow transplantation (ABMT). PBCTs have been performed for individuals with acute nonlymphocytic leukemia (ANLL), acute lymphocytic leukemia (ALL), Hodgkin's disease, non-Hodgkin's lymphoma, brain tumors, multiple myeloma, small-cell lung cancer, testicular cancer, neuroblastoma, breast cancer, and ovarian cancer. PBCTs may be autologous or allogeneic; however, allogeneic PBCTs are currently performed on a limited basis. Certain individuals may require a PBCT rather than BMT if they (a) cannot receive autologous BMT because their marrow is hypoplastic from prior myelosuppressive therapies or radiation to the pelvic bones, (b) have metastatic disease to the marrow, or (c) have conditions that contraindicate general anesthesia.

INDICATIONS FOR TRANSPLANT

Currently, there are numerous diseases, malignant and nonmalignant, that can be treated by HSCT. A summary of the malignant diseases and the appropriate type of transplant are presented in Table 11–1. Severe aplastic anemia (SAA), thalessemia, and severe combined immune deficiencies (SCIDs) are examples of nonmalignant diseases treated with transplantation (Table 11–2).

TABLE 11–1   Major Malignant Diseases Treated with ABMT, PBCT, and Allogeneic Transplants

	ABMT	PBCT	Allografts
Solid Tumors			
Breast	X	X	
Lung (small cell)	X	X	
Lung (non-small cell)	X	X	
Neuroblastoma	X	X	
Testicular/germ cell	X	X	
Ovarian	X	X	
Colon	X		
Melanoma	X		
Sarcoma	X		
Gliomas	X	X	
Hematologic Malignancies			
ANLL	X	X	X
ALL	X	X	X
Chronic myelogenous leukemia (CML)	X	X	X
Hodgkin's disease	X	X	X
Lymphoma			
Non-Hodgkin's lymphoma	X	X	X
Multiple myeloma	X	X	X

Source: Copyright 1995 Immunex Corporation, All Rights Reserved. This table has been licensed exclusively for noncommercial, educational purposes by the American Cancer Society.

TABLE 11–2   Nonmalignant Diseases Treated with Allogeneic Transplants

Aplastic anemia
Fanconi anemia
Paroxysmal nocturnal hemoglobinuria
Wiskott-Aldrich syndrome
Thalassemia
Severe combined immune deficiencies
Hereditary storage disorders
Osteopetrosis
Radiation exposure/injury

THE TRANSPLANT PROCESS

The transplant process is similar whether a patient receives an autologous, allogeneic, or syngeneic transplant and whether the patient receives BM or PBCs. There are several phases in the treatment process: evaluation for eligibility, admission to the unit, conditioning regimen, infusion of the stem cells, recovery, discharge, and rehabilitation.

Patient Evaluation and Preparation

The first phase of the transplant process involves a comprehensive evaluation on an outpatient basis to determine the patient's eligibility for transplantation. During this phase the patient will undergo a clinical evaluation and a laboratory evaluation. The clinical evaluation involves histocompatability tissue typing, bone marrow biopsy and aspiration, appropriate scans, electrocardiogram (ECG), cardiac ejection fraction, complete history and physical examination, pulmonary function tests, chest x-ray, and appropriate consultations (e.g., psychosocial). Numerous tests may be included as part of the laboratory evaluation, such as complete blood count with differential, chemistry profile, viral screen, hepatitis screen (non-A, non-B; A, B, C), herpes titer, HIV antibody test, or **human chorionic gonadotropin (HCG).** Additional preparation may include placement of a central venous catheter and harvesting or stem cell pheresis. Patients may tolerate transplantation better if they are in the early stages of disease and are young. Many transplant centers have an age limit (50–65) beyond which patients are ineligible for transplantation. Patients may also be ineligible for transplantation if they have significant organ abnormalities (e.g., heart, lungs, kidney).

Collection of Marrow Cells

The procedure for collecting bone marrow cells is the same whether the source is the transplant patient or a donor. The cells are obtained during a procedure called a *bone marrow harvest* and under sterile conditions in an operating room. With the patient under general or spinal anesthesia, the marrow is aspirated in 2- to 5-mL aspirates from the posterior iliac crests using a large-bore needle. Approximately 10 to 15 mL/kg of body weight are collected, or a total of approximately 500 to 1,000 mL, to ensure engraftment. This often requires 150 to 200 aspirates to harvest sufficient marrow.

Once the cells are collected, they are placed in a heparinized tissue culture medium and filtered through a series of fine mesh screens to prevent any bone or fat particles from being infused into the patient. For an allogeneic transplant the marrow cells are processed and placed in bags and then infused into the patient within several hours of the procedure. For an autologous transplant the marrow cells are collected during a period of remission (or a time prior to the administration of chemotherapy and radiation), possibly purged of residual malignant cells, and then cryopreserved (frozen) for reinfusion at a later date. Generally, a 90% viability is maintained throughout cryopreservation, and cells may be successfully stored for many years.

Collecting and Mobilizing Peripheral Blood Stem Cells (PBSCs)

It is now known that PBSCs do engraft as marrow cells, but they are 10 to 100 times less concentrated than bone marrow cells. Thus, more volume is needed to collect an appropriate number of cells for engraftment. PBSCs are obtained by a process called *apheresis* using a cell separator machine. This procedure is performed on an outpatient basis and is generally painless. Prior to apheresis a procedure called *mobilization* is conducted with chemotherapy and/or colony-stimulating factors to stimulate the production of PBSCs.

PBSCs are collected via a central venous catheter and separated by apheresis using a cell-separator machine. During the collection, the blood is withdrawn and separated. The red blood cells, platelets, and plasma are returned to the patient, and the stem cells are retained. Each session will last an average of 2 to 4 hours. Most patients require multiple sessions (2–10) over days to weeks in order to collect the appropriate number of cells for engraftment.

Potential complications include those associated with central venous catheter placement, hemothorax, venous thrombosis, line infection, and catheter occlusion or malfunction. Additionally, the patient may experience tingling, chills, and lightheadedness during the pheresis session.

Autologous Purging Techniques

Even though the bone marrow cells or PBSCs are collected while the patient is in remission, microscopic amounts of malignant cells may persist. Thus, the cells may be **purged** to remove all malignant cells before they are infused. Purging remains controversial. This process does have disadvantages, including profound aplasia and prolonged thrombocytopenia, which may leave the patient at increased risk for infectious and bleeding complications.

Hospital Admission

Transplant patients are generally admitted 1 day prior to the initiation of the conditioning regimen. During this phase the transplant team ensures that the patient is thoroughly informed and has consented to the transplant. Informed consent is crucial, because once the conditioning regimen has been given the patient is unable to discontinue treatment.

Upon admission the patient is placed in a protective isolation room. The two main types of isolation are (1) high efficiency particulate air (HEPA) filters and positive air pressure used in conventional hospital rooms, and (2) laminar air flow (LAF) rooms equipped with HEPA filters in which a plastic barrier separates the sterile patient zone from the outer zone.

The admission phase is often overwhelming for the patient and family. Adequate opportunity should be provided for questions and support during this phase of transplantation.

Conditioning Regimen

The next phase of the transplant process involves physiologically preparing the patient to receive the transplant. The terms *conditioning, preparation, and ablation* are used to describe this process. The **conditioning regimen** is given in order to (a) prepare room for the transplanted cells to engraft, (b) suppress the host's immune system in order to allow acceptance of an allogeneic graft, or (c) eliminate malignant disease.

There is no single conditioning regimen used exclusively for transplantation. Conditioning regimens are comprised of various combinations of chemotherapy and/or radiation in differing doses and schedules based on the specific needs of the patient. The specific combinations of chemotherapy and/or radiation depend on the underlying disease, type of transplant, and prior therapy received by the patient. The choice of chemotherapy agents will also, in part, depend on pharmacologic factors (e.g., cell cycle specificity, pharmacodynamics, pharmokinetics, drug interactions, and overlapping toxicities). The chemotherapy agents are usually administered by central venous catheter (CVC) or mouth. For some chemotherapeutic agents and radiation there are cumulative doses beyond which no further treatment is administered.

If radiation is given as part of the conditioning regimen, it is usually given as total body irradiation (TBI) to immunosuppress the patient, for antileukemic effect, or to prepare space for the cells to engraft. TBI is administered in fractionated doses for a total dose in ranges of 500 to 1,600 cGy.

Infusion of Cells

After receiving the conditioning regimen, the patient is given 1 to 2 days of rest and then receives the infusion of the healthy marrow/stem cells. The actual infusion process is similar to any blood transfusion. Over the years various routes have been used for the infusion of marrow/stem cells: intraperitoneal, intrasplenic, and oral. Today, the route of choice is intravenous (IV). The marrow/stem cells are infused through the CVC over several hours. Once the cells enter the blood stream, they pass through the lung and travel to the marrow cavity and reestablish marrow function in 1 to 4 weeks. Total reconstitution of the immune system will take months to years.

For autologous transplants, the patient's marrow is brought from the freezer in several bags to his or her room and thawed by warming them in a 37° C water bath. Once the cells are thawed, they are infused immediately in order to maintain cell viability. For allogeneic or syngeneic transplants, the cells are obtained from the donor in the operating room and then processed in the laboratory. Once the cells are ready for infusion, they are brought directly to the patient's room and infused via the CVC.

The infusion phase is a critical phase in the transplant process, and it is time and labor intensive. Nurses are responsible for preparing the patient and family for the infusion process and for providing support throughout the infusion. Generally, standing orders and emergency medications for the infusion process are prescribed by the physician or nurse practitioner. Although policies vary among centers, nurses often prepare and infuse the marrow or stem cells.

Side effects of the infusion are rare and often mild. The preserving agent used when freezing autologous bone marrow or peripheral blood stem cells, dimethyl sulphoxide (DMSO), causes many patients to experience an immediate garlic or creamed corn taste. Sucking on hard citrus candies or sipping flavored beverages during and following the infusion of stem cells may help lessen the taste; however, the taste may persist for up to 24 hours and may cause temporary nausea and vomiting. Patients undergoing allogeneic BMT do not experience the garlic taste and smell, because the donor marrow cells are not preserved in DMSO.

Other side effects may occur with the infusion of autologous or allogeneic cells. These may include chills, fever, shortness of breath, tightness in the chest, hypotension, coughing, chest pain, decreased urine output, and malaise. Rare complications consist of anaphylaxis, adult respiratory distress syndrome, renal failure, and cardiopulmonary arrest. Nurses need to frequently monitor patients for (a) signs of a reaction, (b) vital signs, and (c) intake and output. Some side effects may be alleviated by decreasing the rate of the infusion of stem cells.

Most PBC infusions are autologous and follow the same procedure for transfusion as autologous bone marrow cell infusions. The main difference between the infusion of bone marrow cells and PSCs is that the volume of PBCs needed is greater. A patient undergoing PBCT may have 4 to 32 bags of stem cells infused, while a patient receiving autologous bone marrow cells may only have 4 to 8 bags. The major potential complications associated with the reinfusion of PBCs include fluid overload, pulmonary edema, macroscopic hemoglobinuria, and temporary renal dysfunction.

Recovery

The recovery phase begins the first day after the infusion of cells and is called *Day + 1*. During this phase the patient waits for engraftment of the cells and normal blood counts. The recovery period will vary depending upon the patient and type of transplant, and it will last 1 to 4 weeks. During this time the patient is pancytopenic and susceptible to complications. Except for GVHD, which usually occurs with allogeneic transplants, the complications from autologous, allogeneic, and syngeneic BMT and PBCT are similar. Some of the potential acute complications and nursing interventions are displayed in Table 11-3. Physical complications may include myelosuppression and gastrointestinal, cardiac, pulmonary, hepatic, or renal problems. Psychologically and emotionally, patients may experience fluctuating levels of distress, anxiety, depression, and anger. Social complications may arise from isolation. Work and financial issues may also complicate adaptation.

The decision to undergo a transplant is a significant one for any individual. Every aspect of the individual's personal and professional life is disrupted. The

TABLE 11–3 Acute Complications of Transplantation

Acute Complications	*Nursing Interventions*
Myelosuppression	
Anemia	Provide rest, give packed RBCs, check lab values
Granulocytopenia	Prevent infections, check WBC/ANC, give CSFs
Thrombocytopenia	Prevent bleeding, give platelets, check platelet count, use electric razor
Infections	Give antimicrobials and CSFs, isolation
Bacterial	
Viral	
Fungal	
Gastrointestinal	
Mucositis	Oral assessment, oral care, lip lubricant
Nausea/vomiting	Antiemetics on schedule, oral hygiene, hyperalimentation, relaxation, imagery
Diarrhea	I & O, F & E status, antidiarrheal agent
Cardiac	Cardiac monitoring, auscultation, baseline 12 lead EKG, cardiac ejection fraction
Pulmonary	Encourage exercise, incentive spirometer
Interstitial pneumonitis	Lung assessment, give antimicrobials
Pulmonary edema	Diuretics, I & O, weight
Pulmonary infections	Assess for fever and changes in pulmonary status, give antimicrobials
Hepatic	
Veno-occlusive	Maintain F & E balance, decrease effects of ascites, weight
Renal insufficiency	Assess F & E status, weight, I & O, assess BUN/Cr, check for peripheral edema & distended neck veins
Graft-versus-host disease	Assess skin, liver, GI tract, I & O, maintain F & E balance
Psychosocial	Spend time with patient/family, provide hope, listen to concerns, use touch, provide support

CSFs = colony-stimulating factors
I = Intake, O = output
F = fluid, E = electrolyte
GI = gastrointestinal

Source: Adapted from King, C. R. (1995). Peripheral stem cell transplantation: Past, present, and future. In P. A. Buschel & C. H. Yarbro (Eds.), *Bone marrow transplantation: Administrative and clinical strageties* (pp. 187–211); and King, C. R. (1996). New frontiers of chemotherapy. In M. B. Burke, G. M. Wilkes, D. Berg, C. K. Bean, & K. Ingwersen (Eds.), *Cancer chemotherapy* (pp. 75–94). Sudbury, MA: Jones and Bartlett.

future becomes uncertain. The financial burden is overwhelming. Patients and families may have to travel a long distance to the transplant center. Patients are also faced with their own mortality and undergo major changes. This may lead to a wide range of emotions throughout the transplant and recovery. These emotions are often transient but significant. Research in the area of psychosocial issues related to transplantation is limited. It is unclear what are the most effective approaches to assist patients and families in coping with transplantation. It is clear, however, that extensive support from multidisciplinary team members (physicians, nurses, social workers, chaplains, mental health specialists, art therapists, and music therapists) is necessary. It may also be helpful to enlist the help of nonprofessionals through volunteers (e.g., church groups, the volunteer office of the transplant center, or other community resources).

Nurses who care for transplant patients play a vital role in preventing latent effects and providing supportive care. Nurses who care for transplant recipients must understand and recognize the potential acute and long-term complications associated with transplantation. Nurses can be instrumental in encouraging patients to comply with self-care activities such as daily exercise, mouth care, and care of the CVC.

Discharge

The goal of BMT/PBCT is to cure the patient and/or provide him or her with improved quality of life. It is essential that there be a smooth transition for the transplant recipient from the transplant center to the home environment. Planning for discharge should begin weeks prior to the anticipated discharge date. Some transplant centers have a professional discharge planner, while others utilize staff nurses or bone marrow coordinators to anticipate discharge needs. Nonetheless, there must be a liaison between the inpatient and outpatient units to ensure continuity of care. Education is a key component of the discharge process. Nurses are involved in educating patients and families on granulocytopenic precautions, preparation of the home environment, care of the CVC, good hygiene, oral care, appropriate activity and diet, and when to contact health care professionals.

Although each transplant center has specific discharge criteria, there are some general guidelines that patients must meet prior to discharge. Generally patients must (a) be afebrile for at least 48 hours; (b) have been able to tolerate oral medications for at least 48 hours; (c) have nausea, vomiting, and diarrhea controlled with oral medications; (d) have an adequate intake of food and fluids; (e) have an absolute neutrophil count (ANC) of 500 to 1000/mm^3; (f) have a hematocrit greater than 25 to 30%; (g) have a platelet count greater than 15,000 to 20,000/mm^3; and (h) have an adequate home environment and support. Patients will be discharged when they meet the transplant's specific discharge criteria and are medically stable. Many centers discharge patients directly to their homes; others choose to have patients stay in an outpatient setting if they do not meet all of the discharge criteria and no longer require the intensive care of the transplant unit.

Rehabilitation

Transplant patients often describe the postdischarge rehabilitation phase as a roller coaster. Research has shown that some transplant recipients will continue to experience physical and psychological problems that affect their quality of life after transplantation.

All transplant patients are monitored closely during the early posttransplant period. Patients may need daily to weekly examinations in the outpatient clinic. These visits will also include tests such as blood tests, chest x-rays, bone marrow aspirations, or lumbar punctures. Additionally, patients may receive one or more blood transfusions, immunoglobulin therapy, **colony-stimulating factors,** or hyperalimentation during the early posttransplant period. Emphasis will be placed on preventing infections during this early rehabilitation period, since infection is a leading cause of readmissions to the hospital.

Throughout the rehabilitation phase, transplant survivors may experience psychosocial effects. These may range from cognitive dysfunction, sexual dysfunction, occupational disability and discrimination, financial difficulties and insurance problems, to a variety of emotional issues.

Long-term complications are latent effects that occur 100 days or more after the infusion of healthy cells. Most of these complications result from the chemotherapeutic agents and/or the radiation given as the conditioning regimen (Table 11–4). During the first year posttransplant, transplant survivors often suffer physical effects. Their focus is on recovery, necessitating frequent visits to health care providers. After the first year posttransplant, some latent effects may resolve, while others may continue as chronic complications. These chronic complications may be physical (e.g., GVHD) or psychosocial (e.g., emotional distress) (Table 11–4).

NURSING CARE OF THE TRANSPLANT PATIENT

The field of transplantation has changed significantly in the past 3 decades from being an experimental therapy to being an accepted, viable treatment modality for some malignant and nonmalignant disorders. Due to significant changes in tissue typing, blood component therapy, conditioning regimens, colony-stimulating factors, and supportive measures, transplant patients are being discharged earlier and more are surviving long term. The current success of transplantation is, in part, dependent upon the supportive care provided by nurses in a variety of settings (e.g., transplant unit, outpatient clinic, home health care agency). Caring for transplant patients is intensive, challenging work and requires that nurses (a) have a sound knowledge of the transplant process, (b) have experience in caring for immunosuppressed patients, (c) possess skills for managing CVCs, and (d) be able to handle emergencies. The goals of nursing care include preventing and managing the potential and long-term complications associated with transplantation and providing support, hope, and optimism for the patient and family.

TABLE 11–4   Long-Term Complications

Late Complications	Time Posttreatment
Chronic GVHD	Day 100 or later
Skin	
Liver	
GI tract	
Oral	
Vaginal	
Infectious complications	100–365 days
Bacterial	
Fungal	
Viral	
Pulmonary complications	100–400 days
Interstitial pneumonitis	
Pneumocystis carinii	
Cytomegalovirus	
Obstructive disease	
Renal	1 year or later
Radiation nephritis	
Renal insufficiency	
Visual/cataracts	1.5–5 years
Neurologic complication	Weeks to years
Leukoencephalopathy	
Neuropsychological	Weeks to years
Memory loss	
Concentration difficulties	
Thyroid dysfunction	Months to years
Hypothyroidism	
Aseptic necrosis	3 months to 1 year
Retarded growth & development	Months to years
Gonadal dysfunction	Months to years
Sterility	
Ovarian failure	
Secondary malignancies	1–15 years
Psychological complications	Weeks to years
Emotional distress	
Depression	
Body image changes	
Anxiety	
Social complications	Weeks to years
Job discrimination	
Changes in relationships	
Insurance discrimination	
Spiritual effects	
Change in meaning of life	
Feeling indebted	Weeks to years

BIBLIOGRAPHY

Belec, R. H. (1992). Quality of life: Perceptions of long-term survivors of bone marrow transplantation. *Oncology Nursing Forum, 19*, 31–37.

Bortin, M. M., Bach, F. H., van Bekkum, D. W., et al. (1994). 25th anniversary of the first successful allogeneic bone marrow transplants. *Bone Marrow Transplantation, 14*, 211–212.

Bortin, M. M., Horowitz, M. M., & Gale, R. P. (1988). Current status of bone marrow transplantation in humans. *Nat Immun Cell Growth Regul, 7*, 334–350.

Bortin, M, M., Horowitz, M. M., & Rimm, A. A. (1992). Progress report from the International Bone Marrow Transplant Registry. *Bone Marrow Transplantation, 10*, 113–122.

Buchsel, P. C. (1993). Bone marrow transplantation. In S. L. Groenwald, M. H. Frogge, M. Goodman, & C. H. Yarbro (Eds.), *Cancer nursing: Principles and practice* (pp. 393–434). Sudbury, MA: Jones and Bartlett.

Ferrell, B. R., Grant, M., Schmidt, G. M. et al. (Eds.). (1992). The meaning of the quality of life for bone marrow transplant survivors: Part 1. The impact of bone marrow transplantation on quality of life. *Cancer Nursing, 15*, 153–160.

Kessinger, A., Armitage, J. O., Landmark, J. D., & Weisenburger, D. D. (1986). Reconstitution of human hemopoietic cells in a patient with acute leukemia. *Experimental Hematology, 14*, 192–196.

King, C. R. (1995). Peripheral stem cell transplantation: Past, present, and future. In P. A. Buchsel & C. H. Yarbro (Eds.), *Bone marrow transplantation: Administrative and clinical strategies* (pp.187–211). Sudbury, MA: Jones and Bartlett.

King, C. R. (1996). New frontiers of chemotherapy. In M. B. Burke, G. M. Wilkes, D. Berg, C. K. Bean, & K. Ingwersen (Eds.), *Cancer chemotherapy* (pp. 75–94). Sudbury, MA: Jones and Bartlett.

Reiffers, J., Bernard, P., David, B., et al. (1986). Successful autologous transplantation with peripheral blood hemopoietic cells in a patient with acute leukemia. *Experimental Hematology, 14*, 312–315.

Weinberg, P. A. (1991). The human leukocyte antigen (HLA) system, the search for a matching donor, National Marrow Donor Program development and marrow donor issues. In M. B. Whedon (Ed.), *Bone marrow transplantation: Principles, practice and nursing insights.* Sudbury, MA: Jones and Bartlett.

Whedon, M. B. (1991). Allogeneic bone marrow transplantation: Clinical indications, treatment process, and outcomes. In M. B. Whedon (Ed.), *Bone marrow transplantation: Principles, practice and nursing insights* (pp. 20–48; 49–69). Sudbury, MA: Jones and Bartlett.

Whedon, M., & Damianos, F. L. (1993). Nursing care issues in autologous bone marrow transplantation. *Oncology, 7*, 78–88.

12

Alternative and Complementary Methods of Cancer Management

Nancy E. Kane

Billions of dollars are spent each year by the public on questionable alternative and complementary treatments and so-called "cures" for cancer. Estimates are that nearly half of all people with cancer seek such treatments at some point in their illness, either in conjunction with traditional therapies or in place of them. Some of these treatments fall into the category of quackery, while others are more acceptable. A common characteristic is that they have not been thoroughly and successfully tested by the scientific approach. (Figure 12–1 lists critical questions that must be asked in evaluating such treatments.) These methods are promoted as effective in the cure, palliation, or control of cancer, but they have not been tested in acceptable clinical trials. However, the public continues to seek them to meet physical or psychological needs. Recognizing the characteristics of these methods and understanding why people seek them is an important part of the nurse's role.

DEFINITION OF ALTERNATIVE AND COMPLEMENTARY METHODS

The definition of alternative and complementary methods of cancer management, according to the American Cancer Society, is "lifestyle practices, clinical tests, or therapeutic modalities that are promoted for general use for the prevention, diagnosis, or treatment of cancer and which are, on the basis of careful review by scientists and/or clinicians, not deemed to have real evidence of value."

1. Has the treatment been objectively studied and found to be effective?
2. Has the treatment shown potential for benefit that clearly exceeds the potential for harm?
3. Have objective studies been correctly conducted under appropriate peer review to answer these questions, with results published in the scientific peer-reviewed literature?

FIGURE 12–1   Critical Questions to Ask When Evaluating Alternative Therapies

Alternative therapies are unproven or disproven methods; **complementary therapies** are supportive therapies that are used to complement standard treatment.

Some alternative therapies are associated with the health food industry, while others are part of the holistic health movement that has gained popularity in recent years. While some alternative therapies are harmless to the user, others may pose considerable health risks, as documented in medical literature. Because these therapies have not undergone the rigors of scientific testing, their risks may not be fully known to the potential user. The information available regarding many of the alternative therapies is in lay literature and is frequently ambiguous. It often emphasizes the medical establishment's failings and exploits peoples' fears and apprehensions about surgery, chemotherapy, and radiation therapy. Lay literature may be the only source of information available, yet it is incomplete and often misleading because of the lack of supporting scientific data.

CATEGORIES OF ALTERNATIVE AND COMPLEMENTARY METHODS

Most therapies fall into one of the following categories: biological products, devices, herbal concoctions, dietary approaches, megavitamin therapy, and psychological/spiritual approaches (including faith healing and "psychic surgery"). The American Cancer Society, National Institutes of Health, and other sources provide information to the public on many alternative and complementary therapies.

Biological products are claimed to enhance the immune system, thereby supporting the body's ability to fight cancer. Some of these products are derived from animal cells or the patient's own blood or urine. Chemicals with supposed cancer-fighting characteristics are also in this category, even though there is no scientific evidence supporting such claims.

A wide array of mechanical and electrical devices are claimed to possess cancer-fighting properties, including the ability to detoxify the system, "charge" the blood, and other unfounded claims.

Herbal concoctions are currently experiencing popularity. Herbs and plants are, in fact, a valid source of effective cancer chemotherapeutic agents. Most herbs listed in the lay literature, however, have not been scientifically tested to establish their effectiveness, and many herb products contain drugs, which raises questions about safety.

- Fear of death, disability, abandonment.
- Concern about medical costs.
- Loss of hope.
- Anger displaced onto doctor.
- Loss of control.
- Influence of family and friends.
- Perceived lack of effective traditional therapy.

FIGURE 12-2   Reasons for Seeking Alternative
and Complementary Treatments

Dietary approaches and megavitamin therapies represent the belief that cancer and other diseases are caused by improper diets, and, therefore, cancer can be cured by altering the diet. The best-known vitamin therapy for cancer is vitamin C. Adding to public confusion, Nobel prize-winning chemist Linus Pauling publicly advocated the therapeutic use of vitamin C. Even though controlled, scientific studies with vitamin C have repeatedly demonstrated no benefit, it is still purported by many to be an effective cancer treatment.

Psychological approaches are the most popular adjunctive therapies used by patients. Familiar approaches include imagery and visualization. The theory behind these approaches is that they can enhance the immune system. However, no acceptable scientific evidence exists to support this claim. Support groups and other mutual support approaches can have a significant effect on quality of life and overall feelings of well-being. However, there is no definitive scientific evidence that these methods can alter the biological course of cancer.

Patients may use these methods in addition to, or as a complement to, traditional therapies. Many of the psychological methods are used as supportive strategies to assist in coping with the emotional and physical strain of cancer treatment. Many health care providers encourage such practices if they seem helpful and comforting to the patient. However, some of the other therapies, such as megavitamins or special diets, may have potentially serious physical effects if not monitored by a knowledgeable practitioner. Interactions with chemotherapy may create toxic side effects and myriad physical problems. Patients may be encouraged by some alternative therapy practitioners to abandon treatments with a well-established record of effectiveness to pursue methods that have no such record.

WHY PEOPLE USE ALTERNATIVE METHODS

People have been seeking and using alternative therapies since ancient times. The reasons often have to do with fears of disability, death, abandonment, exhaustion of standard therapy options, and the high cost of medical care (Figure 12-2). The diagnosis of cancer creates fears, and hope is difficult to maintain when facing a recurrence of disease or increasing pain. Many search for care providers who create a feeling that more can be done and that hope for a cure is not lost. Cancer patients and their families may experience anger toward the physician who has given them bad news or frustration with the treatment choices that offer no guarantee of a positive outcome. An alternative practitioner may seem to provide such guarantees and foster hope for a cure or remission.

People with cancer often feel out of control. They may feel that they have no input into their treatment decisions; they may not feel that they are part of a decision-making team fighting their disease. The American culture also promotes the power of the individual to make personal decisions. Many feel a need to control the unknown and believe that the right to have answers is absolute. Frustration exists in our society that a cure for cancer has not been found and that conventional therapies are toxic and hard to bear. Additionally, people demand attention to the whole person and are increasingly vocal about the desire to have health care providers show concern for the person who has the disease of cancer. All of these factors may encourage cancer patients to seek health care environments where they perceive that they are part of a team, are treated as a whole person, and feel that their concerns and fears are heard and addressed.

Discussions about alternative therapies often arise when patients are facing the terminal phase of their illness. Patients and their families may feel desperate and frightened if they are told there is nothing else to be done. They may feel abandoned by the health care providers who have been so involved in their care. Shifting the goal of care to palliation may be hard to accept or understand.

Families and friends are susceptible to the same fears and worries experienced by the cancer patient. Their feelings of helplessness and powerlessness can be overwhelming as they watch the person they love cope with the side effects of treatment. Often they share in the decision making about treatments and may feel burdened by this responsibility. Well-intentioned family and friends may bring literature or share stories about unproven methods that they hope will help. Sometimes people with cancer may feel pressured to seek alternative therapies to please family and friends. Family and friends may feel guilty if they do not attempt to try every available alternative.

THE NURSE'S ROLE

Nurses are in an important position when patients and their families are considering or using an alternative method of cancer treatment. Nurses are viewed by consumers as less intimidating than doctors and, therefore, easier to approach with questions. Regardless of the care setting, nurses have opportunities to teach, guide, and support. When exploring this subject, nurses should attempt to understand the patient's motivation for seeking alternative or complementary treatment. Why the patient is seeking such therapies is as important as which methods he or she is using. What needs are not being met by the patient's health care providers or the system? What fears does the patient have about the disease or treatment? Is the family member the person seeking such approaches, or is the patient interested? What does the patient hope to gain or achieve from the therapy? Answers to these and other questions may help the nurse gain a better understanding of what the patient or family needs from the health care team. Initiating a dialogue about these issues helps patients and families feel they are heard and

- Assess patient for use of alternate therapies on a regular basis; encourage full disclosure of specifics of practice.
- Present information in a nonbiased fashion; encourage frank and open dialogue.
- Encourage patient to continue standard therapy in conjunction with alternative treatment.
- Allow patient to make his or her own healthcare choices, but assist in ensuring that the patient is fully informed when making those choices.
- Encourage, as appropriate, use of safe alternative therapies such as visualization and cognitive and distraction strategies.
- Monitor appropriate blood tests as indicated by alternative therapy.
- Answer patient's questions honestly, using accurate information; assist patient to obtain accurate printed information as necessary.

FIGURE 12–3   Nursing Strategies Related to Alternative Therapies

Source: From Montbriand, M. J. (1994). An overview of alternative therapies chosen by people with cancer. *Oncology Nursing Forum, 21*(9), 1552. Printed with permission from the publisher.

supported. Figure 12–3 lists other strategies nurses can use when discussing alternative therapies.

Patients who use alternative therapies may be secretive about it, knowing that the medical establishment may not look favorably upon such activity. A trusting relationship with the nurse can encourage sharing of this information. Once patients understand that it is necessary for the health care team to know about all treatments, ingested or not, so that proper monitoring can be done, they may feel less secretive. Approaching this topic with an unbiased and open attitude is critical. If patients or their families do not feel judged, they will more likely be open and honest and listen to accurate information more willingly.

Encouraging patient participation in decision making is crucial. Anything that helps patients feel a part of their treatment effort may help avoid the use of alternative methods; at the very least, it will encourage disclosure if they do choose to pursue such therapies. Patients ultimately are responsible for their treatment choices; however, helping them to make informed choices is part of the role of the nurse. Including the family in decision making whenever appropriate will also help decrease their feelings of powerlessness or helplessness. Keeping everyone well informed about the disease and treatment will lay a foundation for open dialogue if the subject of alternative therapies arises. The goal of communication is to ensure that patients and families feel listened to, cared for, and supported. Answering questions honestly and objectively will assist in attaining that goal.

Experimental treatments or clinical trials may be appropriately offered by the doctor and accepted by the patient. A second opinion may also increase feelings of control over decision making as well as produce other treatment alternatives. It also may reassure patients and families that the care they have been receiving is in fact standard medical care. Most important, the discussion about quality of life must be faced with candor and compassion.

CONCLUSION

For many, the impetus to seek alternative or questionable therapies is based on the feeling that the quality of their life is not being adequately addressed. These methods are described as alternative or questionable because they have not been proved effective by accepted medical standards. However, this does not necessarily mean that a particular therapy has no therapeutic value. Without proper testing, safety and efficacy cannot be established. The methods of evaluation may be frustrating to the public, but they are designed to protect society from fraudulent claims. Assisting patients to understand this process may help them avoid health complications or loss of funds from the use of alternative therapies.

BIBLIOGRAPHY

American Cancer Society. (1993). *Questionable methods of cancer treatment.* Atlanta: Author.

Cassileth, B. R. (1989). The social implications of questionable cancer therapies. *Cancer, 63,* 1247–1250.

Montbriand, M. J. (1994). An overview of alternative therapies chosen by patients with cancer. *Oncology Nursing Forum, 21,* 1547–1554.

Montbriand, M. J. (1993). Freedom of choice: An issue concerning alternate therapies chosen by patients with cancer. *Oncology Nursing Forum, 20,* 1195–1201.

Walters, R. (1993). *Options: The alternative cancer therapy book.* Garden City Park, NY: Avery Publishing Group.

Yarbro, C. (1993). Questionable methods of cancer therapy. In S. L. Groenwald et al. (Eds.), *Cancer nursing: Principles and practice* (3rd ed., pp. 1536–1552). Sudbury, MA: Jones and Bartlett.

Unit 4

Nursing Management of Patient Responses

13

Myelosuppression

Paula Trahan Rieger

Myelosuppression is a common problem in patients with cancer. It is defined as a decrease in the number of circulating blood cells (white and red blood cells and platelets). **Granulocytopenia** refers to a decrease in the total number of white blood cells; **neutropenia** is a decrease in the number of neutrophils; **anemia** is a decrease in the number of red blood cells; and **thrombocytopenia** is a decrease in the number of platelets. Complications of myelosuppression include infection, fatigue, shortness of breath, bleeding, and hemorrhage. See Table 13–1 for a review of normal blood values.

CAUSES OF MYELOSUPPRESSION

Hematopoiesis is the process by which all formed elements of the blood are produced. In humans, this occurs in the bone marrow, where cells of all lineages proliferate, differentiate, and mature from the **pluripotent stem cell** (see Figure 13–1). Because blood cells have a relatively short life span, the marrow is constantly producing new cells. Billions of red cells, white cells, and platelets are produced per kilogram of body weight daily. The body also has a remarkable ability to increase production of blood cells during times of stress, such as infection or inflammation. Factors important in regulating the process of hematopoiesis include the microenvironment of the bone marrow, interactions between cells, and secreted substances known as **hematopoietic growth factors.**

In patients with cancer, there are several reasons why the bone marrow's ability to produce cells can become impaired, resulting in myelosuppression. One of the primary reasons is cancer treatments such as chemotherapy and radiation therapy. Chemotherapy works by interfering with division of rapidly dividing cells; because the bone marrow is such an active organ, it is often temporarily damaged, and myelosuppression results. Because circulating blood cells are not

TABLE 13-1   Normal Blood Values

Value	Normal Range
White blood cells	4.5–11.0 K/mm³
Polys	40–78% of WBC
Bands	0–3% of WBC
Lymphocytes	14–49% of WBC
Monocytes	1–13% of WBC
Eosinophils	0–9% of WBC
Basophils	0–3% of WBC
Red blood cells	4.60– 6.20 MIL/mm³ (males) 4.2–5.4 MIL mm³ (females)
Hemoglobin (Hb)	14–18 G/dL (males) 12–16 G/dL (females)
Hematocrit (Hct)	40–54 % (males) 38–47% (females)
Platelets	150–400 K/mm³

Note: Values may vary slightly by laboratory.

destroyed, blood counts will usually begin to fall within 1 to 2 weeks following chemotherapy, depending on the type of chemotherapy and the lifespan of the cell. Blood counts generally recover within 2 to 3 weeks. For many chemotherapy agents, myelosuppression is the dose-limiting toxic effect (See Table 13-2). Patients receiving combination chemotherapy may be more susceptible to myelosuppression.

Myelosuppression is a side effect of radiation therapy when the irradiated fields involve major bone marrow production sites such as the pelvis and sternum, or when total body irradiation (TBI) is given prior to bone marrow transplantation. The fall in counts often develops more slowly than is seen with chemotherapy.

The severity of myelosuppression can be affected by age (more pronounced in elderly patients), drug dosage, nutritional status (ability to repair damage from chemotherapy), ability to metabolize the drug (impaired hepatic or renal function), prior treatment (decreased bone marrow reserve), sequestration of drug (slow, prolonged release from sequestration in physiologic effusions) and concomitant administration of steroids (immunosuppressive effect).

Cancers such as **leukemia** or **lymphoma**, which affect the bone marrow, impair the normal production of blood cells. Certain types of solid tumors, such as breast cancer or lung cancer, will metastasize to the bone marrow and can also impair the production of normal cells. The end result in both of these instances is myelosuppression.

COMPLICATIONS RESULTING
FROM MYELOSUPPRESSION

All blood cells perform important functions in the body. An understanding of the function of each type of blood cell provides a foundation for identifying com-

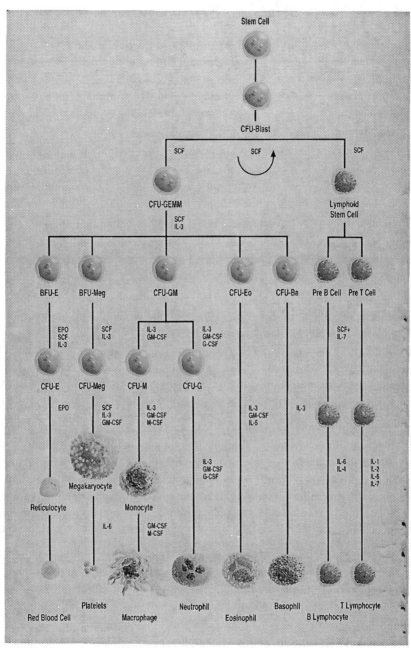

FIGURE 13–1   Hematopoietic Tree

CFU-Blast: colony-forming unit blast; SCF: stem cell factor; CFU-GEMM: colony-forming unit granulocyte, erythrocyte, monocyte, megakaryocyte; IL-3: interleukin-3; BFU-E: burst forming unit erythrocyte; BFU-Meg: burst forming unit megakaryocyte; CFU-GM: colony-forming unit granulocyte macrophage; CFU-Eo: colony-forming unit eosinophil; CFU-Ba: colony-forming unit basophil; EPO: erythropoietin; GM-CSF: granulocyte-macrophage colony-stimulating factor; G-CSF: granulocyte colony-stimulating factor; IL-7: interleukin-7; M-CSF: macrophage colony-stimulating factor; IL-5: interleukin-5; IL-1: interleukin-1; IL-4: interleukin-4; IL-6: interleukin-6.

Source: Figure courtesy of Amgen, Inc., Thousand Oaks, CA.

TABLE 13-2　Myelosuppressive Capacity of Chemotherapeutic Agents*

Mild	Moderate	Severe
Vincristine	Carboplatin (especially platelets)	Busulfan
Bleomycin	Cyclophosphamide	Carmustine
Asparaginase	Dacarbazine	Cytarabine
6-Mercaptopurine	Doxorubicin	Dactinomycin
Ifosfamide	5 Fluorouracil	Etoposide
Steroid hormones	Methotrexate	Lomustine
Cisplatin (moderate doses)	Mitoxantrone	Melphalan
		Nitrogen mustard
		Paclitaxel
		Vinblastine

*Degree of myelosuppression may vary depending on dose and schedule.

plications that result from a decreased number of these cells and determining treatments targeted toward decreasing the severity of these complications.

Granulocytopenia

White blood cells are an important part of the immune system and serve as part of the host defense against infectious agents (bacteria, fungi, and viruses). Neutrophils are important as a first line of defense against bacteria. They move to the site of inflammation and "eat" (phagocytize) bacteria. When white blood cell counts are low, patients are at risk of developing an infection. Research has shown that three key factors are important in predicting the potential of a patient to experience an infectious episode while myelosuppressed. One is the degree of neutropenia. The lower the neutrophil count, the more likely a patient is to become infected. Table 13-3 demonstrates how to calculate the **absolute neutrophil count (ANC)** and the risk of infection associated with various levels of neutropenia. The second key factor is the duration, or length of time, a patient is neutropenic. The longer a patient is neutropenic, the more likely he or she is to become infected. The third key factor is the rate at which the ANC drops, with a more rapid decline elevating risk of infection.

Anemia

Anemia, a decrease in circulating red blood cells (erythrocytes), diminishes the body's ability to carry oxygen to the tissues. Because the average lifespan of a red blood cell is 120 days (versus 12 hours for a neutrophil), anemia tends to develop more slowly in patients receiving chemotherapy. Other, more common causes of anemia in patients with cancer include blood loss, tumor infiltration of the bone marrow, the anemia of chronic disease, and hemolytic anemias. Symptoms experienced by anemic patients vary depending on the severity of the anemia. These may include pallor, weakness, palpitations, syncope, and, in severe cases,

TABLE 13–3 Evaluation of Risk for Infection

Calculation of Absolute Neutrophil Count

$$\frac{\text{Total white blood cell count} \times (\text{\% neutrophils} + \text{\% bands})}{100} = \text{Absolute neutrophil count (ANC)}$$

Level of Neutropenia

ANC (cells/mm³)	Risk for Infection
Greater than 2,000	Not significant
1,500–1,900	Minimal
1,400–1,000	Moderate
900–500	Severe
< 500	Life-threatening

Source: From the National Cancer Institute Criteria for Toxicity Grading.

a systolic murmur. A hemoglobin value of less than 7.0 grams/dL, or hematocrit less than 25%, is generally considered severe anemia.

Thrombocytopenia

Platelets arise in the bone marrow from megakaryocytes, which, when released, break into thousands of tiny platelets. Thrombocytopenia is defined as a circulating platelet count of less than 100,000/mm³. Because platelets perform a vital role in hemostasis, a decrease in their numbers can lead to bleeding and hemorrhage. Platelets assist in this process by sticking to blood vessel walls at the site of injury and forming a plug. They also assist with the conversion of fibrinogen to fibrin, which is important in the formation of blood clots. At any given time, up to one-third of platelets are found in the spleen.

Because platelets have an average life span of 10 days, the platelet **nadir** (low point) is typically seen after the white blood cell nadir. As the platelet count drops, the risk of bleeding increases. The risk is mild with platelet counts between 50,000 and 100,000/mm³, moderate with counts between 25,000 and 50,000/mm³, and severe with counts less than 20,000/mm³. Patients with extremely low platelet counts are at risk for spontaneous hemorrhage, especially of the gastrointestinal tract or the central nervous system.

NURSING MANAGEMENT

The nurse, as a member of the multidisciplinary team, has a crucial role in the management of myelosuppression. Knowledge of the pathophysiology of myelosuppression and interventions targeted toward preventing complications can impede the development of life-threatening complications such as sepsis. Responsibilities of the oncology nurse with respect to myelosuppression include patient assessment and education, along with assisting in treatment.

Assessment

A complete assessment prior to initiation of therapy will serve as a baseline for comparison over the course of therapy and will assist in identifying factors that may determine the degree of myelosuppression. Factors affecting the degree of neutropenia were described earlier. Other factors important in determining a patient's risk for infection include impaired cell-mediated immunity or humoral immunity (resulting from corticosteroid immunosuppressive therapy or hematologic malignancies) or the loss of protective barriers (altered skin and mucous membranes). The degree to which anemia is clinically manifested depends upon how quickly the anemia has developed, the presence of physiological compensatory mechanisms, underlying disease (type of cancer), age, the patient's level of activity, and coexisting medical problems (e.g., cardiac or pulmonary problems). Drugs that inhibit the synthesis of prostaglandins or interfere with platelet function or production will increase the patient's risk of bleeding. Assessment of the patient's medication profile for aspirin-containing drugs and nonsteroidal anti-inflammatory drugs is especially important. These drugs are often found in over-the-counter pain relievers and combination products to treat symptoms of colds and the flu. The pharmacist can be of valuable assistance in identifying these medications and others, such as anticoagulants, that affect this risk. Other factors that influence the risk of bleeding are the duration of neutropenia and infection (high fevers will affect platelet function).

The most common cause of morbidity and mortality in patients with cancer is infection. In the patient with neutropenia, infection can occur from sources outside the body (*exogenous*) or inside the body (*endogenous*). In the majority of cases (over 80%), it is the patient's own natural body flora that cause infections. The most common infective organisms are gram-negative bacilli such as *Escherischa coli* (*E. coli*), *Pseudomonas aeruginosa*, and *Klebsiella pneumonia*, and gram-positive organisms such as *Staphylococcus aureus* and coagulase-negative *Staph* species. Gram-positive organisms are being seen more frequently as a result of the increasing use of indwelling catheters for venous access. Patients who are neutropenic for extended periods of time or receive broad-spectrum antibiotics are at risk of invasive fungal infections, the most common being *Candida albicans*. Causative agents in viral infection include the herpes viruses and cytomegalovirus.

Fever, generally over 38.5°C, is the hallmark, and often only, sign of infection. Other signs of infection include signs of inflammation (redness, heat, swelling, or tenderness), oral lesions or white patches, burning with urination or flank pain, cough or sore throat, nausea, vomiting or diarrhea, or perirectal discomfort. It is extremely important for the nurse to be aware that the hallmark signs of inflammation are often absent when the white count is decreased. A thorough assessment by body system, with special attention to body orifices and catheter insertion sites, is of the utmost importance. Common laboratory tests for the evaluation of infection include a complete blood count with differential, urinalysis, and blood cultures. A chest x-ray is often obtained. Assessment for potential routes of exposure to pathogens, such as air, food, water, catheters, infusions, and equipment and contacts, can assist in developing preventive measures.

The severity of anemia is monitored by the red blood cell count and hemoglobin and hematocrit values. Common symptoms associated with anemia result from a decrease in the delivery of oxygen to the tissues and physiological compensatory mechanisms such as an increased heart rate and shunting of blood to vital organs (See Table 13–4). Alertness to the presence of these symptoms will aid in the early treatment of anemia. Anemia-related fatigue often has a significant impact on the patient's quality of life, but it remains an underrecognized and undertreated problem.

Bleeding or hemorrhage is the major complication associated with thrombocytopenia. Common signs of bleeding include oozing from the gums, bruises, or petechiae (tiny purplish-red spots visible under the skin). Other important assessment parameters include frank bleeding from any body orifice (mouth, nose, vagina, rectum, or urethra) or prolonged bleeding from venipuncture sites or cuts. Signs and symptoms of an intracranial bleed include headaches, blurred vision, disorientation, changes in mental status, and changes in pupil size and reactivity to light. Laboratory parameters used to monitor thrombocytopenia include platelet counts; bleeding times; and, on occasion, testing stools, urine, and emesis for occult blood.

An ongoing assessment, especially during a course of radiation therapy or over multiple cycles of chemotherapy, is important for monitoring complete blood counts and detecting signs and symptoms associated with complications related to myelosuppression. The major complications are infection related to neutropenia, shortness of breath and fatigue related to anemia, and bleeding or hemorrhage related to thrombocytopenia.

Treatment of Myelosuppression

Traditionally, the treatment of myelosuppression has focused on preventive measures and supportive therapies. The introduction of the hematopoietic growth factors, produced through recombinant DNA technology, has significantly altered the supportive therapy of this common problem in patients with cancer.

Measures to prevent infection, summarized in Table 13–4, should be implemented in all myelosuppressed patients. The single most important intervention is frequent and thorough handwashing by all of those who come in contact with the patient. Avoidance of exposure to common pathogens through common routes of transmission can be accomplished through numerous well-established interventions. The use of medications for the prophylactic treatment of infections is somewhat controversial. However, in patients who are severely myelosuppressed or those who are myelosuppressed for extended periods, prophylactic antimicrobial, antifungal, and antiviral medications are often administered.

Fever in a severely neutropenic patient is considered a medical emergency, and progression from a localized infection to sepsis can occur rapidly if antimicrobial therapy is not started promptly. After a thorough evaluation and com-

TABLE 13-4 Nursing Interventions for Myelosuppression

Nursing Intervention	Neutropenia	Anemia	Thrombocytopenia
Assessment	Fever—Monitor vital signs Signs and symptoms of inflammation Signs and symptoms of infection, especially in the following body systems: urinary, pulmonary, integument, and gastrointestinal. Other common sites include the perianal and rectal area, pharynx, mouth, and catheter sites. Factors affecting the degree of myelo-suppression such as: Chemotherapeutic agents Radiation therapy Disease process	Signs and symptoms of anemia Fatigue Pallor Dyspnea Palpitations, angina Alterations in mental status Factors affecting the degree of anemia such as: Cancer treatment Nutritional status	Signs and symptoms of thrombocytopenia Bruises (ecchymoses) Petechiae Bleeding
Prevention and treatment	Institute measures to prevent infection: Practice meticulous handwashing Occupy private room when hospitalized Maintain integrity of skin and mucous membranes Avoid invasive procedures Use sterile technique with all dressing changes Promote adequate nutrition	Institute measures to prevent anemia: Promote adequate nutrition Administer hematopoietic growth factors as ordered Institute measures to treat anemia: Administer transfusions as ordered	Institute measures to prevent bleeding: Alert physician to medications that may alter platelet function Promote measures to avoid constipation (adequate hydration, use of stool softeners, dietary measures such as increased fiber, increase mobility) Use antiemetics to control nausea and prevent retching

Minimize exposure of patient to pathogens Administer hematopoietic growth factors as ordered	Administer hematopoietic growth factors as ordered Implement strategies to manage fatigue	Avoid rectal manipulation with enemas, suppositories, thermometers Avoid intramuscular injections Use soft toothbrush for oral cleansing Cleanse perianal area with sitz bath or irrigation, pat dry Avoid invasive procedures Avoid the use of tourniquets
Institute measures to treat infection: Administer antibiotics and antipyretics as ordered Administer antifungal and antiviral agents as ordered Monitor vital signs regularly Assess for signs and symptoms of sepsis		Institute measures to treat bleeding episodes: Institute measures to control bleeding (direct, firm pressure over bleeding sites until bleeding has ceased, especially after venipuncture or other invasive procedures) Administer platelet transfusions as ordered and perform postplatelet count
Patient education Educate patient on measures to prevent infection: Avoiding crowds or contact with persons with transmissible diseases	Teach the patient measures to manage fatigue related to anemia: Pacing activities	Teach patient measures to prevent bleeding: Avoid activities with the potential for physical injury (contact sports, shaving with a razor, cutting finger or toe nails)

Continued

169

TABLE 13–4 Continued

Nursing Intervention	Neutropenia	Anemia	Thrombocytopenia
Patient education (Contd.)	Avoid sources of stagnant water (humidifiers, water pitchers)	Proper nutritional intake	Be aware of medications that may alter platelet function
	Avoid contact with dogs, cats, birds and other animals	Balancing exercise and periods of rest	Practice oral care with soft toothbrush (chemotherapy toothbrush), avoid flossing
	Maintain good daily personal hygiene (especially mouth and perianal areas)		Take measures to avoid constipation or straining with defecation
	Take measures to maintain skin integrity		Avoid sneezing or forcefully blowing the nose
	Avoid eating fresh fruits or vegetables, or contact with cut or fresh flowers	Teach patient reportable signs and symptoms:	Use water-based lubricants during sexual intercourse
		Dyspnea and palpitations at rest	Avoid wearing constrictive clothing
	Teach patient to monitor a temperature and report a single fever greater than 38.5°C or three fevers in 24 hours greater than 38°C	Chest pain	
		Dizziness	Teach patient reportable signs and symptoms:
		Trouble concentrating	Severe headache or blurred vision
	Teach patient to report promptly signs and symptoms of infection		Episodes of spontaneous bleeding
		Self-administration of epoetin alfa as appropriate	
	Teach patient parameters for the use of antipyretics		Coping strategies to adjust to lifestyle changes occurring as a result of myelosuppression
		Coping strategies to adjust to lifestyle changes occurring as a result of myelosuppression	
	Self-administration of hematopoietic growth factors as appropriate		
	Coping strategies to adjust to lifestyle changes occurring as a result of myelosuppression		

pletion of laboratory tests, empiric therapy is usually started based on the most likely causative agent. The choice of agent will vary depending on the institution and can be modified according to culture results. Historically, patients have been admitted to the hospital for intravenous antibiotics and supportive care until neutrophil counts normalized. Increasingly, regimens that are more cost effective, involving oral or intravenous antibiotics in an outpatient setting, are being evaluated. Criteria are being developed for identifying those patients who might safely be treated on an outpatient basis.

The hematopoietic growth factors are natural body proteins that influence the growth, differentiation, and biological activity of a variety of hematopoietic cells. Several of these substances are now available for the supportive treatment of myelosuppression. White blood cell growth factors include filgrastim (Neupogen®), a single-lineage growth factor affecting neutrophils, and sargramostim (Leukine®), a multilineage growth factor affecting primarily neutrophils and monocytes. In clinical studies, filgrastim has been shown to decrease the period of neutropenia, reduce the incidence of infections as manifested by febrile neutropenia, and decrease the need for intravenous antibiotics in patients with nonmyeloid malignancies following chemotherapy or autologous bone marrow transplantation (see Figure 13–2). Sargramostim is indicated for the acceleration of myeloid recovery following autologous bone marrow transplantation in patients with nonmyeloid malignancies or when marrow engraftment is delayed. It is also approved for the support of older patients with acute myelogenous leukemia following high-dose induction chemotherapy.

In asymptomatic patients with mild anemia, treatment is not generally necessary. As the severity of anemia increases, however, resting cardiac output begins to rise significantly, with an increase in both the heart rate and stroke volume; therapy is then warranted. Traditionally, red blood cell transfusions have been used to treat severe anemia, with the goal of symptomatic relief. Although red cell transfusions are effective, patients are increasingly concerned about the risk of transfusion-transmitted complications such as infection with the hepatitis or human immunodeficiency virus. The availability of erythropoietin in recombinant form (epoetin alfa) has led to new supportive strategies for the treatment of anemia. The production of red blood cells in the body is controlled by erythropoietin. Clinical trials have demonstrated the effectiveness of epoetin alfa (PROCRIT®) in increasing red cell counts, thereby decreasing the need for transfusions in patients with chemotherapy-related anemia. Patients have reported improved energy levels and quality of life as a result of therapy with epoetin alfa.

Patients experiencing thrombocytopenia are often placed on bleeding precautions in an attempt to prevent bleeding or injury (see Table 13–4). Platelet transfusion as a supportive measure is most frequently used for platelet counts of less than 20,000/mm³ or to achieve a platelet count of 50,000/mm³ prior to an invasive procedure. A common problem for patients who have received multiple platelet transfusions, especially from random donors, is the development of antiplatelet antibodies, which diminishes the effectiveness of transfused platelets and can lead to transfusion reactions. Currently, no growth factors have received regulatory (U.S. Food and Drug Administration) approval for the treatment of

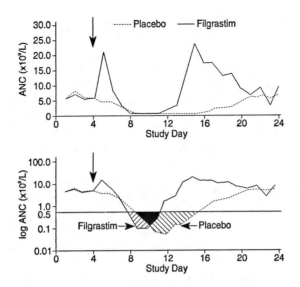

FIGURE 13–2   Differences in Neutrophil Profiles during Cycle 1 of Chemotherapy for Filgrastim Group versus Placebo Group

Median absolute neutrophil count (ANC) in the study groups during cycle 1. The counts are shown on a linear scale (top) and log scale (bottom). The arrow denotes the start of placebo or filgrastim administration. The hatching highlights the degree and duration of neutropenia (counts less than 0.5×10^9).

Source: From Blackwell, S., & Crawford, J. (1994). Filgrastim (r-metHuG-CSF) in the chemotherapy setting. In G. Morstyn & T. M. Dexter (Eds.), *Filgrastim (r-metHuG-CSF) in clinical practice* (Figure 1). New York: Marcel Dekker. Reprinted by courtesy of Marcel Dekker, Inc. (Adapted from Crawford, J. et al. [1991]. Reduction by granulocyte colony-stimulating factor of fever and neutropenia induced by chemotherapy in patients with small-cell lung cancer. *The New England Journal of Medicine, 325,* 164–170. Reprinted by permission of *The New England Journal of Medicine,* copyright 1991 Massachusetts Medical Society.)

thrombocytopenia. Thrombopoietin, a growth factor for platelets, has recently been identified and is now being studied in clinical trials.

Patient Education

Patients with cancer now receive their treatment predominantly as outpatients or at home. Nurses play a primary role in teaching patients and families the knowledge and skills needed to receive treatment safely in these settings. Assessment of the patient's learning needs and any barriers to learning (visual or hearing problems) will aid the development of a teaching plan targeted to the patient's needs. Patients should be aware of how and why myelosuppression occurs as a result of their disease and/or treatment and when it is expected to occur. Awareness of signs and symptoms that should be reported to the health care team is of crucial importance so that complications such as infection or bleeding can be treated promptly. Since infections may be lethal, education should include methods to contact the health care team any time of the day or week. Patients and families should be aware of precautions that they can take to minimize complications associated with myelosuppression. Teaching patients and family members skills such as subcutaneous injection for the administration of growth factors or sterile dressing changes for indwelling catheters should also be considered. Excellent patient education materials such as preprinted pamphlets and videotapes are available that can be individualized to the patient's preferred method of learning. Sources of educational materials include the American Cancer Society, National Cancer Institute, major comprehensive cancer centers, and major pharmaceutical companies. The *Oncology Nursing Forum* also publishes patient education materials.

CONCLUSION

The contributions of nurses are vital in the effective multidisciplinary management of myelosuppression. Awareness of the potential for myelosuppression, thorough assessment of the patient with special attention to symptoms of complications, assisting in the treatment of complications, and educating the patient and caregiver about myelosuppression form the cornerstone of quality care.

BIBLIOGRAPHY

Barton Burke, M., Wilkes, G. M., & Ingerwessen, K. (Eds.). (2nd ed.). (1996). *Chemotherapy care plans: Designs for nursing care*. Sudbury, MA: Jones and Bartlett.

Bodey, G. P., Buckley, M., Sathe, Y. S., & Freireich, E. J. (1966). Quantitative relationships between circulating leukocytes and infection in patients with acute leukemia. *Annals of Internal Medicine, 64*, 328–340.

Chabner, B. A., & Longo, D. L. (Eds.). (1996). *Cancer chemotherapy and biotherapy: Principles and practice* (2nd ed.). Philadelphia: Lippincott-Raven.

Dorr, R. T., & Von Hoff, D. D. (Eds.). (1994). *Cancer chemotherapy handbook* (2nd ed). Norwalk, CT: Appleton & Lange.

Hays, K. (1990). Physiology of normal bone marrow environment. *Seminars in Oncology Nursing, 6*, 3–8.

Kuck, A. W., Itano, J., & Matthews, L. V. (Eds.). (1994). *Care of the patient experiencing cancer-related bone marrow suppression*. (Computer-assisted instruction). Pittsburgh: Oncology Nursing Society. Published and distributed by Williams and Wilkins.

Maxwell, M. B., & Maher, K. E. (1992). Chemotherapy-induced myelosuppression. *Seminars in Oncology Nursing, 8*, 113–123.

Pizzo, P. A. (1993). Management of fever in patients with cancer and treatment-induced neutropenia. *New England Journal of Medicine, 328*, 1323–1332.

Rieger, P. T., & Haeuber, D. (1995). A new approach to managing chemotherapy-related anemia: Nursing implications of epoetin alfa. *Oncology Nursing Forum, 22*, 71–81.

Rostad, M. (1991). Current strategies for managing myelosuppression in patients with cancer. *Oncology Nursing Forum, 18*(2 Suppl.), 7–15.

Tenenbaum, L., & Leshin, D. (1994). Hematopoietic alterations associated with chemotherapy and biotherapy. In L. Tenenbaum (Ed.), *Cancer chemotherapy and biotherapy: A reference guide* (2nd ed., pp. 223–239). Philadelphia: W. B. Saunders.

14

Common Clinical Problems

Anna R. Du Pen
Joan T. Panke

Pain and symptom management are central to the nursing care of cancer patients. From diagnosis to death, a patient is likely to experience pain, nausea, fatigue, and many other symptoms that affect quality of life and have a significant impact on the patient's ability to fight the disease. Perhaps no other area of cancer treatment can be impacted so greatly by nursing as control of these symptoms.

PAIN

Pain affects over half of cancer patients at some time during the disease course. "Alteration in comfort" is one of the most frequently cited of all nursing diagnoses. With today's pain management techniques 95% of pain can be controlled, and nursing plays a significant role in making that relief a reality. Cancer pain is a result of tumor growth or of cancer-treatment-related sequelae (Figure 14–1).

Pain Assessment

One of the most critical components of the nurse's role in managing pain is assessment. The most significant pieces of information are the location, intensity, and quality of the pain. Many choices the physician makes in determining the best treatment option are dependent on these three pieces of information. Pain intensity not only is valuable in assessing patients, but also is an excellent marker for whether or not the pain is controlled and how much relief the patient is getting. If the patient states that the pain is a 7 on a scale of 0 to 10 prior to pain medicine and then after an hour the intensity level drops to a 2, the patient has achieved a clinically significant improvement as a result of the intervention. The quality of pain is also important for treatment planning. For example, a patient

FIGURE 14-1   Causes of Treatment-Related Pain

Chemotherapy-Related Pain	**Postsurgical Pain**
Oral mucositis	Postmastectomy
Peripheral neuropathy	Postnephrectomy
Acute and chronic herpetic pain	Postthoracotomy
Osteonecrosis secondary to steroids	Post radical neck dissection
Pseudorheumatism	Stump and phantom limb pain
Radiation-Related Pain	**Procedure-Related Pain**
Osteoradionecrosis	Bone marrow biopsy
Myelopathy	Bone biopsy
Brachial plexopathy	Lumbar puncture and spinal headache
Lumbar plexopathy	Venipuncture
Radiation-induced peripheral nerve tumors	

Source: From Campa, J. A. III, & Payne, R. (1993). Pain syndromes due to cancer treatment. In R. Patt (Ed.), *Cancer pain* (p. 42). Phildelphia: Lippincott. Reprinted with permission.

with a "burning" component will often have specific drugs used to assist in relieving the pain from damaged nerves. Other factors that either relieve the pain or make the pain worse are equally important to assess in the patient with pain. Consistent use of a pain assessment tool will greatly facilitate pain management.

Pain Management Techniques

Pain management often requires a variety of approaches to achieve relief. Analgesic drugs are the most frequently used therapy, but other techniques such as physical and psychological modalities also play a significant role.

Analgesic Drug Therapy   The World Health Organization (WHO) provides practitioners with a basic "ladder" approach to pain management. Mild pain is treated with nonopioid analgesics, such as acetaminophen, the nonsteroidal anti-inflammatory drugs (NSAIDS), and a variety of drugs known as adjuvant analgesics. The NSAIDS have been shown to be particularly effective in treatment of bone metastasis pain. **Adjuvant** drugs are drugs for which the principle indication is other than for analgesia, but that have secondary effects of creating analgesia. A good example are the tricyclic antidepressants, which have a proven efficacy in the treatment of nerve damage pain, such as the peripheral neuropathy associated with some chemotherapy agents.

Moderate levels of pain are treated with mild opioid and adjuvant therapy. Severe pain is treated with strong opioid and adjuvant therapy. The use of opioids, or narcotics, often raise questions about addiction. **Addiction** is defined as a psychological dependence. The addicted patient takes opioids to experience the euphoric or sedative effects of the agent, and not for the pain-relieving effect. The opioid addict is consumed with obtaining and habitually using opioids. Addiction in the cancer patient is extremely rare (< 1%). However, a physiological process called tolerance is believed to be the result of chronic opioid use.

TABLE 14-1 Around-the-clock Opioid Analgesics for Moderate to Severe Chronic Cancer Pain

Generic Name	Approximately Equal Dose / Schedule	24-hour Oral Total	Oral-to-IV Dose Ratio	24 hour IV Dose	Hourly IV Dose
Morphine					
Immediate release	30 mg q 4 hrs	180 mg	3:1	20 mg	2.4 mg/hr
Controlled release	90 mg q 12 hrs	180 mg	3:1	20 mg	2.4 mg/hr
Hydromorphone	7.5 mg q 4 hrs	45 mg	5:1	9 mg	.375 mg/hr
Methadone	20 mg q 6 hrs	80 mg	2:1	40 mg	1.6 mg/hr
Levorphanol	4 mg q 6 hrs	16 mg	1:1	16 mg	.6 mg/hr
Demerol	not recommended for chronic use				
Transdermal fentanyl	50 mcg patch q 72 hrs	parenteral not generally used for chronic administration			
Oxycodone					
Controlled release	Studies indicate controlled release oxycodone has twice the bioavailability of controlled release morphine (e.g., oxycontin 30 mg = MS contin 60 mg).				

Recommendations for Conversion from Mild-to-Moderate Opioids to Controlled-Release Oxycodone

Daily dose of Opioid/Combination Products (e.g., Percocet®, Tylox®, Vicodan®)	Starting Dose of Oxycodone Controlled Release*
1–5 tablets or capsules per day	10–20 mg q 12 hr
6–9 tablets or capsules per day	20–30 mg q 12 hr
10–12 tablets or capsules per day	30–40 mg q 12 hr

*Data from Purdue Frederick Company

Tolerance occurs when a larger dose of opioid is required to maintain the same level of analgesia for the same level of pain. Increasing dose requirements in the patient with progressive disease that produces increased pain intensity should not be confused with the tolerance phenomenon.

Opioids are the primary agents in the treatment of severe pain. Morphine is the standard drug of choice in this category, and all other opioids are equated to it in efficacy (see Table 14–1). Whenever a patient requires transfer from one medication to another, the **equianalgesic** chart is utilized to prevent under- or over-dosing. Medication should be given in amounts sufficient to control the pain and at regular intervals appropriate to the duration of action of the drug.

Cancer pain can be acute, chronic, intermittent, or a combination of all of these. Patients with acute pain such as postsurgical or **procedural pain** should be treated aggressively over the short term, and the dose should be tapered down as the level of pain decreases. Patients who require medication for chronic pain need a baseline level of analgesia provided by scheduled medication on an around-the-clock basis. Intermittent pain is often termed *breakthrough* pain. It may last from a few seconds to a few hours. It may or may not have an event that precipitates it. These patients often need extra or "rescue" doses to control breakthrough pain. The rescue dose of medication should be equianalgesic to 10% to 30% of the dose the patient receives in 24 hours. When patients require more than three rescue doses in a day, consideration should be given to adjusting their around-the-clock dose or maximizing the adjuvant analgesics.

Physical Modalities   Physical methods of relieving pain can be effective in some patients. Both heat and cold can be helpful. Be careful not to use excessive heat because of the risk of burns. Try alternating heat with cold. **Transcutaneous electrical nerve stimulation (TENS)** may offer relief, or the more simple strategies of rubbing the skin around the affected area with a rough towel or loofah may also provide some relief. Consultation with a physical therapist may be helpful. Many patients benefit from a simple exercise program, which can prevent muscle stiffness that accompanies inactivity.

Cognitive Modalities   Cognitive techniques also have their place in pain management. Stress and pain are known to exacerbate one another. Unrelieved pain can be very stressful, and stress associated with cancer can exacerbate pain. The use of stress-reducing techniques can be a potent adjunct to the pain management plan. Simple self-hypnosis exercises, progressive muscle relaxation, guided imagery, and biofeedback are some of the techniques commonly employed to help manage pain.

Nontraditional and Complementary Methods   There are many nontraditional therapies available for cancer pain management, some with merit documented in controlled studies and many others with little data to support them. Massage is a therapy that may benefit patients with significant myofascial pain, and the services of licensed massage therapists are beginning to be covered by some third-party payers. However, massage should be used with extreme caution in patients with bone metastases, who are prone to pathological fractures. Practitioners spe-

TABLE 14–2 Antiemetics Used for the Treatment of Chemotherapy-Induced Nausea and Vomiting

Class	Agent	Action	Side Effects	Route
Benzamides	Metoclopramide	CTZ and periphery (dopamine and serotonin antagonist)	Mild sedation Dystonic reactions Restlessness	IV
Benzodiazepines	Lorazepam	CNS	Mild sedation Dose-related memory loss	Oral and IV
Butyrophenones	Haloperidol Droperidol	CTZ (dopamine antagonist)	Akathisia Sedation Dystonic reactions	IV
Cannabinoids	THC Dronabinol Nabilone	Cerebral cortex	Moderate sedation Dizziness Ataxia Orthostatic hypotension Dry mouth Dysphoria	Oral
Corticosteroids	Dexamethasone Methylprednisone	Prostaglandin inhibitor Useful in combination with other antiemetics	Generally mild	Oral and IV
Phenothiazines	Prochlorperazine	Dopamine antagonist in CTZ	Orthostatic hypotension Those similar to butyrophenones and metoclopramide	Oral, IV, and IM
Serotonin antagonists	Granisetron Ondansetron	Selectively blocks serotonin (5-HT$_3$) receptors of the gut and visceral afferent nerves	Mild headache Transient transaminase elevation	Oral and IV

Source: Adapted from Ettinger, D. S. (1995). Preventing chemotherapy-induced nausea and vomiting: An update on a review of emesis, *Seminars in Oncology,* 22(4: 10), 6–18.

cializing in acupuncture, herbal medicine, immunotherapy, and other alternative medicines also offer treatment plans for patients with cancer-related pain. Patients often seek out these therapies, but clear outcome data are not available. Patients should be counseled that these nontraditional and complementary therapies may be helpful in combination with traditional therapies when their physician has approved their use. (See Chapter 12 for more discussion.)

Pediatric Pain

Pediatric pain management requires special attention to assessment techniques and to pediatric pharmacologic doses; however, most concepts of adult pain management apply equally to the pediatric population. Assessment in young children may rely to a large degree on observation, physiological indicators, and report by "proxy" of attendant caregivers. Older children are able to self-report pain with special tools such as the "happy face–sad face" scale or the "poker chip" method of quantifying pain. Procedure-related pain can be particularly problematic in children. The use of anesthetic creams prior to attempting placement of intravenous lines is helpful. Many centers have pediatric anesthesiologists who specialize in assisting with pain management. Nursing responsibilities include working with the child and the parents in establishing a pain assessment plan and working together to assure optimal relief.

NAUSEA AND VOMITING

Nausea and vomiting are frequently the most distressing side effects of cancer and its treatment. Causes of nausea and vomiting include the effects of radiation and chemotherapy, obstruction of the gastrointestinal tract by tumor growth and metastasis, constipation, metabolic abnormalities, and stress. These side effects are described as *anticipatory, acute,* or *delayed.* Regardless of the onset of symptoms, steps to prevent and control nausea and vomiting help patients maintain quality of life during treatment.

Patients receiving chemotherapy experience acute nausea and vomiting resulting from irritation of the gastrointestinal tract or stimulation of specific receptor sites in the central nervous system. Nausea and vomiting may be evident shortly after treatment and may last 24 hours. Patients receiving cisplatin, however, report delayed emesis even when symptoms are controlled during the first 24 hours. Patients undergoing radiation therapy to the stomach, abdomen, and brain may develop nausea and vomiting or gastritis from damage to the epithelial lining and accumulation of waste products from cell destruction. Onset of symptoms may occur within 6 hours following radiation treatment and may persist for 3 to 6 hours. Delayed or persistent nausea and vomiting occurs after the initial 24 hours of treatment.

A combination of antiemetic agents appears to be most successful for prevention and treatment of nausea and vomiting. Examples of antiemetic agents include metoclopramide, dexamethasone, prochlorperazine, lorazepam, and antihistamines (Table 14–2). Antiemetic therapy is usually based on the ematogenic potential of the chemotherapy agent being used or whether the field of radiation may produce nausea and vomiting. Many of these agents have associated side effects that can be bothersome in spite of their effectiveness in controlling nausea and vomiting. The 5-Ht3 antagonists (ondansetron/Zofran® and granisetron/Kytril®) are particularly effective in decreasing nausea and vomiting and are associated with fewer side effects. Antacids may afford additional relief of symptoms.

Nursing responsibilities include assessing the patient's pattern of nausea and vomiting, noting onset, aggravating factors, and duration. Because of the incidence of **anticipatory nausea** and vomiting, it is recommended that antiemetics be given before initiation of therapy. Antiemetic treatment should be continued on an around-the-clock schedule after starting cancer treatment according to the anticipated length of symptoms. Afterwards, antiemetics should be available on an as-needed basis.

Relaxation, distraction, and guided imagery also help alleviate nausea and vomiting. For patients experiencing anticipatory nausea and vomiting, these techniques can be particularly beneficial. Dietary measures to reduce these side effects include a soft, bland diet low in fat and sugar. Frequent, small meals are often best tolerated. If nausea and vomiting become severe, a liquid diet and intravenous fluids may be indicated. Maintaining an adequate fluid intake will prevent dehydration.

Nursing interventions include assessment, implementation, and evaluation of antiemetic therapy. Instruct patients and family to report persistent nausea and vomiting. Effective antiemetic therapy includes frequent reassessment to ensure that symptoms are kept to a minimum.

BOWEL DYSFUNCTION

Oncology patients can exhibit the full spectrum of altered bowel function from severe diarrhea to constipation and complete bowel obstruction. Bowel dysfunction can occur with chemotherapy, with radiation therapy, and from tumor involvement.

Diarrhea can be a side effect of various chemotherapeutic agents, radiation therapy to the abdomen, antibiotics, and **graft-versus-host disease.** Surgical resection of the bowel may lead to diarrhea, as can hyperosmolar dietary supplements or tube feedings, inflammation of the bowel, and "seepage" around a fecal impaction. Clinical effects of diarrhea may include fluid and electrolyte loss, fecal incontinence, and the development of severe perianal irritation. Treatment of diarrhea depends on the etiology, but it may include antidiarrhea and opioid agents (Lomotil®, Imodium®, codeine, tincture of opium), aluminum-containing antacids (Amphogel®, Basalgel®), bulk-forming agents (Metamucil®), the avoidance of high dietary fiber and other bowel stimulants, and the restriction of oral intake to rest the bowel.

Constipation can result from impairment of peristaltic activity by neurotoxic chemotherapy, opioid analgesics, immobility, changes in eating habit, dehydration, hypercalcemia, and neurogenic phenomena secondary to metastatic disease (e.g., spinal cord compression). Constipation can be managed by preventive techniques, including the elimination of causative factors, or by judicious use of stool softeners, laxatives, or both. Patients at risk for constipation (particularly those on chronic opioids) should be started on a prophylactic bowel regimen that includes a high-fiber diet, increased fluid intake, bulk-forming agents, laxatives, and stool softeners.

Partial or complete bowel obstruction occurs most frequently in patients with advanced abdominal malignancies or those with adhesions caused by prior surgery or radiation therapy. Neurotoxicity from chemotherapy and impaction from severe opioid-induced constipation and ileus can also lead to signs of obstruction. These symptoms can be insidious in onset and produce only intermittent symptoms. Abdominal pain, nausea, and vomiting are common symptoms. Patients may be treated conservatively with nasogastric suction and restriction of all oral intake. Other extreme cases require surgical intervention to relieve the obstruction.

MUCOSITIS

Mucositis is a side effect that interferes not only with patient comfort, but with adequate intake of food and fluids as well. Frequent assessment and teaching of preventative measures and reporting of symptoms help decrease discomfort and avoid potential infection.

Inflammation and ulceration of mucosal surfaces along the gastrointestinal tract are potential side effects of certain chemotherapeutic agents and radiation therapy. While chemotherapy may cause systemic mucositis, radiation therapy generally affects the specific site within the treatment field. In the mouth and oropharynx, stomatitis and esophagitis may occur after chemotherapy or after radiation of the head and neck. Xerostomia, or dry mouth, may be a further complication for patients receiving radiation for head and neck cancer. Infection and poor nutritional status may compound mucositis and impede healing.

Nursing responsibilities include assessing the oral mucosa at least daily, and more frequently as mucositis occurs. Instruct patients to report changes in taste, changes in sensation (burning or tenderness), difficulty swallowing, bleeding gums, and the appearance of lesions. Seek recommendations from other services including nutrition, infectious disease, and pain management. Equal attention to assessing the rectal and vaginal mucosa for bleeding, discharge, and discomfort should be incorporated into the nursing care plan.

Preventative measures and treatment for oral mucositis are centered on meticulous oral hygiene. Brushing and flossing are recommended unless bleeding is a risk, in which case substitute tooth sponges or gauze. Rinsing with sodium bicarbonate and water or warm saline before and after each meal and at bedtime helps keep the mouth clean. Teach patients to avoid commercial mouthwashes, tobacco, alcohol, extremes in food and fluid temperature, and spicy or acidic foods.

Encourage sufficient fluid intake of greater than 3 liters per day. Antibiotics, antifungals, and antivirals may be indicated to treat mucositis and superinfections. Topical and systemic analgesics can relieve pain associated with eating and swallowing. Preparations containing a combination of medications aid in both symptom relief and healing. These preparations may include topical anesthetics such as viscous lidocaine and dyclonine hydrochloride and soothing agents such as diphenhydramine and sucralfate.

For rectal and vaginal mucositis, instruct patients to avoid both chemical and physical irritants such as tampons, suppositories, and thermometers. If the patient is neutropenic or if the mucosa is impaired, intercourse should be avoided. The perineum should be washed with soap and water after each urination and bowel movement, taking care to pat or air dry. Sitz baths provide soothing relief. Assess for diarrhea and constipation, which may aggravate mucositis.

FATIGUE

Patients undergoing chemotherapy or radiation therapy for cancer treatment often experience fatigue. Fatigue can be attributed to multiple factors, including the resulting waste products from tumor breakdown or from the tumor's competing for nutrients. An increased metabolic rate due to tumor growth or infection rapidly depletes energy. Anemia, poor nutrition, infection, depression, pain, and the effects of some medications may compound the problem. Because of the many potential contributing factors, it is often difficult to determine the cause and the proper course of treatment of fatigue.

Fatigue may be temporary or it may persist over the course of treatment. Even after therapy is completed, fatigue may continue for several months. For the cancer patient struggling to continue with work and family responsibilities along with activities of daily living, this side effect has a significant impact on quality of life.

The attempt to determine potential causes of fatigue guides treatment choices. Physical causes such as anemia and nutritional deficits are corrected when possible. Efforts should be made to determine whether fatigue is related to depression, and antidepressant treatment should be initiated if appropriate. Review of the patient's medications may reveal whether causes of fatigue point to drug interactions or side effects.

Pain often causes fatigue, and medications used to treat pain may cause sedation. Pain medication should not be reduced in order to decrease sedation, because the patient will most likely become fatigued from the pain itself. Sedation associated with opioid analgesics often decreases beginning 72 hours after initiating the medication. If sedation persists, stimulants such as methylphenidate (Ritalin®) and dextroamphetamine may decrease drowsiness.

Practical approaches to reducing fatigue include allowing for adequate periods of rest throughout the day. The patient may find that although certain activities need limiting, a normal routine is possible. Dietary measures include eating complex carbohydrates, which provide more energy than sweet or processed foods.

Adequate fluid intake should be encouraged. Prednisolone is often used for patients with advanced cancer to boost energy and increase appetite. Relaxation and distraction techniques also help the patient combat fatigue.

Education of the patient and family members regarding potential fatigue during chemotherapy or radiation therapy should begin before treatment is initiated. Steps to relieve fatigue may be taken to keep the patient as active and involved in work, social, and family activities as possible. Involving the patient and family in planning strategies to battle fatigue help the patient best meet his or her needs.

ALOPECIA

Hair loss (alopecia) can be a devastating physical and emotional event for the cancer patient. Various chemotherapeutic agents, as well as cranial irradiation, may cause thinning or complete loss of the patient's hair. This is the result of the cytotoxic treatment's disruption of the mitotic activity of the hair follicle, which weakens the shaft and causes the hair to break. Scalp hair is primarily affected, although loss of pubic, axillary, and facial hair may also occur. Initial loss of hair usually begins 2–3 weeks after treatment, and regrowth occurs within 8 weeks of cessation of therapy. In patients receiving cranial radiation doses greater than 4,500 rads, hair loss may be permanent.

Proactive patient and family education should occur whenever hair loss is anticipated. An early purchase of a wig may be helpful. Patients vary in their responses to hair loss and altered body image. Nurses can assist patients in understanding their feelings and in using a variety of head coverings. The American Cancer Society's program *Look Good, Feel Better* is an example of specific assistance available to support patients.

DYSPNEA

Severe dyspnea is perhaps one of the most distressing symptoms for patients and families, particularly when it occurs in the home care setting. While tumors in the lung tissues, either primary or metastatic, are most often associated with dyspnea, many other etiologies exist. Pleural effusion and fibrotic changes in the lung parenchyma from radiation or chemotherapy are frequent causes of dyspnea. Impingement on lung tissue by engorged lymphatics, loss of functional lung tissue after surgical resection, pericardial effusion, congestive heart failure, and anemia are all likely sources to be considered.

Chemotherapy, radiation therapy, or surgery may be indicated to treat dyspnea when the tumor itself is suspected of causing dyspnea. Patients with recurrent pleural effusions will require thoracentesis and possibly instillation of sclerosing agents to prevent reaccumulation of fluid. Antibiotics, diuretics, bronchodilators, and steroids may also be used to alleviate dyspnea. Nondrug therapy may be initiated, including relaxation training and breathing exercises, positioning to facilitate ventilation, psychosocial support, and controlling room temperature and circulation. Oxygen therapy is helpful in ameliorating dyspnea that is associated with hypoxemia. Opioids and sedatives may be used to palliate tachypnea and "air hunger" symptoms in the terminally ill.

CONCLUSION

Pain, nausea, and myriad other symptoms often accompany a cancer diagnosis. Careful nursing assessment greatly assists the physician in the development of effective treatment strategies. The nurse's role includes ongoing evaluation of treatment to assure optimal comfort for patients as they move through the cancer experience. When nurses work together with medicine, pharmacy, nutrition, physical therapy, and other disciplines, control of pain and other symptoms can be effectively accomplished.

BIBLIOGRAPHY

American Pain Society. (1992). *Principles of analgesic use in the treatment of acute and cancer pain* (3rd ed.). Skokie, IL: Author.

Canty, S. L. (1994). Constipation: A side effect of opioids. *Oncology Nursing Forum, 21,* 739–745.

Curtis, E. B., Krech, R., & Walsh, T. D. (1991). Common symptoms in patients with advanced cancer. *Journal of Palliative Care, 7,* 25–29.

Coyle, N., Cherny, N., & Portenoy, R. (1995). Pharmacologic management of cancer pain. In D. B. McGuire, C. H. Yarbro, & B. R. Ferrell (Eds.), *Cancer pain management* (2nd ed., pp. 89–130). Sudbury, MA: Jones and Bartlett.

Ettinger, D. S. (1995). Preventing chemotherapy-induced nausea and vomiting: An update and a review of emesis. *Seminars in Oncology, 22* (4, Suppl. 10), 6–18.

Held, J. L. (1994). Cancer care: Managing shortness of breath. *Nursing 94, 24,* 31.

Jacox, A., Carr, D. B., Payne, R., et al. (1994). Management of cancer pain. *Clinical practice guideline.* AHCPR Pub. No. 94–0592. Rockville, MD: Agency for Health Care Policy and Research, U.S. Department of Health and Human Services, Public Health Service.

Roberts, D. K., Thorne, S. E., & Pearson, C. (1993). The experience of dyspnea in late-stage cancer: Patients' and nurses' perspectives. *Cancer Nursing, 16,* 310–320.

Skalla, K. A., & Lacasse, C. (1992). Patient education for fatigue. *Oncology Nursing Forum, 1*(10), 1537–1541.

15

Vascular Access Devices and Ambulatory Pumps Used in Cancer Treatment

Dawn Camp-Sorrell

The increased need for intravascular access in the care of patients with cancer is responsible for the diversity of currently available long-term **vascular access devices (VADs)** and ambulatory pumps. Movement of care from the inpatient setting to the outpatient setting has stimulated the race for manufacturers to develop the best VAD and ambulatory pump. The care of various types of VADs is similar in many ways—for example, in the need for education and the need for aseptic technique when handling the catheter. However differences and controversies exist in care related to flushing techniques, clamping the catheter, withdrawing blood samples, and managing complications. VADs are indicated for patients needing long-term infusions of fluids, blood, and medications; total parenteral nutrition, or obtaining blood samples. Although over the past 2 decades the manufacturers of VADs have greatly improved their designs, the two major complications continue to be occlusion and infection. This chapter provides an overview of long-term VADs and ambulatory pumps available for use in treating patients with cancer.

OVERVIEW OF VADS

Three types of long-term VADs are currently available: peripherally inserted central catheters (PICCs), tunneled catheters, and implantable ports. The basic design of all VADs is similar; however, each VAD available offers distinct advantages and disadvantages (see Table 15–1). VADs are constructed of silicone or

TABLE 15-1 Advantages and Disadvantages of VADs

Type of VAD	Advantages	Disadvantages
PICCs	No danger of chest injury on insertion Economical placement Easy to remove RN can insert No puncturing of skin after insertion Not a surgical procedure to place External portion can be repaired Dual lumens available	Restricts activities Body image affected Difficult to perform self-care Routine daily to weekly maintenance May not be sutured to anchor May collapse with blood withdrawal Must have occlusive dressing in place at all times
Tunneled catheters	Tunnel with Dacron cuff to anchor in subcutaneous tissue Can be used for central venous pressure monitoring No puncturing of the skin after placement Triple-lumen catheter available External portion can be repaired Additional antimicrobial cuff available Easy to remove	Requires physician to place May require physician to remove Surgical procedure for placement Daily to weekly site care Body image may be affected Restricts some activities Higher maintenance requirements
Implanted ports	Double-lumen catheter available Minimal maintenance care Minimal interference with activities Body image less affected	Requires physician to place Requires physician to remove Surgical procedure for placement Higher initial placement cost Requires puncturing of the skin to access Can interfere with MRI, CT scan, or radiation procedures

Abbreviations: RN, registered nurse.

Source: From Winslow, M., Trammell, L., & Camp-Sorrell, D. (1995). Selection of vascular access devices and nursing care. *Seminars in Oncology Nursing, 11*(3), 168. Reprinted with permission.

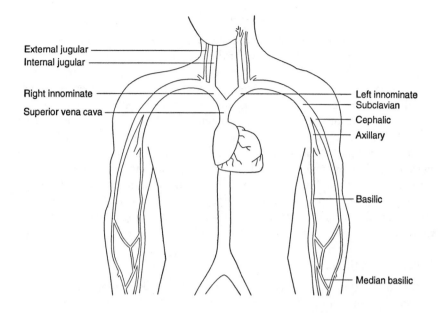

FIGURE 15–1   Venous System for Catheter Placement

polyurethane materials, which are considered biocompatible and thromboresistant. All VADs are radiopaque to allow for visualization under fluoroscopy or radiographic views, to determine placement after insertion or any time malposition is suspected. The distal tip of the catheter after insertion is located in the superior vena cava or above the junction of the right atrium (see Figure 15–1). Once inserted, the distal tip position must be confirmed by fluoroscopy or radiograph. Generally VADs have an open distal tip, except for the Groshong® catheter, which is designed with a closed distal tip with a three-way valve.

All VADs can be used immediately after placement for bolus injections or continuous intravenous infusions for any type of fluids, medications, nutritional supplements, and blood components in all patient settings. Although smaller-gauge VADs may not yield blood upon withdrawal, all VADs are designed to be used for obtaining blood samples. VADs are available in single-, double-, or triple-lumen designs to accommodate all access needs.

Peripherally Inserted Catheters

Descriptions of the use of peripherally inserted central catheters (PICCs) are found in the literature as early as 1912. However the PICC became recognized as a viable means for intravenous therapy in the early 1980s in neonatal intensive care. Since that time, adaptations to the design have made it ideal for use with all patient populations needing a long-term device. Numerous PICCs are available in single- and double-lumen designs that can be left inserted up to 3 months or longer. An advantage to selecting the PICC is that specially trained registered nurses can insert the device at the bedside without the patient's undergoing a surgical procedure. The PICC is the most economical VAD to insert, including the catheter cost and placement. When the PICC is no longer need-ed, the device can be easily removed at the bedside or in a clinic.

One of the major disadvantages of selecting a PICC is ensuring that the nurs-ing personnel maintain the specialized skill of inserting these devices. Although this skill is recognized by all State Boards of Nursing as an invasive procedure that a registered nurse can perform, standards for educational requirements or clinical competency have not been established. The majority of PICCs placed are not sutured to the skin after insertion; therefore, care of the catheter must be meticulous. The insertion site for PICCs is in the antecubital area, which may limit the patient's activity and pose difficulty in caring for the catheter (e.g., flushing and dressing changes). Even though PICCs are available in numerous gauges from 23 to 16, the catheter can collapse easily during aspiration for blood samples.

Tunneled Catheters

Tunneled catheters were originally designed in the 1970s for long-term adminis-tration of parenteral nutrition, especially for pediatrics. Since that time numer-ous design changes have been made to increase the ease of insertion and use. The tunneled catheter is the only VAD available in a single-, double-, or triple-lumen design. A Dacron cuff is located on the catheter to secure the device within the subcutaneous tissue approximately 2 inches from the exit site and to minimize the risk of ascending bacteria within the tunnel. An additional Vita® cuff is avail-able that has silver ions to kill bacteria for an additional 4 to 6 weeks after place-ment. Unfortunately, current studies have not shown a significant decrease in infection with use of the Vita® cuff. With the exception of the Groshong® catheter, which does not require clamping, all tunneled catheters are available with attached clamps.

Tunneled catheters are devices that can be used for months to years as long as they are cared for adequately. In emergency situations, the catheter can be used to measure central venous pressure to determine whether the patient needs hemodynamic monitoring. Tunneled catheters are available in larger gauge sizes from 14 to 18 as well as smaller sizes ranging from 20 to 23. Insertion of this device is a surgical procedure; however, removal can be performed at the bedside. The costs of tunneled catheters and their placement are significantly greater than the costs of PICCs.

Implantable Ports

The concept of an implantable port began with the introduction of the Ommaya® shunt in 1972. In 1982 the first port was developed in an attempt to decrease the occurrence of infection and to lessen the negative body image that can occur with other VADs. Ports are available in a variety of designs with a sep-tum that can be accessed from the top, side, or a 360-degree approach. Each port has a portal body manufactured from plastic, polyurethane, titanium, or a com-bination of these materials. Ports are the only devices that are designed to access the peritoneal, arterial, venous, or epidural body systems through the portal septum. Septums are designed to withstand 500 to 2,000 needle punctures. Denser septums have been designed to grip the needle tighter to decrease the risk of needle dislodgment. Larger septums are available to provide more surface area for access to minimize potential scar tissue build-up from repeated access.

Within the portal body is a reservoir varying in volumes of 0.5ml to 2ml. Below the reservoir is a plastic or metal needle stop that serves as the base of the portal body. Suture holes are available around the base of the portal body to suture the port to the fascia layer. Ports are available in a one-piece design in which the catheter is permanently attached to the port or as a two-piece design in which the catheter is permanently attached during surgical placement. Ports are available with large- and small-gauge catheters that can be used for months to years.

Although the port is the most expensive device to place, no maintenance supplies are required because the port is completely under the skin. Port placement and removal are performed in the surgical suite, although the antecubital port can be placed and removed in the angiographic area or physician's office. The antecubital port comes with a sensor wire catheter tracking system that eliminates the need for fluoroscopy. There are reports in the literature that implantable ports, especially titanium ports, may interfere with magnetic resonance imaging (MRI), CT scans, or radiation therapy procedures.

PATIENT SELECTION

The vast array of devices available demands specialized knowledge in selecting the appropriate VAD and providing care to the device. Nurses are in a perfect position to continually assess the need for a VAD based on the frequency of access and the condition of the patient's veins. Ideally, VAD selection is a multidisciplinary decision with consideration of the different types of VADs available, the condition of the patient's peripheral veins, and the anticipated frequency of access. VAD selection should be based on: (a) the patient's needs as well as his or her ability to care for the device, (b) cost considerations of insertion and maintenance, (c) type of intravenous therapy, and (d) availability of support systems.

PICCs are not suited for high-fluid-volume infusions, rapid bolus infusions, hemepheresis, or hemodialysis. The patient must have adequate cephalic or basilic veins for inserting a PICC for a limited need of intravenous therapy. Patients who have had a radical neck dissection, mastectomy, radiation to the chest, or inability to cannulate the neck veins; are cachectic; or are unable to undergo a surgical procedure are appropriate candidates for a PICC. For tunnel catheters or PICCs, the patient or a significant other must be able to perform catheter maintenance procedures.

Tunneled catheters are an appropriate choice for patients undergoing intensive intravenous therapies such as bone marrow transplant or high-dose chemotherapy that will result in a prolonged nadir. Obese patients usually require a tunneled catheter because the antecubital veins are not easily palpable or the chest has a large amount of adipose tissue, making port access difficult.

Implantable ports are appropriate for children who continue to be active despite intravenous therapy. Geriatric patients who have poor dexterity, making maintenance care for a PICC or tunneled catheter impossible, are excellent candidates for a port. Patients must have ample area of the anterior chest for an implantable port; this excludes patients with fungating chest tumors. Patients requiring bimonthly or monthly intravenous therapy for a solid tumor not resulting in a prolonged **nadir** or not needing triple-lumen catheters are appropriate candidates for an implantable port. Implantable ports are the best selection if the patient enjoys swimming activities, since tunneled catheters or PICCs may limit participation.

A major disadvantage of a port is that the skin must be punctured after implantation with a noncoring needle. Some patients may be "needle phobic," thus requiring the selection of another VAD. Additionally, the noncoring needles may be difficult to obtain in some geographic areas, or nurses may not have the knowledge or skill to access the port.

MAINTENANCE CARE

Controversy continues about the care for patients with VADs (see Table 15–2). While much research is in progress, current results have not conclusively resolved these clinical practice issues. The purpose of flushing VADs is to clean residue such as fibrin or debris that adheres to the internal catheter or inside the port reservoir. The lowest concentration of heparin flush should be used; however, the amount and frequency still warrants further research. To date, studies investigating the efficacy of normal saline flushes have mainly focused on short-term peripheral catheters. What is known is that it is important to maintain a pulsing motion to promote a more turbulent flow and to use positive pressure when instilling the flush to prevent retrograde of blood. Specific guidelines on maintenance care are available from the VAD manufacturer and should be followed.

Pressure on the VAD should never exceed 25 to 40 pounds per square inch (psi). Smaller-gauge syringes such as 1 ml will create pressure exceeding these limits. The current recommendation is to use syringes greater than 3 ml to flush or administer bolus injections. To prevent introduction of microorganisms, injection ports and luer junctions are cleansed before accessing. After appropriate skin preparation, implanted ports are accessed aseptically with a noncoring needle. Gloves are worn during the procedure, but in some cases, particularly with immunosuppressed patients, masks and gowns also may be used.

Tunneled catheters, PICCs, and accessed implantable ports require frequent dressing changes. The basic steps in dressing changes include washing hands, removing the old dressing, washing hands, cleansing the site, covering the site with an occlusive sterile dressing, and anchoring the catheter. Cleansing agents that can be used include alcohol, betadine, hydrogen peroxide, or soap and water

TABLE 15-2 Care of VADs

VAD	Flushing Routine*	Bolus Flushing	Dressing/Cap Changes	Blood Withdrawal (Discard Method)
Tunneled catheters	1 mL to 3 mL daily to weekly with HS** Maintain positive pressure	Before and after med with 5 mL of compatible solution	Remove old dressing Use aseptic technique Inspect site Cleanse site from catheter outward Cover site with occlusive dressing Change injection caps every 5–7 days	Withdraw 3–5 mL of blood and discard Withdraw blood samples Flush with 5–10 mL of NS, then HS or resume fluids
PICCs	1 mL to 2 mL daily with HS** Maintain positive pressure	As above	As above plus Pull old dressing upward to remove If skin closure dressings are used, change during dressing change	
Ports	2.5 to 5 mL of HS** every month	As above	As above	

Abbreviations: HS, heparin solution; NS, normal saline.
*Flush all lumens.
**Groshong catheters use 5 mL of NS flush weekly.

Source: From Winslow, M., Trammell, L., & Camp-Sorrell, D. (1995). Selection of vascular access devices and nursing care. *Seminars in Oncology Nursing, 11*(3), 170. Reprinted with permission.

followed by the application of a gauze or transparent dressing. The frequency of changes, type of dressing, type of cleansing agent, and use of ointment remains controversial and warrant further research. The studies that have been conducted lacked the inclusion of all variables such as the patient's diagnosis, educational preparation for dressing changes, personnel performing the dressing change, type of VAD, cleansing agent protocol, type of dressing, and type of intravenous therapy. Injection caps are usually changed weekly or more often, depending on the frequency of access.

BLOOD WITHDRAWAL

Different blood withdrawal techniques can be used to obtain blood specimens. The most common method is the discard technique, whereby 3 to 10 ml of blood are discarded, the specimen is obtained, and the catheter is flushed. The amount of discard and the best technique still warrant further research. Caution always should be used when obtaining blood specimens for coagulation studies or certain drug levels, because heparin, aminoglycosides, digioxin, aminophylline, and phenytoin have been found to be absorbed into the catheter material, resulting in erroneous values. Alternative methods to obtain blood samples for these tests are peripheral or finger lancet collection. Vacutainer needles are gaining popularity in obtaining blood samples because of the reduced risk of contamination and blood exposure to the personnel. However, a vacutainer may cause too much pressure on a PICC or Groshong® catheter, which may cause the catheter to collapse.

COMPLICATIONS

Despite the significant design changes and the newer catheter materials, infection and occlusion remain the major complications of VADs. Infection occurs as a result of bacteria adhering to and multiplying on the catheter surface or the skin. The patient's body reacts to the device as a foreign body by forming a fibrin sleeve around the catheter. This sleeve is a perfect place for organisms to adhere, resulting in an infection. Organisms enhance their adherence by producing an extracellular "slime." This slime acts as a barrier that protects embedded organisms from antibiotics, phagocytic neutrophils, macrophages, and the body's own antibodies. Conventional antibiotics are administered to rid the body of the infection; however, the bacteria within the slime are not killed, and therefore the infection recurs. The most common types of organisms are coagulase-negative staphylococci, Staphylococcus aureus, and Candida.

There are several potential sources of VAD infection. The VAD insertion or exit site serves as an area where organisms can migrate along the external surface of the PICC or tunneled catheter causing an infection. The catheter hub provides the means for organisms to travel along the internal surface of the VAD from manual manipulation, for example, during flushing or drug administration.

Hematogenous seeding can occur (e.g., from the gastrointestinal tract) and adhere to the fibrin on the surface of the catheter. The infusate could be contaminated with bacteria. The rougher surfaces of the catheter will increase the attachment of organisms and predispose thrombus formation, which further promotes organism colonization.

When an infection is suspected, blood cultures should be drawn peripherally and from all lumens of the VAD to determine the source of the infection. When organisms are greater from the VAD than from the peripheral culture, the source is determined to be from the VAD. Treatment of the infection depends on the extent of the infection (local versus systemic), the organism, and the physical condition of the patient (see Table 15–3). Exit site infections are the least serious and are treated locally with antimicrobial ointment and with oral antibiotics without removing the VAD. Tunnel infections usually require removal of the catheter and the initiation of intravenous antibiotics. Uncomplicated systemic infections are treated with intravenous antibiotics and usually respond without removing the VAD. Complicated systemic infections are associated with septic thrombosis or deep-seated infections requiring removal of the device and intravenous antibiotics for up to 4 weeks.

Controversy remains about when to remove the device and the type of antibiotic therapy. Usually the VAD is removed in the following circumstances: (1) the patient is clinically unstable; (2) the infectious source is fungi, gram-negative bacilli, or pseudomonas; (3) the patient continues to be symptomatic 2 to 3 days after beginning antibiotics; or (4) there is a complicated intravascular focus such as endocarditis or septic thrombosis. If the VAD is not pulled, there is a 20% chance that the infection will recur, compared with only a 3% risk of recurrence if the VAD is removed.

VADs often exhibit partial occlusion, in which the catheter flushes easily but blood cannot be aspirated. A total occlusion occurs when the catheter cannot be flushed and blood cannot be aspirated. Other signs of total occlusion include the development of collateral circulation, arm and neck edema, and external jugular distention. After VAD insertion, the catheter becomes encased with fibrin, beginning at the venotomy site and growing down to the catheter tip. Normally the body's fibrinolytic system is activated to contain and lyse the clot. However, extensive or chronic endothelial injury perpetuates fibrin clot formation, leading to a partial or total occlusion. Other causes for occlusion are precipitation formation, catheter malposition, pinch-off syndrome, catheter fracture, or a defect in the catheter.

Treatment of an occlusion begins with gently irrigating the catheter with normal saline in an attempt to flip the fibrin off the catheter tip (see Figures 15–2 and 15–3). Having the patient change positions or cough and deep breathe may facilitate moving the catheter tip off the vein wall. A thrombolytic agent such as Urokinase® can be used in an attempt to dissolve the clot. Usually the clot will be dissolved within 1 hour after Urokinase® instillation. If the catheter does not open, a venogram or catheter gram should be performed to ascertain the cause of the occlusion. Although a chest x-ray can be obtained to assess the catheter tip

TABLE 15–3 Types of VAD Infections

Type/Location	Symptoms/Signs	Diagnosis	Management
Local Exit site Insertion site	Erythema Pain Exudate Fever	+ Blood cultures from VAD + Culture from exit/insertion site	Evaluate for altered skin integrity because of dressing, tape, cleansing solution, or ointment Use alternative cleansing or dressing technique Oral antibiotics; IV in immunosuppressed
Port pocket	As above Cellulitis	+ Culture from port pocket fluid + Blood culture from port	As above If + culture for *stapholococcus aureus*, remove port If symptoms persist for more than 48 hrs, remove port and pack pocket with antibiotic-soaked gauze Remove port with cellulitis
Tunneled	As above Induration Tenderness of tract Cellulitis	+ Blood culture from VAD + Culture from expressed tunnel exudate	Remove catheter with local cellulitis IV antibiotics for 24 hrs. If symptoms persist, remove catheter
Systemic (septicemia) Colonized thrombi Colonized fibrin Intraluminal Extraluminal Sludge	Enhanced venous pattern Edema Discomfort Signs of sepsis Fever, chills Continuous infections Chills or hypotension with VAD flushing	+ Culture from tip of catheter + Venogram shows fibrin or thrombus + Blood cultures with 15 or more colonies of an organism + Blood culture from VAD 5–10 times greater than peripheral culture	IV antibiotics infuse via each lumen to eradicate infection Antibiotic lock technique Fibrinolytic therapy with IV antibiotics Remove VAD if symptoms or + culture persist for more than 48–72 hrs. Remove VAD for + *bacillus* or *candida* cultures

Source: From Rumsey, K., & Richardson, D. (1995). Management of infection and occlusion associated with vascular access devices. *Seminars in Oncology Nursing, 11*(3), 178. Reprinted with permission.

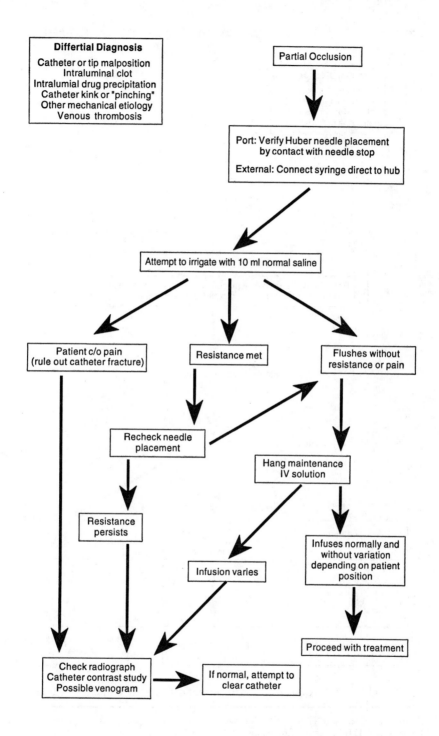

FIGURE 15–2 Evaluation and Treatment of Partial Catheter Occlusion

Source: From Alexander, H. R. (1994). *Vascular access in the cancer patient.* Philadelphia: Lippincott, p. 170. Reprinted with permission.

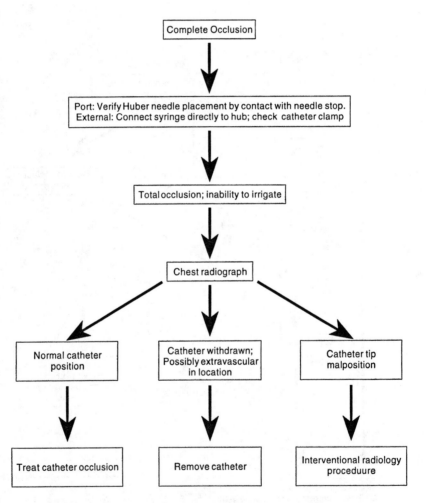

Differential Diagnosis

Catheter or tip malposition
Intraluminal clot
Intraluminal drug precipitation
Catheter kink or "pinching"
Access needle malposition
Other mechanical etiology

Complete Occlusion

Port: Verify Huber needle placement by contact with needle stop.
External: Connect syringe directly to hub; check catheter clamp

Total occlusion; inability to irrigate

Chest radiograph

| Normal catheter position | Catheter withdrawn; Possibly extravascular in location | Catheter tip malposition |
| Treat catheter occlusion | Remove catheter | Interventional radiology proceduure |

FIGURE 15–3   Evaluation and Treatment of Complete Catheter Occlusion

Source: From Alexander, H. R. (1994). *Vascular access in the cancer patient.* Philadelphia: Lippincott, p. 171. Reprinted with permission.

location, a catheter gram is necessary to determine the nature of the obstruction. During a catheter gram, radiograph contrast medium is injected into the catheter. An obstruction will show a deflection of the smooth jet stream of the dye.

AMBULATORY PUMPS

Ambulatory pumps are an important means for drug delivery in cancer therapy. Pump designs vary in reliability, precision, safety, simplicity of use, and power source. The three major types are peristaltic, syringe driven, and elastomeric. More than 600 models are available to safely deliver intermittent or continuous intravenous therapy. Although ambulatory pumps are similar, each type has unique advantages and disadvantages, which are outlined in Table 15–4. Peristaltic pumps operate in a rotary or linear mechanism. The linear mechanism allows appendages to move fluid forward in a wavelike motion within the intravenous tubing. The rotary mechanism uses a cam within a cylinder to rotate the tubing, squeezing the fluid forward. Syringe pumps have a simple design of a disposable syringe in which the plunger is pushed forward by a spring-powered or electronically controlled device. Elastomeric pumps have a balloon that acts as a membrane when filled with fluid. As the balloon deflates by gravity or exerted positive pressure, the fluid is forced out of the system.

Because ambulatory pumps can be used with all types of VADs, specific criteria must be assessed prior to pump selection. The patient or significant other must be able to learn the pump operation and alarm features and troubleshoot problems. The type of drug therapy influences the pump selection, because large-volume infusions such as total parenteral nutrition can not be delivered by a syringe-driven or elastomeric pump. Cost of the pump and proposed therapy must be reviewed, since, for example, current Medicare guidelines will not reimburse for the use of elastomeric pumps or certain intravenous medications. The patient's physical characteristics, such as visual acuity or manual dexterity, must be assessed to determine his or her ability to manipulate the pump.

EDUCATION

Previously, the care of VADs and ambulatory pumps was provided by the nurse. In this era of health care change, however, maintenance care and monitoring for potential complications is often the responsibility of the patient and/or a significant other. Prior to beginning the educational process, factors that affect learning must be assessed, such as age, physical status, emotional status, educational level, and stress level. Most manufacturers of VADs and pumps provide written material and videos to facilitate the teaching process. Maintenance care and potential problems must be discussed, followed by a return demonstration to ensure that the teaching is completed.

TABLE 15–4   Advantages and Disadvantages of Different Types
of Ambulatory Infusion Pumps

Type of Device	Advantages	Disadvantages

Syringe	Lightweight and portable
	Cost-effective
	Ease of patient use
	Excellent for antibiotics and
	  pain management
	No dose calculations
	Little or no maintenance
	Visualize drug flow
	Alarms
		Device can fracture and break if
		  dropped
		Limited volumes
		Not for large-volume infusions
		Drug stability factor
		Requires adequate manual dexterity
		  to work with syringe and tubing
		Free-flow risk

Elastomeric	Lightweight, portable, &
	  concealable
	Ease of patient use
	Excellent for antibiotics
	No programming
	No maintenance
	Reservoir and tubing attached
		Difficult to fill
		Admixture considerations
		Drug stability factor
		Calculate concentrations and
		  volumes
		Limited infusion rates
		Not for large-volume infusions
		Reimbursement concerns
		Cost prohibitive in long-term
		  therapies

Peristaltic	Provides intermittent and
	  continuous infusions
	All types of infusion therapy
	Alarm systems
	Wide range of infusion rates
	  and volumes
		Requires programming
		Carrying pouch heavy when full
		Upstream occlusion
		Free-flow risk
		Labor intensive

Source: From Rapsilber, L., & Camp-Sorrell, D. Ambulatory infusion pumps: Application to oncology. *Seminars in Oncology Nursing, 11*(3), 217. Reprinted with permission.

CONCLUSION

VADs and ambulatory pumps are indispensable in the management of patients with cancer. The newer technology has allowed for cancer treatments and supportive care to be administered safely and effectively. Nursing research must be conducted to scientifically determine the best means of caring for VADs as well as for managing complications. Nurses involved in the care of these devices must be aware of standards established and remain up to date with advances described in the research literature.

BIBLIOGRAPHY

Alexander, H. R. (1994). *Vascular access in the cancer patient*. Philadelphia: Lippincott.

Baranowski, L. (1993). Central venous access devices: Current technologies, uses, and management strategies. *Journal of Intravenous Nursing, 16*(3), 167–194.

Boothe, A. (1995). Vascular access in the oncology patient. *Surgical Oncology Clinics of North America, 4*(3) 377–568.

Camp-Sorrell, D. (1995). Advances in access devices for chemotherapy and pain management. *Seminars in Oncology Nursing, 11*(3), 153–229.

Centers for Disease Control and Prevention. (1995). *Draft guideline for prevention of intravascular device-related infections*. Washington, D.C.: Department of Health and Human Services.

Fulton, J. S. (1993). Vascular and related access devices. *Nursing Clinics of North America, 28*(3), 850–984.

Raad, I., Luna, I., Khalil, A. M., Costerton, J. W., Lam, C., & Bodey, G. P. (1994). The relationship between the thrombolitic and infectious complications of central venous catheters. *Journal of the American Medical Association, 27*, 1014–1016.

16

Nutritional Support

Gail M. Wilkes
Tracy Yemma

Malnutrition is a major cause of morbidity and mortality in patients with cancer. It can result from nutritional effects of the cancer itself or from the toxicities of antitumor therapies (surgery, chemotherapy, radiation therapy, and biological therapy). Treatment can cause mild, transient nutritional changes in the patient, such as mucositis from chemotherapy, or it may lead to severe, permanent nutritional problems, as is the case with abdominal resection. Nutritional problems require ongoing assessment, counseling, and intervention.

NUTRITIONAL EFFECTS OF CANCER

Anorexia, the loss of appetite, is a frequent problem for patients with cancer. Changes in hypothalamic function or in taste, the development of food aversions, early satiety, and the psychological stress of the cancer diagnosis have been suggested as causes of anorexia. Ultimately, they affect the patient's ability to consume enough nutrients to maintain a normal weight. In addition, anorexia is one of the most challenging symptoms of advanced cancer for patients, families, and health care providers.

Cancer **cachexia,** a complex metabolic problem, is seen in the majority of patients with advanced cancer. Cachexia is characterized clinically by anorexia, early satiety, weight loss, electrolyte and water abnormalities, and a progressive weakening of vital functions. The various factors contributing to this problem are shown in Figure 16–1. The tumor itself is responsible for initiating cachexia; only by controlling the disease can the syndrome be reversed.

The weight loss seen in cachexia is the result of a negative balance between caloric intake and expenditure. However, decreased intake cannot entirely

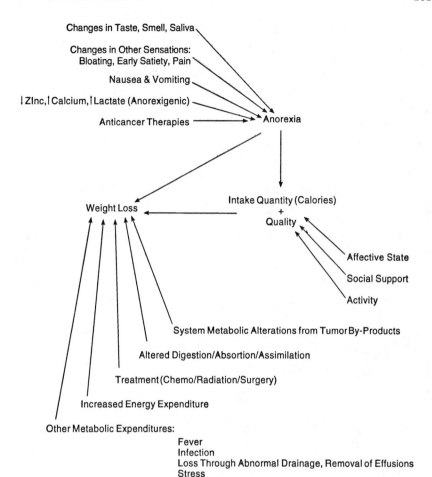

Changes in Taste, Smell, Saliva

Changes in Other Sensations:
Bloating, Early Satiety, Pain

Nausea & Vomiting

↓Zinc, ↓Calcium, ↓Lactate (Anorexigenic)

Anticancer Therapies

Anorexia

Weight Loss

Intake Quantity (Calories)
+
Quality

Affective State

Social Support

Activity

System Metabolic Alterations from Tumor By-Products

Altered Digestion/Absortion/Assimilation

Treatment (Chemo/Radiation/Surgery)

Increased Energy Expenditure

Other Metabolic Expenditures:

Fever
Infection
Loss Through Abnormal Drainage, Removal of Effusions
Stress

FIGURE 16–1   Factors Influencing Weight Loss in Cachexia

Source: From Lindsey, A. M. (1986) Cancer cachexia: Effects of the disease and its treatment. *Seminars in Oncology Nursing, 2,* 1929. Reprinted with permission of W. B. Saunders Company.

explain the progressive weight loss manifested in patients with cancer. The body's normal response to decreased food intake is the lowering of the basal metabolic rate (BMR). Although it is rarely seen, some patients with cancer exhibit a significant increase in BMR and total energy expenditure, possibly as a result of tumor growth and host metabolic alterations. However, not all patients with cancer manifest increased energy needs.

Poor utilization of nutrients, another major cause of cancer cachexia, involves altered metabolism of glucose, protein, and fat. Cachectic patients' inability to gain weight and increase their lean body mass despite adequate nutritional support is due partly to these metabolic changes.

The etiology of electrolyte disturbances is usually complex and tumor specific. Weight loss and increased catabolism cause additional sodium and potassium losses. Gastrointestinal (GI) tract obstruction or increased intracranial pressure from tumor growth can cause vomiting, resulting in fluid and electrolyte losses. Small-bowel fistulas can result in major losses of sodium, bicarbonate, potassium, magnesium, and zinc.

Patients with hepatic or cardiac metastases or obstruction of the urinary, lymphatic, or venous tracts will also have fluid and electrolyte imbalances. Hormone-secreting tumors that impair renal function cause similar changes. For example, **small-cell carcinomas of the lung** and hypothalamic tumors both result in inappropriate secretion of antidiuretic hormone, water retention, and hyponatremia. The **adrenocorticotropic hormone** produced by some tumors also causes fluid and electrolyte abnormalities.

Bone destruction or hormonal changes can cause alterations in calcium metabolism. Hypocalcemia also occurs as a result of malnutrition; however, when this is coupled with hypoalbuminemia, the ionized part of the total calcium remains normal. **Hypercalcemia** is associated with parathyroid tumors, primary tumors of the breast or thyroid that metastasize to the bone, and multiple endocrine adenomatosis.

A patient's fluid needs increase with fever or with any GI disturbance, such as vomiting or diarrhea. Patients with advanced cancer exhibit increased intracellular and extracellular water content. This water retention may partially obscure an actual loss of lean body mass and mislead the observer who uses the patient's weight as an index of nutritional status.

NUTRITIONAL EFFECTS OF TREATMENT

Treatment modalities used to control cancer can have an adverse effect on the already impaired nutritional status of the patient. This is of great concern since it has been shown that there are increased morbidity and mortality and decreased response to treatment in malnourished patients undergoing cancer treatment. Therefore, it is important to optimize the nutritional status of patients receiving cancer treatment.

Surgery

Radical surgery of the head and neck regions frequently results in impaired mastication and swallowing. Fat malabsorption, gastric stasis secondary to vagotomy, and diarrhea may occur after esophagectomy. In addition to hypoglycemia and malabsorption, dumping syndrome is common following partial gastrectomy and gastrojejunostomy. **Dumping syndrome** is a complex reaction, probably due to an excessive, rapid emptying of the contents of the GI tract. Symptoms include nausea, weakness, sweating, palpitation, varying degrees of syncope, often a sensation of warmth, and sometimes diarrhea occurring after the ingestion of food. Patients with this syndrome require careful nutritional management to prevent chronic deficiencies of iron, calcium, and the fat-soluble vitamins.

TABLE 16–1 Nutritional Consequences of "Radical" Resection

Organs Resected	Nutritional Sequelae
Oral cavity and pharynx	Dependency on tube feedings
Thoracic esophagus	Gastric stasis (secondary to vagotomy)
	Fat malabsorption
	Gastrostomy feedings in patients without reconstruction
Stomach	Dumping syndrome
	Fat malabsorption
	Anemia
Small intestine	
Duodenum	Pancreatobiliary deficiency with fat malabsorption
Jejunum	Decrease in efficiency of absorption (general)
Ileum	Vitamin B_{12} malabsorption and bile salt absorption
Massive (> 75%)	Fat malabsorption and diarrhea; vitamin B_{12} malabsorption; gastric hypersecretion
Colon (total or subtotal)	Water and electrolyte loss

Source: From Lawrence, W., Jr. (1977). Nutritional consequences of surgical resection of the gastrointestinal tract for cancer. *Cancer Research, 37,* 2379. Reprinted with permission of Cancer Research, Inc.

Patients generally experience substantial sodium and water losses immediately after ileostomy. The losses usually decrease within 7 to 20 days, approaching the range seen in otherwise healthy individuals on stable diets. Patients who have had massive small-bowel resection (leaving a functional small bowel of 3 feet or less) have serious long-term problems with maintenance of adequate nutrition. Total pancreatectomy and the resulting absence of pancreatic digestive enzymes lead to diabetes mellitus, as well as malabsorption of fats, proteins, fat-soluble vitamins, and minerals. Nutritional problems resulting from radical surgeries are shown in Table 16–1.

Radiation

Side effects of radiation treatment are site and dose dependent. Other influencing factors include preexisting medical conditions (e.g., colitis, diverticulitis, alcohol and tobacco abuse) and concurrent chemotherapy administration. Not all side effects occur for each and every patient; they depend on the anatomical site being radiated, the magnitude of the dose, and the presence of other influencing factors.

One type of radiation treatment that often compromises nutrition is radiation to the head and neck. Radiation injury to the salivary glands, oral mucosa, oral musculature, and alveolar bone may be manifested as **xerostomia** (mouth dryness), loss of taste ("mouth blindness"), **mucositis** (inflammation of the mucous membrane), oral infection, and production of thick, viscous saliva. Injury to the alveolar bone may result in the late occurrence of **osteoradionecrosis,** and dental caries may be a late effect of earlier side effects. The consistency of food should be adjusted for patients with viscous mucus to facilitate swallowing. When swallowing is impossible, enteral or total parenteral nutrition may be necessary. Residual mucous often settles into the throat and sinuses, causing nausea. Additional effects, including mouth sores, **dysphagia,** or nausea and vomiting, may make eating painful or unpleasant, exacerbating anorexia. Radiation damage to the esophagopharyngeal area may also lead to reduced oral intake, dysphagia, and **odynophagia,** or painful swallowing.

The small-bowel epithelium is very sensitive to radiation. Changes in intestinal function as a result of pelvic or abdominal radiotherapy include enterocolitis and diarrhea. Potential late/chronic side effects of radiation to the pelvis or abdomen include stricture formation and fistulas. Symptoms of this damage, such as abdominal pain, nausea, vomiting, and malabsorption, threaten adequate oral intake and nutritional status.

Please refer to Chapter 8 for additional discussion of this treatment modality and Chapter 14 for a complete discussion of management strategies.

Chemotherapy

Most of the effects of chemotherapy on nutrition are the result of interference in normal cellular activities. The effects produced depend on the type of drug, dosage, duration of treatment, rates of excretion, and individual susceptibility. Again, not all patients experience the side effects described. Among the most common effects of chemotherapy are diarrhea, nausea, and vomiting. Diarrhea and vomiting can lead to fluid and electrolyte imbalances and, if prolonged, dehydration and metabolic alkalosis. Persistent vomiting or diarrhea mandate nutritional intervention. Other common alimentary tract problems caused by chemotherapeutic agents include altered taste and smell, mucositis, stomatitis, and constipation.

Please refer to Chapter 9 for further information on this treatment modality.

DEVELOPMENT OF THE CARE PLAN

Protein malnutrition is frequently seen in hospitalized patients with cancer. This can interfere with the response to treatment and affect the patient's overall quality of life. The goals of nutritional care are to prevent or correct nutritional deficiencies and minimize weight loss. A team approach is critical to successful assessment and management.

The first step in planning nutritional care of the patient is an assessment of nutritional status. Although the assessment may consider several factors, it is performed primarily to determine the degree to which the patient's need for nutrients is being met by his or her food intake. Table 16–2 outlines the components of the nutritional assessment. This assessment serves as the basis for a care plan that includes monitoring, evaluation, and education. Perhaps most important is the comparison of present to usual body weight and then comparison of

TABLE 16–2 Components of the Nutritional Assessment

Medical History	*Physical Examination*
Duration and type of malignancy	General appearance
Frequency, type, and severity of complications (infections, draining lesions, etc.)	Condition of hair
Type and duration of therapy	Condition of skin
Specific chemotherapeutic agents used	Condition of teeth
Radiation sites	Condition of mouth, gums, and throat
Antibiotics used	Edema
Other drugs used	Performance status
Surgical procedures performed (site, type, date)	Identification of nutritionally related problems (fistula, pain, stomatitis, xerostomia;
Side effects of therapy (diarrhea, anorexia, nausea and vomiting)	infection, constipation, diarrhea, nausea and vomiting, obstruction)
Concomitant medical conditions (diabetes, heart disease, liver failure, kidney failure, infection)	

Dietary History	*Socioeconomic History*
24-hour recall of foods eaten, including snacks	Number of persons living in the home (ages and relationships)
Composition of food taken in 24 hours (calories and protein, caffeine, liquor)	Kitchen facilities
Time of day meals and snacks eaten	Income
Past or current diet modifications	Food purchased by
Self-feeding ability	Food prepared by
Physical activity	Patient's comprehension level
Use of oral supplements	
Special cancer diet	Amount spent on food per month
Vitamins, minerals, or other supplements	Outside provision of meals
Modifications of diet or eating habits as a result of treatment or illness	
Foods withheld or given on the basis of personal, cultural, or religious grounds (kosher, vegetarian, etc.)	
Food preferences	
Food allergies or intolerances	

Anthropometric Data	*Biochemical Data*
Height	Hematocrit
Weight	Hemoglobin
Actual weight as percentage of ideal	Serum albumin (prealbumin if available)
Weight change as percentage of usual	Serum transferrin
Triceps skinfold measurement	Creatinine
Actual triceps skinfold as percentage of standard	Creatinine height index
Midarm circumference	Total lymphocytes
Midarm muscle circumference	Delayed hypersensitivity response—skin testing
Actual midarm muscle circumference as percentage of standard	Nitrogen balance
	Blood urea nitrogen
	Sodium, potassium, carbon dioxide, chloride
	Glucose

Source: Modified from Skipper A., Szeluga, D. J., Groenwald, S. L. (1993). Nutritional disturbances. In S. L. Groenwald, M. H. Frogge, M. Goodman, & C. H. Yarbro (Eds.), *Cancer nursing: Principles and practice* (pp. 620–643). Sudbury, MA: Jones and Bartlett Publishers. Reprinted with permission.

current to ideal body weight. A weight loss of 34% of ideal body weight is incompatible with life.

Optimally, the dietitian reviews information from the patient's chart and conducts the full assessment. However, when dietitian services are limited or unavailable, nurses should draw upon their own knowledge of nutrition to collect and review patient data and identify patients who are at high risk for nutritional problems. Nurses can then arrange consultations between the dietitian and these high-risk patients and ensure that the entire health care team is involved in each patient's nutritional care.

Because it may be difficult for nurses caring for patients with cancer to perform comprehensive assessments, use of the Subjective Global Assessment (SGA) tool, which was modified by Ottery to reflect nutritional needs, is rapid and efficient. The patient is asked to answer questions about weight change, food intake, presence of gastrointestinal symptoms during the prior 2 weeks, and functional capacity over the prior month. The nurse (or physician or dietitian) completes the final three sections on (1) history of disease-related nutritional requirements, (2) physical examination (loss of subcutaneous fat, muscle wasting, presence of edema/ascites), and (3) an SGA rating as to whether the patient is well nourished, moderately or potentially malnourished, or severely malnourished. This tool is shown in Figure 16–2. Reassessments should be performed 2 to 4 weeks after each intervention, and the nutritional plan should be modified as needed, according to the patient's response.

NUTRITIONAL INTERVENTION AND COUNSELING

Whenever possible, the GI tract should be used for feeding the patient. Figure 16–3 illustrates an algorithm of optimal nutritional support and intervention developed by Ottery. Table 16–3 lists several suggestions for increasing oral intake of regular foods; there are also many medical nutritional products that can be used to augment reduced food intake. These products are usually high-calorie and/or high-protein liquid preparations that can supplement regular meals, be taken between meals, or serve as meal replacements. In addition, protein-fortified drinks or double-strength milk (one-quarter to one-third cup nonfat dry milk mixed with one cup fluid milk served cold) can add protein and calories to the diet.

It is not unusual for patients to develop lactase deficiency following chemotherapy or abdominal radiation. Symptoms may include bloating, cramping, or gas 1 to 3 hours after eating milk products. Restricting milk products eliminates an excellent source of calories and protein. These patients may benefit from the use of Lactaid®, an enzyme added to milk or used with milk products to break down the lactose. Patients may use Lactaid milk, pills, or drops. Lactose pills, sold as "milk digestants," are sold in some health food stores. Dairy Ease also sells pills.

Printed resources, such as cookbooks and guides to increasing intake, are available through the American Cancer Society, the National Cancer Institute,

Subjective Global Assessment (SGA) of Nutritional Status

(To the patient: please check the box or fill in the space as indicated in the next four sections.)

A. History

1. Weight change:
In summary of my current and recent weight:
I currently weigh about ____ pounds
I am about ____ feet ____ inches tall
A year ago I weighed about ____ pounds
Six months ago I weighed about ____ pounds
During the past two weeks, my weight has
☐ decreased   ☐ not changed   ☐ increased

2. Food Intake:
As compared to my normal, I would rate my food intake during the past month as:
☐ unchanged
☐ more than usual
☐ less than usual
I am now taking: ☐ little solid food
☐ only liquids ☐ only nutritional supplements
☐ very little of anything

3. Symptoms: *During the past two weeks, I have had the following problems that kept me from eating enough (check all that apply):*
☐ no problems eating
☐ no appetite, just did not feel like eating
☐ nausea   ☐ vomiting
☐ constipation   ☐ diarrhea
☐ mouth sores   ☐ dry mouth
☐ pain (where?) _____
☐ things taste funny or have no taste
☐ smells bother me
☐ other _____

4. Functional capacity: *Over the past month, I would rate my activity as generally:*
☐ normal, with no limitations
☐ not my normal self, but able to be up and about with fairly normal activities
☐ not feeling up to most things, but in bed less than half the day
☐ able to do little activity and spend most of the day in bed or chair
☐ pretty much bedridden, rarely out of bed

(The remainder of this form will be completed by your doctor, nurse, or therapist. Thank you.)

A. History (continued)
    5. Disease and its relation to nutritional requirements
        Primary diagnosis (specify) _____
        (stage, if known) _____
        Metabolic demand (stress) ☐ no stress ☐ low stress ☐ moderate stress ☐ high stress

B. Physical *(for each trait specify: 0 = normal, 1 = mild, 2 = moderate, or 3 = severe)*
____ loss of subcutaneous fat (triceps, chest)   ____ muscle wasting (quadriceps, deltoids)
____ ankle edema   ____ sacral edema   ____ ascites

C. SGA rating *(select one)*
☐ A = well nourished   ☐ B = moderately (or suspected of being) malnourished
☐ C = severely malnourished

FIGURE 16–2   Subjective Global Assessment (SGA) of Nutritional Status

Source: Reproduced with permission from Ottery, F. (1994). Oncology patient-generated Subjective Global Assessment (SGA) of Nutritional Status. *Nutritional Oncology, 1*(2) 9.

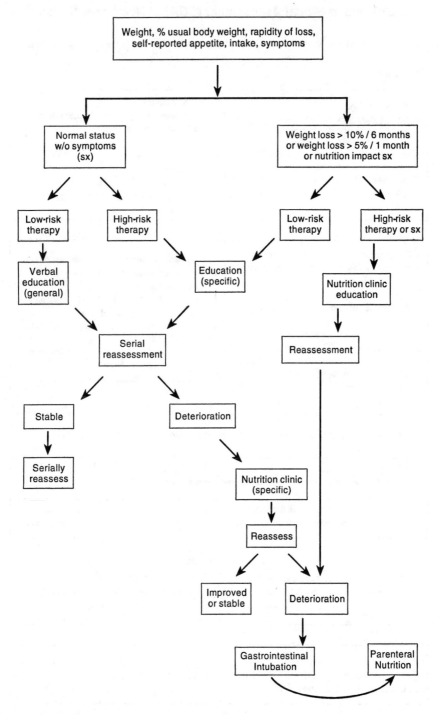

FIGURE 16–3 Algorithm of Optimal Nutritional Support and Intervention

Source: Reproduced with permission from Ottery, F. D. Rethinking nutritional support of the cancer patient: The new field of nutritional oncology. *Seminars in Oncology, 21*(6) 774.

and nutritional product companies. They can be helpful for patients who are attempting to increase their oral intake. These guides provide variety and ideas for patients or family members preparing foods.

ENTERAL AND PARENTERAL FEEDING

Patients who are unable to eat adequately for extended periods may benefit from enteral or parenteral feedings. The general rule of thumb is "If the gut works, use it."

Enteral Feeding

Formula characteristics and the patient's medical status must be reviewed before an enteral formula is recommended by the nutritionist and selected by the physician or nurse specialist. Formula characteristics to be considered include digestability of nutrients, osmolality, viscosity, nutritional completeness, ease of use, cost, and taste, if it is to be taken orally. Formula osmolality and rate of delivery are major factors in the patient's tolerance of the tube feeding.

Formula types fall into four major categories. *Complete products* are essentially meal replacements that require digestion and a relatively intact capacity for intestinal nutrient absorption. *Chemically refined products* require minimal or no enzymatic activity prior to absorption and are designed specifically for patients with digestion problems or severe malabsorption. Some products are indicated for patients with pancreatic cancer who have pancreatic exocrine insufficiency. Some may also reduce intestinal damage caused by some chemotherapeutic agents or abdominal radiation. *Modular products* may be combined to form an individualized feeding solution or used in conjunction with other tube feeding products to boost calorie or protein intake. *Specialty products* are designed for patients with hepatic or renal failure or trauma. These products vary considerably in terms of their specific amino acid, carbohydrate, and fat content and are used to tailor nutrient intake to the metabolic abnormalities that accompany major stress or organ failures.

Parenteral Nutrition

Parenteral nutrition is defined as the intravascular administration of macronutrients, vitamins, minerals, and trace elements, either peripherally or through a central line. Patients who are receiving aggressive treatment or are experiencing severe, reversible symptoms, cannot be sustained by the oral route, and are not candidates for tube feeding may benefit from this alternate support. This technique is referred to as **total parenteral nutrition (TPN), hyperalimentation, or intravenous hyperalimentation.** Either partial or total nutritional support may be provided. Indications for TPN are listed in Figure 16–4.

Dextrose and amino acid solutions should be infused daily. Fat emulsions should be used at least twice a week to provide essential fatty acids. Most patient care settings have developed policies and procedures for parenteral nutrition. It is important for the health care team and patient and family to have clear goals

TABLE 16–3 Symptom-Specific Nutrition Plans for Patients with Cancer

Symptom	Etiologies	Nutrition Plan
Anorexia	Radition; chemotherapy; metabolic or psychologic problems associated with chronic disease	• Suggest brisk walk before meals as tolerated. • Offer small, frequent, high caloric-density feedings. • Adjust meal size to appetite. • Enhance or minimize food odors. • Create a relaxed, pleasant eating atmosphere. • Suggest small amounts of alcohol before meals.
Alterations in taste/smell	Radiation; chemotherapy; metabolic problems; medications	• Avoid offensive foods. • Experiment with seasonings and food combinations. • Enhance or minimize food odors. • Serve foods at room temperature.
Mouth dryness	Radiation; chemotherapy; medications	• Puree or liquefy foods. • Use artificial salivas. • Add sauces, gravies, and juices. • Serve liquids with meals. • Experiment with food temperature.
Dysphagia/odynophagia (painful swallowing)	Radiation; chemotherapy	• Modify foods to a soft consistency. • Avoid highly seasoned, spiced, or acidic foods. • Adjust food temperature to tolerance.
Early satiety	Surgery; anorexia; tumor involvement	• Encourage 1/3–1/2 calories at breakfast, when early satiety is at its lowest point. • Offer small, frequent, high caloric-density feedings. • Limit liquids with meals. • Minimize intake of low caloric-density foods and liquids. • Exercise between meals.

Nausea/vomiting	Multifactorial	• Eat dry, bland foods (e.g., crackers, toast) before meals.
		• Avoid offensive foods.
		• Minimize food odors.
		• Shorten food preparation time.
		• Consume larger portions when nausea subsides.
		• Eat bland, easy-to-digest meals several hours before treatment.
		• Eat and drink slowly.
		• Identify best-tolerated foods; avoid poorly tolerated foods, such as fatty, spicy, overly sweet, or strongly flavored foods.
		• Have someone else prepare meals.
		• Use single servings or convenience items.
		• Suggest small, frequent meals.
Stomatitis/mucositis (mouth sores)	Radiation; chemotherapy	• Avoid acidic, salty, or spicy foods.
		• Avoid extremes in food temperature.
		• Suggest soft foods.
Diarrhea	Surgery; chemotherapy; radiation; tumor involvement; medications; bacterial infection; malabsorption	• Use low-residue diet during acute phase.
		• Increase fluid consumption.
		• Increase potassium intake.
		• Avoid gas-producing foods and beverages.
		• Adjust lactose intake to level of tolerance; eliminate it if necessary.
Constipation	Chemotherapy; medications; low-residue diet; inadequate intake	• Increase residue as tolerated.
		• Increase fluid consumption.
		• Increase physical activity as tolerated.

Source: Adapted from Ross Products Division, Abbott Laboratories, Columbus, Ohio, from "Symptom Specific Nutrition Plans for Patients with Cancer," *Dietary Modifications in Disease,* 1983, p. 15. Used with permission.

Nonfunctional GI tract
 obstruction
 ileus
 bowel resection
 stomatitis
 dysphagia treatment
Therapeutic bowel rest
 fistulae
 radiation or chemotherapy-induced enteritis
Hypermetabolism when gut cannot be used
 fever, infection
 major surgery
 bone marrow transplant
Malnutrition when gut cannot be used
 malabsorption
 need for rapid repletion

FIGURE 16–4   Indications for Total Parenteral Nutrition

for parenteral nutrition, because this form of nutrition may become an "extraordinary treatment" and give rise to an ethical dilemma when used to support an individual for whom there is no hope for recovery or improvement.

PHARMACOLOGICAL MANAGEMENT OF ANOREXIA

While no pharmacological intervention has been shown to extend life in patients with anorexia and cachexia, certain agents have been shown to increase appetite, leading to weight gain. Studies using megesterol acetate have shown that this agent can cause increased appetite and weight gain representing lean body mass, and that these patients have improved quality of life.

CONCLUSION

Nutrition is a critical dimension in the care of persons with cancer. It is important for nurses to include a nutritional assessment in their initial patient assessment and to reassess patients after nutritional interventions have been made. Finally, it is important for the nurse to collaborate with other health care team members and to advocate for effective nutritional management. The multidisciplinary team, including the nutritionist, nurse, and physician, is critical to the success of nutritional assessment and intervention.

BIBLIOGRAPHY

Bruera, E. (1992). Current pharmacologic management of anorexia in cancer patients. *Oncology, 6,* 125–132.

Curtas, S., Chapman, G., & Meguid, M. M. (1989). Evaluation of nutritional status. *Nursing Clinics of North America, 24,* 301–313.

Davidson, B., Laan, R.V., Hirschfeld, M., et. al. (1990). Ethical reasoning associated with the feeding of terminally ill elderly cancer patients. *Cancer Nursing, 13,* 286–291.

Grant, M. M. (1986). Nutritional interventions: Increasing oral intake. *Seminars in Oncology Nursing, 2,* 36–43.

Irwin, M. M. (1986). Enteral and parenteral nutrition support. *Seminars in Oncology Nursing, 2,* 44–54.

Kern, K. A., & Norton, J. A. (1988). Cancer cachexia. *Journal of Parenteral and Enteral Nutrition, 12,* 286–298.

Lindsey, A. M. (1986). Cancer cachexia: Effects of the disease and its treatment. *Seminars in Oncology Nursing, 2,* 1929.

Ottery, F. D. (1994). Cancer cachexia: Prevention, early diagnosis, and management. *Cancer Practice, 2,* 123–135.

Ottery, F. D. (1994). Rethinking nutritional support of the cancer patient: The new field of nutritional oncology. *Seminars in Oncology, 21,* 770–778.

Skipper A., Szeluga, D. J., & Groenwald, S. L. (1993). Nutritional disturbances. In S. L. Groenwald, M. H. Frogge, M. Goodman, & C. H. Yarbro (Eds.), *Cancer nursing: Principles and practice* (pp. 620–643). Sudbury, MA: Jones and Bartlett.

17

Oncologic Emergencies

Brenda K. Shelton

People with cancer are at risk for life-threatening medical emergencies caused by complications of the disease itself or its treatments. These emergencies are grouped according to the mechanism of injury: (a) obstructive or compressive disorders; (b) metabolic disorders; and (c) disruptions of hematologic/immunologic function. Oncologic emergencies can be the initial manifestation of a malignancy, occur during the treatment phase, or occur with progressive disease. Nurses who know which patients are at risk can promote early detection and treatment of oncologic emergencies. The most common emergencies associated with specific types of cancer are shown in Table 17–1. Early intervention decreases morbidity and may help the patient regain functional status. In all oncologic complications, treatment of the underlying cause is crucial in preventing recurrence.

GENERAL NURSING CONSIDERATIONS

Nursing interventions for patients with oncologic emergencies include periodic assessment of changes in the patient's status, administration of treatments, education, and emotional support. Many oncologic emergencies are completely reversible if treatment is administered promptly. Assessments and physical care vary with the type of emergency and the stage of the patient's disease. If the oncologic complication is the first manifestation of disease, the patient's anxiety about symptoms may be compounded by the shock of the new cancer diagnosis. The nurse needs to provide information as well as emotional support during this period. Nurses caring for people with cancer can identify populations at risk for developing these complications, participate in early detection, and collaborate in the management of care once the emergency has been diagnosed. A summary of

214

TABLE 17-1 Oncologic Emergency and Tumor Type

Emergency	Bone	Brain	Breast	Colorectal	Esophagus	H/N	Kidney	Lung	Melanoma	Ovary	Pancreas	Prostate	Stomach	Leukemia	Lymphoma	Myeloma
Leukostasis	—	—	—	—	—	—	—	—	—	—	—	—	—	D,P	—	—
Disseminated intravascular coagulation (DIC)	—	P	P	P	P	—	P	D,P	P	P	D,P	D,P	—	D,P	P	—
Hypercalcemia	D,P	—	T,P	P	—	—	D,T,P	D,P	—	—	D,P	T,P	—	D,P	D,P	D,P
Neoplastic cardiac tamponade	—	—	P	—	P	P	—	P	P	—	P	—	—	T,P	D,T,P	P
Sepsis	—	—	T	—	—	—	—	T	T	T	T	—	—	D,T,P	D,T,P	D,T,P
Spinal cord compression	D,P	P	P	P	—	—	P	P	P	P	P	D,P	—	P	D,P	P
Superior vena cava syndrome	—	—	D,P	—	D,P	D,P	P	D,P	P	—	—	—	—	—	D,P	—
Syndrome of inappropriate ADH (SIADH)	—	D,T,P	T	—	—	—	P	D,P	T	—	D,P	—	—	T	T	T
Tumor lysis syndrome	—	—	—	—	—	—	—	T	—	—	—	—	—	T	T	—

D = at diagnosis
T = during treatment
P = with progressive disease

Source: Adapted from Shelton, B. K. (1994). Cancer critical care: Past, present and future. *Seminars in Oncology Nursing, 10*(3), 150–151.

the common oncologic emergencies addressed in this chapter and their associated nursing diagnoses is provided in Table 17–2.

DISORDERS OF OBSTRUCTION OR COMPRESSION

Oncologic complications resulting from tumor mass may cause compression, destruction, or invasion of the tissues surrounding the tumor. This may occur from primary or from metastatic tumors, and it usually involves solid tumors. These disorders are definable by scopic or radiographic procedures that detect and localize the invasion of the tumor into other body tissues. The most effective management of obstructive disorders is surgical **debulking;** however, many patients have unresectable tumors or other contraindications to surgery, necessitating other treatment options. Typical obstructive emergencies are superior vena cava syndrome, spinal cord compression, neoplastic cardiac tamponade, and leukostasis.

Superior Vena Cava Syndrome

Superior vena cava syndrome (SVCS) is a disorder of venous congestion caused by obstruction of venous drainage in the upper thorax. The superior vena cava is particularly vulnerable to obstruction because of its thin walls, low venous pressure, and anatomic location. It is surrounded by lymph nodes and enclosed in a rigid compartment formed by the mediastinum, sternum, and right main stem bronchus. Enlarged lymph nodes or local tumor extension can compress and obstruct the vena cava extrinsically or by direct invasion of the tumor into the lumen of the vessel. Thrombus formation accompanying tumor compression or a permanent indwelling venous access device is another risk factor for SVCS.

The hallmarks of the clinical presentation of SVCS are manifestations of venous congestion in the upper body. The onset of symptoms is often slow and progressive, with individual variation of each symptom. Patients commonly present with shortness of breath, headache, visual disturbances, facial edema, swelling of the trunk and upper extremities, and less frequently with chest pain, cough, and dysphagia. Physical examination may reveal thoracic and neck vein distention, tachypnea, conjunctival edema, and altered level of consciousness.

The diagnosis of SVCS is made by suspicious clinical findings, chest radiograph and chest **computerized tomography (CT).** A venogram will ascertain whether there is an accompanying thrombus in the vena cava.

Radiation and/or chemotherapy are the most common treatments for SVCS. Treatment is based on the history and size of the tumor, its responsiveness to treatment, and any prior treatment. Radiation therapy is usually the best method of reducing the size of a tumor. **Lymphomas** are more radiosensitive than **carcinomas,** and in these cases symptomatic relief can usually be attained within 3 to 4 days after the start of radiation therapy, with objective improvement occurring within 7 to 14 days. Chemotherapy is used with radiation to treat chemosensitive tumors; it is administered first to reduce the tumor or limit lung tissue expo-

TABLE 17–2 Oncologic Emergency and Nursing Problems

	Altered Mental Status	Seizure Precautions	Decreased Cardiac Output	Altered Oxygenation	Altered Tissue Integrity	Altered Fluid Balance	Altered GI Elimination	Altered GU Elimination	Pain
Superior vena cava syndrome	X	X	X	X	X	X	—	—	X
Spinal cord compression	—	—	—	—	—	—	X	X	X
Neoplastic cardiac tamponade	X	—	X	X	—	X	—	—	—
Leukostasis	X	X	X	X	—	—	—	—	—
Hypercalcemia	X	X	—	—	—	X	X	X	—
SIADH	X	X	—	—	—	X	—	X	—
Tumor lysis syndrome	X	X	X	X	—	X	—	X	—
Disseminated intravascular coagulation	X	X	X	X	X	—	—	X	X
Sepsis	X	X	X	X	X	X	—	X	—

Source: Adapted from Shelton, B. K. (1994). Cancer critical care: Past, present and future. *Seminars in Oncology Nursing, 10*(3), 153.

sure to radiation. Chemotherapy alone may be used against tumors that are extremely sensitive to the effects of cytotoxic drugs (e.g., small-cell carcinoma) or when the mediastinal tissues have already been irradiated to maximum tolerance. Airway assistance, steroids, diuretics, and thrombolytics or anticoagulants may be used adjunctively to decrease local inflammation and edema and to treat intraluminal thrombosis.

Nursing management of acute SVCS includes maintaining airway patency, monitoring fluid and electrolyte balance, and monitoring vital signs and level of consciousness. Patients should be observed for respiratory stridor. Changes in mental status should be noted immediately, as they may indicate progressive central nervous system (CNS) involvement. Nurses should avoid accessing veins of the involved extremity (or extremities) because of the potential for venous stasis, phlebitis, and thrombosis.

Spinal Cord Compression

Spinal cord compression (SCC) is a disorder caused by direct pressure on the spinal cord with compromised vascular supply to the area, resulting in spinal cord infarct or vertebral collapse. Approximately 5% to 10% of people with metastatic disease develop spinal cord compression.

The earliest symptom of SCC is localized or radicular back pain, often preceding other symptoms by several months. More than 90% of patients with SCC experience back pain, which can be exacerbated by manual palpation of the affected area. Most patients experience weakness in the lower extremities by the time SCC is diagnosed. Approximately one-half of patients also exhibit sensory and autonomic dysfunction at diagnosis. The location of symptoms depends on the site of compression and the nerves involved. Sensory deficits include numbness and paresthesias; autonomic dysfunction is generally associated with a poorer prognosis. Bladder dysfunction begins with hesitancy and incomplete voiding and progresses to urinary retention. Constipation is an early indication of bowel problems, but sphincter control is lost as the cord compression worsens. SCC can also affect sexual function. Because of the nonspecific nature of the early complaints, health care personnel should have a high index of suspicion for SCC in patients complaining of back pain and weakness and having a history of malignancy.

Patients with SCC symptoms require a thorough neurologic evaluation. A **magnetic resonance imaging (MRI)** scan has replaced the myelogram as the diagnostic test of choice for confirmation of the diagnosis of SCC because it precisely identifies the location of all lesions.

Successful treatment of SCC depends on early diagnosis and treatment. Permanent nervous system damage occurs if therapy is not begun immediately. The choice of treatment is dictated by the type and location of the tumor, rapidity of symptom onset, and the patient's overall prognosis. Recent research suggests that radiation therapy is the best treatment for SCC because response rates are equivalent to those obtained with surgery, but result in lower rates of morbidity. Radiation treatments are begun as soon as the diagnosis is confirmed to prevent irreversible neurological deficits. Steroids are administered concomitantly to reduce local edema and improve neurological function.

Surgical decompression, such as partial resection of the tumor or laminectomy, is performed less frequently than radiation. It is used for patients with rapidly progressing dysfunction, for those with radioresistant tumors, or for those who have had previous maximal radiation to the involved area. Some residual tumor may remain after surgery, so radiation is generally administered to prevent tumor regrowth and optimize neurological function.

After surgery, nurses should monitor the restoration of neurological function, provide comfort measures, and ensure hygiene. Because the spine is unstable, a logrolling method is used to move the patient and a back brace may be ordered. If radiation is given postoperatively, the incision line should be carefully monitored because radiation impairs wound healing. Patients receiving treatment to the thoracic spine may experience **dysphagia** (difficulty in swallowing); topical anesthetics and dietary modifications may be helpful in alleviating this situation.

Pericardial Effusion/Cardiac Tamponade

Malignant infiltration of the pericardium causes inflammation, resulting in increased production of pericardial fluid. **Pericardial effusion** (accumulation of fluid in the pericardial sac) impedes the return of venous blood, hinders diastolic filling, and reduces stroke volume. **Cardiac tamponade** occurs when the amount and pressure of the pericardial fluid exceed the venous pressure of blood returning to the heart, leading to no cardiac inflow or outflow of blood. When this condition develops gradually, the pericardium can compensate by stretching to hold up to 1 liter of fluid and still maintain cardiac output. With rapidly developing effusions, compensation does not occur, and a smaller volume of fluid impairs cardiac output. Tumor involvement and radiation side effects can cause the pericardium to become fibrotic, leading to constrictive pericarditis. If constriction is severe, tamponade can occur without fluid accumulation.

The signs and symptoms of progressive pericardial effusion can be divided into three stages (see Table 17–3). Early symptoms of neoplastic cardiac tamponade are nonspecific and include dyspnea, cough, hepatomegaly, pain, orthopnea, cyanosis, venous distention, and leg edema. As cardiac function is further compromised, signs of ventricular failure are apparent: hypotension with cold, clammy skin; decrease in pulse pressure; thready pulse; and distended neck veins. As the pericardium becomes less able to compensate, blood pressure measurements will reveal increasing pulsus paradoxus, a pressure that decreases markedly with inspiration.

Pericardial effusion can be confirmed by an echocardiogram, but it is suspected when the heart size exceeds half the diameter of the chest on a chest radiograph. An emergency pericardiocentesis is performed in cases of critical cardiac compromise or cardiac arrest. Other interventions to manage recurrent pericardial effusions include placement of an indwelling catheter, balloon pericardotomy, placement of a pericardial window, and pericardectomy. Unless the original cause of the effusion is treated, the fluid will reaccumulate. Sclerosing agents may

TABLE 17-3 Stages of Progressive Pericardial Effusion

Stage I		Stage II		Stage III	
Clinical Findings	Pathophysiological Correlates	Clinical Findings	Pathophysiological Correlates	Clinical Findings	Pathophysiological Correlates
Subjective Asymptomatic	Hemodynamic compensatory mechanisms effective	Subjective Dyspnea, shortness of breath with exertion, fatigued, lightheaded Fullness, heaviness felt in chest Abdominal discomfort	Decreased cardiac output and arterial blood pressure Compression of heart Increased right ventricular pressure causes venous stasis in liver and splanchnic veins	Subjective Dyspnea, shortness of breath at rest, orthopnea Cough, hoarseness, dysphagia Retrosternal chest pain Anxiety, apprehension	Decreased cardiac output Impingement of effusion on bronchi, esophagus, and laryngeal nerves Compression of heart Progressive hypoxia
Objective Mild tachycardia (100 beats per minute)	Maintaining cardiac output	Objective Tachycardia (>100 beats per minute) Occasional pulsus paradoxus Mild peripheral edema and abdominal distension	Maintaining cardiac output Inspiratory fall in arterial systolic pressure Venous/visceral congestion	Objective Tachycardia (>100 beats per minute) Pulsus paradoxus Jugular venous distension, ascites Hypotension Impaired consciousness Pale, cyanotic appearance Muffled heart sounds, friction rub	Decreased cardiac output Inspiratory fall in arterial systolic pressure Venous congestion Decreased systolic pressure and increased diastolic pressure Progressive hypoxia Peripheral vasoconstriction Distension of pericardial cavity

Source: Mangan, C.M. (1992). Malignant pericardial effusions: Pathophysiology and clinical correlates. Oncology Nursing Forum, 19, 1215–1223. Reprinted with permission.

be instilled to adhere the pericardial sac to the heart and prevent reaccumulation of fluid.

Leukostasis

Leukostasis refers to hyperviscosity and microcirculatory occlusion with high circulating numbers of white blood cells. The syndrome occurs in newly diagnosed or recurrent aggressive acute leukemia patients when white blood counts, including blast cells, exceed 100,000/mm³. The pulmonary and neurologic systems are the most likely affected; however, renal failure, splenic infarction, and bowel infarction may occur.

Signs and symptoms of leukostasis are those of thrombosis and ischemia of the involved organ system and are often rapid in onset. Mental status changes, seizures, or focal neurologic deficits occur with microcirculatory occlusion of cerebral vessels. Pulmonary manifestations include dyspnea, labored breathing pattern, hypoxemia, and diffuse diminished breath sounds followed by infiltrates with bronchial breath sounds.

The diagnosis of leukostasis is usually made by exclusion, although CT scans help identify diffuse microcirculatory hemorrhage indicative of leukostasis. The chest radiograph initially shows hypoventilation from disuse atelectasis of the alveoli, but later demonstrates infiltrates compatible with pneumonia.

Leukostasis is treated by immediate anticancer chemotherapy. The white blood count can be halved by a single **leukopheresis** treatment, reducing the immediate life-threatening risk of leukostasis. If leukopheresis is unavailable, exchange transfusions are employed. Leukopheresis is usually repeated daily for 2 to 3 days, until the chemotherapy has its peak effects. Low-dose cranial radiation (approximately 100–300 cGy) is sometimes used; it is thought to destroy malignant cells and stabilize cell membranes.

Nurses caring for acute leukemic patients should recognize patients at high risk for this syndrome and perform frequent neurologic and pulmonary assessments. Any changes from baseline are reported and are likely to precipitate more aggressive medical interventions.

METABOLIC DISORDERS

Metabolic disorders associated with malignancy may be **paraneoplastic**—arising from intrinsic tumor characteristics—or related to treatment. There are a multitude of rare symptom constellations caused by tumors, many with unknown mechanisms. The more common problems are electrolyte disruptions such as hypercalcemia, syndrome of inappropriate antidiuretic hormone secretion (SIADH), and tumor lysis syndrome.

Hypercalcemia

Hypercalcemia is defined as a serum calcium greater than 11 mg/dl. It is the most common oncologic emergency, occurring in 10% to 20% of cancer patients. The three most common causes of hypercalcemia are (1) bone destruction by malignant infiltration of the bone, (2) tumor production of parathormone (PTH)-like hormone substances, and (3) tumor production of prostaglandins. All of these factors enhance bone resorption of calcium, leading to bone demineralization and serum hypercalcemia. Common malignant diagnoses predisposing patients to hypercalcemia are breast cancer, prostate cancer, renal cell cancer, small-cell lung cancer, multiple myeloma, lymphoma, and leukemia. Other factors that may contribute to hypercalcemia are dehydration, immobilization, fractures, and renal insufficiency. Medications such as the thiazide diuretics, lithium carbonate, and estrogens may also place a patient at risk for hypercalcemia.

Hypercalcemia can cause gastrointestinal, cardiac, neuromuscular, and renal dysfunction. The clinical manifestations vary and are usually proportional to the degree of hypercalcemia and the rate of its development (Table 17–4).

The goal of medical management of hypercalcemia is to reduce bone resorption of calcium and increase renal excretion of calcium. Primary treatment usually includes vigorous hydration using normal saline to restore fluid volume and increase glomerular filtration. Diuretics such as furosemide are given during hydration to promote renal excretion of calcium; however, thiazide diuretics are not recommended, because they depress calcium excretion. Rapid-acting agents to lower the serum calcium are employed if hydration and diuretics are ineffective. Pamidronate disodium is a bisphosphonate used to decrease osteoclast activation and bone resorption. Mithramycin is an antineoplastic agent that lowers calcium by inhibiting PTH, but it must be used with caution because of its effects on platelets and on renal and liver function. Other agents used to control hypercalcemia are gallium nitrate, etidronate, glucocorticoids, and calcitonin.

Nurses play a key role in identifying patients at risk for developing hypercalcemia, evaluating changes in hypercalcemia-related symptoms, administering medical therapy, and monitoring treatment side effects. Although encouragement of mobilization and promotion of weight bearing can prevent further long-bone demineralization, patients with bone involvement are at risk for developing pathological fractures and may need to modify their physical activity.

Syndrome of Inappropriate Secretion of Antidiuretic Hormone

The syndrome of inappropriate secretion of antidiuretic hormone (SIADH) is caused by release of excessive antidiuretic hormone (ADH) from the posterior pituitary gland. ADH modifies the permeability of the distal collecting tubules in the kidney, causing water retention and decreased serum osmolality.

The most common disease-related cause of SIADH is the ectopic production of ADH by tumor cells. Infections, tumors, and other disorders of the central nervous system can also cause SIADH by directly stimulating the hypothalmus and posterior pituitary. The lungs contain ADH receptors that can be stimulated by pneumonia, chronic obstructive lung disease, tumors, or mechanical ventilation. Both cyclophosphamide and vincristine have also been associated with development of SIADH.

Patients with SIADH have variable symptoms that depend on the degree of fluid retention and hyponatremia. Table 17–5 shows symptoms associated with

TABLE 17-4   Symptoms of Hypercalcemia

System	Mechanism	Signs and Symptoms
Gastrointestinal	Depressed smooth muscle contractility causes delayed gastric emptying and decreased intestinal motility	Early: nausea, vomiting, anorexia, constipation Late: obstipation and ileus; weight loss
Neuromuscular	Depressed excitability of neurons	Early: lethargy, drowsiness; restlessness, mood changes Mild: mental status changes, poor calculation, decreased attention span, somnolence Late: psychotic behavior, marked confusion, slurred speech, stupor, coma
	Impaired electrical conduction and cell membrane permeability in skeletal muscles	Early: muscle weakness, fatigue Late: profound muscle weakness, hypotonia
	Prostaglandin-mediated bone resorption	Bone pain
Renal	Interference with action of ADH on renal collecting tubules → inability to concentrate urine and then volume contraction followed by ↓ glomerular filtration rate	Early: polyuria Mild: polydipsia Late: prerenal azotemia
Cardiovascular	Impaired electrical conduction and cell membrane permeability, altered intracellular metabolism; arterial vasoconstriction	Early: hypertension Mild: sinus bradycardia, prolonged PR interval, shortened QT interval, dysrhythmias, especially in digitalized patients Late: prolonged QT interval due to widened T wave, coving of ST segment, AV block, asystole.

Source: Lang-Kummer, J.M. (1994). Hypercalcemia. In S. E. Groenwald, M. H. Frogge, M. Goodman, & C. H. Yarbro (Eds.), *Cancer nursing principles and practice* (3rd ed., p. 528). Sudbury, MA: Jones and Bartlett.

mild, moderate, and severe hyponatremia. Patients present with weight gain without edema, anorexia, nausea, vomiting, and CNS manifestations.

Both serum and urine diagnostic laboratory studies are evaluated for evidence of SIADH. Hallmark serum laboratory values are hyponatremia and hypoosmolarity. Due to fluid retention and serum dilution, hypokalemia, hypocal-

TABLE 17–5 Signs and Symptoms of SIADH

Severity (Sodium Level mEq/L)	Symptoms	Signs
Mild (125–135)	Lethargy Fatigue Short-term memory deficit Inappropriate behavior Oliguria Peripheral edema	Decreased serum sodium Decreased serum osmolarity Increased urinary osmolarity Increased urinary sodium Mild dilutional electrolytes

Moderate (118–124)	Confusion/disorientation
	Weakness
	Somnolence—
	  difficulty to arouse
	Hallucinations
	Tremors
	Weight gain
		Same as above but also:
		  Dilutional hypokalemia
		  Dilutional hypocalcemia
		  Decreased urinary
		    aldosterone
		Total body edema (anasarca)
		Pulmonary crackles

Severe (112–117)	Obtundation/coma
	Seizures
	Inability to protect airway
	  and mobilize secretions
		Diminished breath sounds,
		  crackles, gurgles
		Gallops and murmurs
		Increased JVP

Source: Shuey, K. M. (1994). Heart, lung, and endocrine complications of solid tumors. *Seminars in Oncology Nursing*, 10(3), 185.

cemia, and hypomagnesemia also occur. The urine shows increased urinary sodium and increased urinary osmolarity.

In mild to moderate cases, restricting fluids to 500 to 1000 cc a day corrects the hyponatremia. For patients with more severe symptoms, administration of hypertonic saline and furosemide will rapidly correct the fluid and electrolyte imbalance. Demeclocycline, which blocks the renal tubule response to ADH, may be used to manage chronic SIADH.

Tumor Lysis Syndrome

When patients with rapidly dividing or therapy-sensitive tumors receive cytotoxic chemotherapy or radiotherapy, large numbers of tumor cell membranes rupture, releasing the intracellular contents into the bloodstream. This complication is called **tumor lysis syndrome (TLS)** and is characterized by elevated levels of uric acid, potassium, and phosphate; decreased levels of calcium; and metabolic acidosis. The clinical signs and symptoms and usual management strategies for TLS are included in Table 17–6. The most common malignancies to develop TLS are leukemia, lymphoma, and small-cell lung cancer; however other large tumors have been associated with the disorder. The risk of TLS is increased in individuals with renal insufficiency, since they are unable to excrete the toxic wastes rapidly.

The combination of hyperuricemia and severe electrolyte disturbances can cause renal failure and cardiac arrest. Urate crystals precipitate within and obstruct the renal tubules, causing uric acid nephropathy. Patients at increased risk for developing TLS should be identified before the initiation of therapy. Symptoms of electrolyte disturbances may occur as early as 6 hours after treatment initiation, but generally begin within 24 to 48 hours. Acute tumor lysis syndrome generally resolves within 4 to 7 days after treatment is initiated, as long as renal function is adequate and electrolyte abnormalities have been corrected.

Electrolytes, uric acid, and renal function are measured before treatment begins and are closely monitored during therapy. High-risk patients are vigorously hydrated to dilute the potassium and phosphate and decrease the concentration of uric acid in the urine. Because uric acid is more soluble and less likely to precipitate in alkaline urine, sodium bicarbonate is added to IV fluids. Diuretics are administered along with hydration measures to promote excretion of potassium and phosphate. Allopurinol, a drug that decreases uric acid levels by interfering with purine metabolism, is used prophylactically in high-risk patients.

DISRUPTIONS OF HEMATOLOGIC OR IMMUNOLOGIC FUNCTION

The hematologic and immunologic systems are greatly affected by both the malignancy and the treatment. Infection, bleeding, and anemia occur in more than 90% of cancer patients. The most specific to oncologic processes are disseminated intravascular coagulation and septic shock.

Disseminated Intravascular Coagulation

Disseminated intravascular coagulation (DIC) is a hematologic disorder characterized by rapid formation of fibrin clots in the microcirculation, consumption of clotting factors, and stimulation of fibrinolysis, or clot degradation. The syndrome manifests as simultaneous clotting and bleeding. The first symptoms of DIC are usually skin and soft tissue thromboses and hemorrhage seen as demarcation cyanosis, petechiae, ecchymosis, and oozing from injection and surgical sites. Organ dysfunction from circulatory impairment leads to mental status changes, oliguria, and slowed gastrointestinal motility. Frank bleeding from any body orifice occurs with clotting factor depletion and can result in hypotension and tachycardia. A summary of bleeding and clotting symptoms associated with DIC is provided in Figure 17–1.

In cancer patients, DIC is often subclinical and chronic in nature, with the etiology related to tumor growth, invasion into normal tissue, or procoagulants produced by tumors. There may be few manifestations of bleeding until the disorder is severe or widespread. DIC is confirmed by suspicious clinical signs and

TABLE 17-6 Signs and Symptoms/Management of Tumor Lysis Syndrome

Clinical Situation	Possible Intervention or Medication	Usual Dose	Rationale	Additional Information
Hyperkalemia	Kayexalate	60 cc	Cation-exchange resin that binds with potassium, promoting its excretion.	Can be given p.o. or as an enema.
	Glucose & insulin	$D_{50}W$ 50 cc IV 10 u Reg Insulin IV	The glucose will raise plasma insulin levels, levels, causing an intracellular shift of potassium. The insulin prevents hypoglycemia.	This causes a rapid decrease in serum potassium, but is only a temporary measure because the potassium is now intracellular and will cross the cell membrane again.
	Diuretics: Furosemide (Lasix)	10–200 mg IV	To promote the excretion of potassium.	If unable to achieve results with Lasix®, other diuretics may need to be tried (i.e, Bumex® 1–5mg IV; Diuril® 250–600mg IV, alone or in combination).
	Hemodialisys	—	Rapid removal of metabolic toxins	—
Hyperuricemia	Allopurinol	600 mg loading dose followed by 300 mg/day	To inhibit the conversion of nucleic acids to uric acid.	Possible side effects include skin rashes and GI upset. Also may potentiate the action of 6-mercaptopurine and azathioprine.
	Hydration with sodium bicarbonate	Add 50–150 mEq $NaHCO_3$ to each liter of fluid	Will produce an alkaline urine. Uric acid is more soluble in an alkaline setting, therefore preventing precipitation and crystallization.	
	Diuretics	See above	A brisk urine output will aid in the excretion of uric acid.	See above.
	Hemodialysis	—	Rapid removal of metabolic toxins.	—

Hyperphosphatemia	Phosphate-binding agents. (1) Amphojel® (2) Alu-caps®	(1) 30 cc every 4–6 hours (2) 1,900 mg every 4–6 hours	Binds with phosphorous, thereby promoting its excretion and lowering serum levels.	
	Glucose and insulin	See above	See above. This will also cause a shift of phosphorous.	See above
	Diuretics	See above	Also promotes excretion of phosphorous.	See above
	Hemodialysis	—	Rapid removal of metabolic toxins	—
Hypocalcemia	Calcium Carbonate	650mg 1–4 times per day	Given to decrease the cardiac and neuromuscular symptoms associated with hypocalcemia.	Given based on serum levels and symptoms.
	Calcium Gluconate	1 amp = 1 gm		
	Hemodialysis	—	Rapid removal of metabolic toxins.	—

Source: Violette, K. (In press). Tumor lysis syndrome. In B. K. Shelton & S. Stecker (Eds.), *Oncology critical care nursing*. Sudbury, MA: Jones and Bartlett.

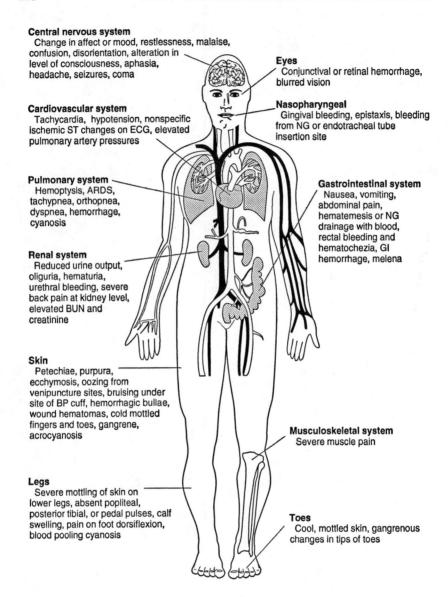

Central nervous system
Change in affect or mood, restlessness, malaise, confusion, disorientation, alteration in level of consciousness, aphasia, headache, seizures, coma

Eyes
Conjunctival or retinal hemorrhage, blurred vision

Nasopharyngeal
Gingival bleeding, epistaxis, bleeding from NG or endotracheal tube insertion site

Cardiovascular system
Tachycardia, hypotension, nonspecific ischemic ST changes on ECG, elevated pulmonary artery pressures

Pulmonary system
Hemoptysis, ARDS, tachypnea, orthopnea, dyspnea, hemorrhage, cyanosis

Gastrointestinal system
Nausea, vomiting, abdominal pain, hematemesis or NG drainage with blood, rectal bleeding and hematochezia, GI hemorrhage, melena

Renal system
Reduced urine output, oliguria, hematuria, urethral bleeding, severe back pain at kidney level, elevated BUN and creatinine

Skin
Petechiae, purpura, ecchymosis, oozing from venipuncture sites, bruising under site of BP cuff, hemorrhagic bullae, wound hematomas, cold mottled fingers and toes, gangrene, acrocyanosis

Musculoskeletal system
Severe muscle pain

Legs
Severe mottling of skin on lower legs, absent popliteal, posterior tibial, or pedal pulses, calf swelling, pain on foot dorsiflexion, blood pooling cyanosis

Toes
Cool, mottled skin, gangrenous changes in tips of toes

FIGURE 17–1   Clinical Presentation of DIC

Source: Allen, M.A. (1993). Disseminated intravascular coagulation. In J. E. Wright & B. K. Shelton (Eds), *Desk reference for critical care nursing* (p. 1192). Sudbury, MA: Jones and Bartlett.

symptoms and laboratory test findings. Laboratory tests reflect the pathophysiologic process of excessive clot formation followed by excessive clot lysis, with thrombocytopenia occurring first, followed by hypofibrinoginemia and prolonged prothrombin time. The definitive diagnosis of DIC is made with elevation of fibrin degradation products (FDPs) that occurs as clots lyse. Other coagulation studies are less sensitive, but they are likely to be abnormal as well.

Heparin administration is the primary treatment for DIC because it inhibits thrombin activity. It is given by continuous infusion until DIC is controlled. Identification and treatment of the underlying cause are crucial to preventing recurrence. Concurrent administration of platelets, packed red blood cells, fresh frozen plasma, and cryoprecipitate helps to achieve hemostasis until the underlying coagulopathy is corrected.

Septic Shock

Oncology patients whose immune systems are suppressed by the disease or by treatment toxic to the bone marrow are at a greater risk for life-threatening infections. The most common source of infection since the development of effective prophylactic antibiotic regimens is gram-positive organisms; however, gram-negative bacteria, fungi, parasites, and viri may also cause infection in the immunocompromised host. Many patients with septic shock never demonstrate positive cultures confirming the infectious source.

Pathogenic toxins produced by microbes cause local damage to the endothelial lining of capillaries and activate clotting factors and the complement system. These mechanisms trigger vasodilation and blood pooling in peripheral vascular beds. Subsequent reduction of the circulating blood volume leads to inadequate tissue perfusion and shock.

Fever is an early sign of infection, and, because there are insufficient white blood cells for an adequate immune response, it may be the only indication of infection. Early symptoms of impending shock are irritability; confusion; chills; tachycardia; tachypnea; weak peripheral pulses; hyperglycemia; excessive thirst; nausea; warm, dry skin; and diastolic hypotension. As shock progresses, cool skin becomes cold and clammy, and there is peripheral edema; oliguria; and deterioration of neurological, respiratory, or cardiac function.

Since the immune defense system is dysfunctional, early detection and management of septic shock are essential for the patient to recover from this infection. Most febrile, neutropenic patients will already be receiving prophylactic antibiotic therapy; untreated patients are started on broad-spectrum antimicrobials with any sign of an infection. Medical management of septic shock generally includes administration of fluids to expand the dilated vascular pool and vasoactive drugs to enhance vasoconstriction and maintain cardiac output. Respiratory support and management of metabolic acidosis may also be important aspects of care for these patients.

Nurses caring for patients with impending septic shock are required to constantly evaluate the patient's circulatory status through vital sign monitoring, measurement of central venous pressure, and intake and output measurements. Vigilant physical examination by the nurse may reveal potential infection sources that may influence the treatment plan.

CONCLUSION

The identification of high-risk patients and key signs and symptoms of oncologic emergencies are essential responsibilities of the nurse caring for cancer patients. Most oncologic emergencies are reversible or can be palliated with early intervention. This overview of the more common oncologic complications provides a basis from which to build an individualized plan of care for each cancer patient.

BIBLIOGRAPHY

Baker, G. L., & Barnes, H. J. (1992). Superior vena cava syndrome: Etiology, diagnosis, and treatment. *American Journal of Critical Care, 1*(1), 54–64.

Barry, S. (1989). Septic shock: Special needs of patients with cancer. *Oncology Nursing Forum, 16*(1), 23–27.

Batcheller, J. (1992). Disorders of anti-diuretic hormone secretion. *AACN Clinical Issues in Critical Care Nursing, 3*, 370–378.

Batcheller, J. (1994). Syndrome of inappropriate antidiuretic hormone secretion. *Critical Care Nursing Clinics of North America, 6*(4), 687–692.

Colman, R. W., Rubin, R. N. (1990). Disseminated intravascular coagulation due to malignancy. *Seminars in Oncology, 17*(2), 172–186.

Harnett, S. (1989). Septic shock in the oncology patient. *Cancer Nursing, 12*(4), 191–201.

Held, J. L., & Peahota, A. (1993). Nursing care of the patient with spinal cord compression. *Oncology Nursing Forum, 20*(10), 1507–1514.

Kaplan, M. (1994). Hypercalcemia of malignancy: A review of advances in pathophysiology. *Oncology Nursing Forum, 21*(6), 1039–1069.

Mangan, C. M. (1992). Malignant pericardial effusions: Pathophysiology and clinical correlates. *Oncology Nursing Forum, 19*(8), 1215–1223.

Stucky, L. A. (1993). Acute tumor lysis syndrome: Assessment and nursing implications. *Oncology Nursing Forum, 20*(1), 49–57.

Wilson, J. K. V., & Massaryk, T. J. (1989). Neurologic emergencies in the cancer patient. *Seminars in Oncology, 16*(6), 490–503.

18

Sexuality, Sexual Dysfunction, and Cancer

Margaret Barton Burke

As cancer survival rates have improved, issues concerning survivors' quality of life have received increased attention. One area of quality of life that is affected by cancer and its treatment modalities is sexuality.

Sexuality is a comprehensive term defined by the World Health Organization as an integration of the physical, psychological, and social aspects of sexual beings in ways that are positively enriching and enhance personality, communication, and love. Sexuality involves more than the sex act and reproduction; it encompasses who and what we are as a male or female, how we get that way, how we feel about it, and how we deal with each other about it. An individual's sexuality consists of sexual drive, sexual activities, intimacy and physical closeness, expressions of maleness and femaleness, and gender identity. Influencing factors include societal norms, religious background, and culture, as well as health and illness.

One aspect of sexuality, sexual dysfunction, can be experienced by cancer patients as a side effect of their disease or treatment. Research literature suggests that from 20% to 90% of cancer patients experience sexual problems either as a consequence of the disease itself or as a side effect of treatment. Sexual difficulties include loss of desire, inability to reach orgasm, or a decrease in the intensity of orgasm on the part of both sexes due to **dyspareunia** and decreased vaginal sensitivity in women and erectile dysfunction and impaired ejaculatory ability in men.

BARRIERS TO ASSESSING SEXUAL FUNCTION AND DYSFUNCTION

Despite the prevalence of sexual dysfunction in cancer patients, nurses often neglect or disregard this area of clinical practice. Barriers to intervention appear to stem from implicit assumptions about sexuality on the part of both the patient and the nurse as well as lack of information regarding changes in sexual function and advances in the field of sexual therapy for this patient population.

The assumptions the nurse brings to the nurse–patient interaction may not be at a conscious level. Quite often the subject of a patient's sexuality is not broached by the nurse due to perceptions such as "The patient is too sick from the side effects of treatment," or "It is too early in the diagnostic process to discuss the topic of sex," or "If sexual function is really a problem, the patient will bring it up." The same types of assumptions may be made by the patient, who may think, "What will my nurse think if I bring up the subject of sex at this point in my treatment?" or "Maybe there is no help available for my sexual problems, so it is better not to ask questions." If this failure to communicate continues, the nurse may unwittingly convey another unspoken message, that any sexual dysfunction experienced by the patient is permanent and cannot be treated, and that the patient and partner must deal with changes on their own.

One way to avoid such misunderstandings is to obtain a sexual history during the initial nurse–patient interaction. Gentle, clear questions about the patient's sexual functioning prior to and since diagnosis and treatment will convey the nurse's willingness to discuss this subject openly. Incorporating some basic questions into the review of systems can introduce the topic and serve as a starting point for more detailed inquiry.

The following simple questions, identified by Lamb and Woods, may eliminate the discomfort on the part of either the nurse or the patient to discuss the subject:

- Has your surgery (radiation therapy, chemotherapy or biotherapy) changed the way you see yourself as a man (woman)?
- Has the cancer or its treatment affected your sexual function?

If the answer to either of these questions is affirmative, specific details can be elicited.

Another, more subtle assumption or bias pervades the manner in which sexual assessments are conducted by health providers. That is *heterocentricity*, the presumption that the person being treated has a sexual partner who is a member of the opposite sex. Assumptions about sexual orientation may be evident in the questions asked of patients. Such bias can be minimized by becoming comfortable in asking open-ended questions such as "Tell me about who you live with"; "Tell me about the importance of sexuality in your life"; or "Are you sexually active? With men, women or both?" rather than asking "Are you gay or straight?" or "Do you have a boyfriend or girlfriend?" Moreover, marital status does not necessarily reveal information about the role of sexuality in a patient's life. Single individuals may be highly active sexually and may be more concerned about changes in sexuality and sexual function than their married counterparts.

1. Recognize that sexuality is a basic human need.
2. Gather adequate physiological knowledge to counsel a patient with a specific sexual problem.
3. Recognize your own feelings about human sexuality.
4. Recognize your feelings about heterosexuality, homosexuality, and bisexuality.
5. Include discussions of sexuality in a nursing history as a natural part of the assessment.
6. Understand the language of sex: Your vocabulary may not be the same as your patient's colloquialisms.
7. Be careful not to impose your morality, or spiritual or sexual biases on your patient.
8. Do not force the patient to talk about sex or sexual concerns.
9. Do not assume that once the topic has been discussed that the issue is ended.
10. Do not assume that there is only one way to convey sexual information, i.e., an instructional pamphlet.
11. Remember the needs of the partner.
12. When possible, discuss the topic of sex and sexuality with both partners simultaneously; this assures that both the patient and partner have been given the same information.
13. It may be necessary to change positions and develop new ways of pleasuring each other after treatment for cancer.
14. Teach the patient and partner to deal with any bowel, bladder, or general hygiene concerns and need for lubrication or appliances before sexual relations.
15. Explore new zones of pleasure and the use of fantasy as a way of increasing pleasure.
16. Do not make sex an all or nothing experience. Remember that human relationships, including sexual ones, are a matter of compromise.

FIGURE 18–1 Sexual Counseling Guidelines

Knowing the patient's sexual orientation is not nearly as important as assessing for limitations to the patient's usual sexual practices. Nonjudgmental inquiries about sexual behavior will help minimize the bias of the assessment and can make the patient feel more comfortable revealing information about his or her sexuality.

Figure 18–1 lists sexual counseling guidelines for nurses who are unaccustomed to this area of clinical practice. Nurses are in an ideal position to assess patients' sexual concerns, provide reassurance and education, and refer for treatment when necessary.

SEXUAL DYSFUNCTIONS RELATED TO CANCER AND ITS TREATMENTS

Cancer and its treatments can alter sexual function directly, indirectly, or both. The direct effects on sexual function are seen when the tumor involves the sex or reproductive organs, requiring such surgical procedures as vaginectomy, prostatectomy, or penectomy. Surgery, chemotherapy, and radiation therapy may contribute to sexual dysfunction by altering ovarian or testicular function, and infertility may become an issue for both men and women.

Less severe changes, such as bleeding or pain during intercourse, can have both direct and indirect effects on sexuality. Changes in body image from a mastectomy or the creation of an ostomy, along with consequent distraction or preoccupation with bodily functions, may make the patient unable to relax and enjoy sex. Treatment side effects such as malaise, fatigue, and nausea and vomiting may reduce sexual drive and desire, while alopecia can make a patient feel less sexually attractive. Cancer and its treatment can affect the sexual response by either increasing or decreasing libido through the masculinizing or feminizing effects of treatment.

Indirect effects on sexual function may occur secondary to diagnosis and treatment. These sequelae may contribute to psychological reactions and changes in social roles. Cancer-related weakness and debility may be associated with a decrease in sexual drive. This loss of libido may also be a secondary reaction to sexual dysfunction, or it may be a symptom of depression (see Chapter 19). Additionally, medications used in conjunction with cancer treatment may affect sexual functioning or responsiveness. Table 18–1 lists the potential effects of specific cancers on sexual function, fertility, and partner relationships, along with implications for clinical practice.

NURSING INTERVENTIONS

In addition to the substantive clinical information given in Table 18–1, nursing interventions should focus on open communication between the patient and nurse. The key to successful nursing intervention in the areas of sexuality and sexual dysfunction is to give patients permission to discuss their concerns openly in a safe environment. A classic intervention, the PLISSIT model, is featured in Figure 18–2. It offers four levels of intervention depending on the nurse's comfort level with the subject matter. It is recommended that discussions of potential sexual problems begin at the time of diagnosis, letting patients know they have *permission* to discuss the subject whenever necessary.

Assessment is the key to identifying problems or issues related to sexuality. An initial evaluation includes questions about the patient's current state of sexual functioning, a history of past sexual experiences, and an assessment of current relationships. This also provides an opportunity to offer *limited information* about the sequelae of disease, treatment, and sexual dysfunction. A more thorough evaluation (Figure 18–3) would cover family background, attitudes toward sex, and an exploration of the patient's concept of the impact of cancer on sexual functioning. After taking a sexual history, the nurse can offer *specific suggestions* or a referral for more *intensive therapy*. It is a good idea to bring up the subject again during treatment. However, for some patients the posttreatment phase is the optimal time for a more thorough exploration of sexual concerns.

TABLE 18–1 Effects of Cancer on Sexuality, Sexual Function, Fertility, Partners, and Clinical Implications

Site	Dysfunction: Organic	Dysfunction: Psychological	Effect on Fertility	Impact on Partner	Comments	Implications for Clinical Practice
Cervix	Treatment of in situ with cone biopsy will not cause dysfunction. Radical hysterectomy will shorten the vagina 1/3 to 1/2; this may be appreciable but usually is not.	Sometimes.	No, with cone biopsy for in situ stages; yes, with hysterectomy and/or XRT.	Sometimes (partner may feel he can "catch cancer" or be affected by its treatment, especially XRT.	XRT to the pelvis will cause thickening of the vagina and may cause stenosis and/or fistula formation and dyspareunia.	Deep pelvic thrusts may be painful, and sexual positions may have to be modified to avoid discomfort. Water-soluble lubricants on a woman's thighs, which are then adducted during intercourse, can create the sensation of a deep vagina. Alternative position: vaginal penetration from behind between closely adducted thighs. Vaginal dilators or frequent intercourse may prevent stenosis. Polyglycol-based, water-soluble lubricants are recommended.
Uterus	Total abdominal hysterectomy with pelvic node dissection usually causes no dysfunction. XRT to the pelvis will cause thickening of the vagina if this is included in the fields.	Sometimes.	Yes, with either XRT or surgery.	Sometimes.	Due to lack of literature on female sexual response, it is very difficult to determine between physical and emotional dysfunction.	Menopausal changes of sudden onset in previously asymptomatic women include vaginal dryness and hot flashes. Vaginal lubricants of the polyglycol-based, water-soluble type are suggested.
Ovary	In premenopausal women, bilateral oophorectomy will result in menopausal symptoms.	Sometimes.	Yes (except with cases of unilateral oophorectomy).	Sometimes.	Dyspareunia can occur. Germ cell ovarian tumors usually occur in one ovary. An oophorectomy of the affected ovary should maintain fertility by preserving the uterus and other ovary.	If premenopausal, treatment of menopausal changes including vaginal dryness and hot flashes. Vaginal lubrication is suggested. Chemotherapy may cause alopecia, nausea, vomiting, and fatigue, minimizing desire for sexual intercourse.

Continued

TABLE 18-1 Continued

Site	Dysfunction: Organic	Dysfunction: Psychological	Effect on Fertility	Impact on Partner	Comments	Implications for Clinical Practice
Vulva	Simple vulvectomy can result in introital stenosis. Radical vulvectomy includes removal of the clitoris.	Usually.	No; patient is often post-menopausal.	Usually.	Radical vulvectomy can cause a decrease in ROM of lower extremities.	Postoperative perineal numbness may impair arousal. After clitorectomy there may be a decrease in or absence of orgasms.
Breast	The absence of fore-play using nipple stimulation for arousal may cause some difficulties.	Usually.	Dependent upon treatment used.	Usually.	If oophorectomy and hormonal manipulations are utilized, this can affect all aspects of sexuality.	Chemotherapeutic agents may cause ovarian failure with hot flashes and vaginal dryness. Vaginal lubricants should be used. Mastectomy: prosthesis and lingerie may conceal the surgical site. Alternative positions for intercourse may be suggested to keep breast or scar out of sight. To prevent unrealistic expectations after breast reconstruction, a drawing or photograph of how the new breast might look should be shown prior to the reconstruction.
Prostate	Total prostatectomy results in impotence. Simple prostatectomy usually results in retrograde ejaculation.	Usually.	Usually.	Usually.	Bilateral orchiectomy or hormonal manipulations can result in erectile failures and ejaculation difficulties. If estrogen treatment is initiated, gynecomastia may result.	At biopsy: erectile difficulties, erectile failure, complete loss or reduced amount of seminal fluid. After surgery: erectile difficulties, retrograde ejaculation. With systemic therapy: malaise, weight loss, anemia, and pain. Impotence treatment: intracavernosal injections of prostaglandin E1, papaverine, and phentolamine; vacuum erection devices; vascular surgery; penile implants, either semirigid or inflatable.

Site						
Testicular	Nerve damage due to retroperitoneal lymph node dissection usually results in retrograde ejaculation and can cause impotence.	Usually.	Sometimes, if unilateral; always, if bilateral. Suggest utilization of sperm bank prior to chemotherapy and retroperitoneal lymph node dissection.	Usually.	Hormonal aberration (especially decrease in androgen) will cause a decrease in libido and may cause impotence, retarded ejaculation, and a decrease in sexual responsiveness.	Retroperitoneal lymphadenectomy has a significant negative impact on sexual functioning and fertility due to difficulty with ejaculation. Reduced semen volume may occur from radiation scatter to the prostate and seminal vesicles. Higher radiation doses may cause greater erectile and orgasmic difficulties. Impotence treatment: see prostate cancer.
Bladder	Local—seldom: In male, radical cystectomy involves removal of bladder, urethra, and prostate; therefore, he is impotent. In female, cystectomy usually includes urethra, uterus, and anterior vagina.	Usually.	Always with XRT; this cancer is most common in older males.	Usually.	The development of continent urostomies has made the use of the ostomy bag unnecessary in many cases. Wearing a cummerbund, decorative stoma covering, or underwear with the crotch cut out may help.	In females: there is limited research. Bladder cancer in women has similar sequelae to gynecologic cancers receiving an anterior pelvic exenteration with a narrow vagina. Dyspareunia resulting from vaginal tightness and lack of lubrication. In males: inadequate or brief erections can occur in almost all men. Orgasm, if experienced, is less intense and without ejaculation.
Colon/Rectum	Usually; nerve damage in males negatively affects erectile ability.	Usually; especially with formation of an ostomy.	None; except with XRT and chemotherapy.	Sometimes.	Women sometimes have a hysterectomy with the operative procedure. With ostomies and external collection devices, specific suggestions about emptying appliance before engaging in sex can relieve anxiety about leaks and odors.	Anterior resection is a surgical procedure with better sexual outcomes than abdominoperineal resection. Women report more positive sexual outcomes than men regardless of the surgical approach.

Continued

TABLE 18–1 Continued

Site	Dysfunction: Organic	Dysfunction: Psychological	Effect on Fertility	Impact on Partner	Comments	Implications for Clinical Practice
Hodgkins lymphoma/ non-Hodgkins lymphoma	The disease process and the effects of the therapy may decrease sexual drive and ability.	Sometimes.	Yes, with XRT to the pelvis without shielding of the gonads; chemotherapy will decrease sperm and ova maturation.	Usually.	Patients on chemotherapy alone should be using some form of contraception. The effects of chemotherapy on sperm counts and ova maturation is not totally understood.	Further research is needed to sort out multiple variables and their influence on sexuality in Hodgkins and non-Hodgkins' lymphoma survivors.
Leukemia	The disease process and associated blood counts with chemotherapy may affect ability to have an erection.	Sometimes.	Chemotherapy affects sperm count and ova maturation; but they may rebound after cessation of treatment.	Usually.	Extensive fatigue often diminishes sex drive and function.	Most frequent sequelae include poor body image, decreased sexual drive and satisfaction. Further research is needed to sort out multiple variables and their influence on sexuality in leukemia survivors.

Note: Chemotherapy, radiation, and analgesics all are associated with generalized feelings of malaise. This can have a profound effect on feelings of self-esteem, self-worth, sexuality, and libido. All these factors should be taken into consideration when assessing the sexual needs and/or problems of cancer patients and their families.
XRT = radiation therapy   ROM = range of motion

Source: Adapted from Andersen, B. L., & Lamb, M. L. (1995). Sexuality and cancer. In G. P. Murphy, W. Lawrence, & R. E. Lenhard (Eds.), *American Cancer Society textbook of clinical oncology* (2nd ed., pp. 699–713). Atlanta, GA: American Cancer Society; Lamb, M. L., & Woods, N. F. (1981). Sexuality and the cancer patient. *Cancer Nursing, 4,* 138–139; and Halfin, V., Morgantaler, A., Barton Burke, M., & Goldstein, I. (1996). Sexuality and cancer. In R. Osteen (Ed.), *Cancer Manual.* Framingham, MA: American Cancer Society.

(P) Permission: Give *permission* to be sexual when undergoing or recovering from treatment or when living with the disease.

(LI) Limited Information: Provide factual *information* about the effects of the disease and treatment on sexuality, sexual function, and fertility. Basic information about sexual function may be necessary. Common areas of concern may be the capacity for continued performance (e.g., full erections, ejaculation, orgasm), fertility, or possible interferences such as pain and fatigue.

(SS) Specific Suggestions: Provide *specific strategies* for managing sexual activity. Examples include setting the context for sex so that it is optimal for comfort and arousal (e.g., choosing times when rested, emptying urinary pouches), ways to decrease discomfort or conserve energy (e.g., different coital positions), or activities in lieu of intercourse (e.g., body massage, masturbation).

(IT) Intensive Therapy: Refer to *sexual therapy* or *psychotherapy* to manage sexual dysfunctions, permanent sexual disabilities, distress from the sexual changes, or marital distress. Such problems require mental health professionals who are experienced in many intervention strategies.

FIGURE 18–2   The PLISSIT Model

Source: Adapted from Annon, J. (1974). *The behavioral treatment of sexual problems. I.* Honolulu: Kapiolani Health Services; and Andersen, B. L., & Lamb, M. A. (1995). Sexuality and cancer. In G. P. Murphy, W. Lawrence, & R. E. Lenhard (Eds.), *American Cancer Society textbook of clinical oncology* (2nd ed., pp. 699–713).

Because the sexual partner plays a pivotal role in sexual recovery after cancer treatment, it is recommended that partners be included when the problem is assessed and in subsequent discussions on the subject. Patients who are unable to have regular intercourse as a consequence of their disease or treatment may still experience touch, intimacy, and pleasure in a variety of ways, provided both partners are sufficiently motivated, open-minded, and flexible. Figures 18–4 and 18–5 offer patient education tools for nurses to use with their patients, both male and female.

LONG-TERM EFFECTS OF CANCER TREATMENT IN CHILDHOOD

Large numbers of cancer survivors are adults who have been cured of childhood cancers. In both males and females, sexual dysfunction can result from surgical intervention, chemotherapeutic agents, and radiation dosage, frequently causing delayed gonadal effects.

Although some adult survivors of childhood cancer choose to have families of their own, this population is found to be less likely to attempt a pregnancy. Among female survivors of acute lymphocytic leukemia and Hodgkin's disease

Database
- *Social History:* education, occupation, parental roles, religious beliefs and practices.
- *Social Unit:* partnered, married, living together, group living arrangement, duration, children, problems/concerns.
- *Medical/Surgical/Psychiatric:* problems and/or medications.
- *Obstetrical/Gynecological Information:* number of children, abortions, vaginal deliveries, menstruation (frequency, duration, regularity), contraceptives, problems regarding menopause.
- *Sources of Sex Education:* books, films, workshops, formal courses.

Sexual Attitudes, Desire, and Practices
- *Autosexual:* early sex education, age started, masturbation/masturbatory history, feelings regarding this activity, most sensual areas on the body (mouth, ears, neck, breasts, penis, vagina, clitoris).
- *Desire for Sexual Experience:* increased, decreased, fluctuations/changing patterns, feelings about sexual adequacy, feelings about femininity/masculinity, body size, appearance (hair, breasts).
- *Sexual Interaction with Partner*
  - Preliminaries of lovemaking: initiation, extent of communication, characteristics of love play; behaviors that detract from the overall erotic encounters; sexual norms between partners; extracoital options.
  - Erectile functioning: quality of erections, situations that precipitate erectile failure, satisfaction with penile size.
  - Facility for vaginal lubrication: sufficient time for lubrication, rapidity of lubrication, changes in patterns of lubrication, vaginal pain during penetration.
  - Orgastic capacity: how climax is achieved, masturbation, manual/oral manipulation by partners, vaginal/rectal penetration, description of and frequency of climax or orgasm, change in quality of the experience, concern over partner reaching climax, situations that inhibit orgastic attainment
- *Extramarital/Extracouple Experience:* frequency, duration.

FIGURE 18–3   Sexual Assessment Model

Source: Copyright 1996 by Margaret Barton Burke. All rights reserved. Used with written consent of the author.

who become pregnant, the frequency of adverse pregnancy outcomes has not been particularly increased. In contrast, risk for adverse outcomes does appear to be increased in certain treatment groups, such as those who have undergone abdominal irradiation for Wilms' tumor (Halfin, Morgantaler, Barton Burke & Goldstein, 1996).

Ongoing follow-up and assessment of childhood cancer survivors will identify any long-term reproductive, psychosexual, or other sequelae. It is hoped that such information will lead to treatment modification, resulting in reduced sequelae and optimizing patients' quality of life.

The diagnosis of cancer has undoubtedly affected your life in many ways. It has forced you to deal physically with various tests and treatments and emotionally with the many lifestyle changes that treatment can produce. Cancer care may include surgery, chemotherapy, biotherapy, and radiation therapy; it may also involve the use or withdrawal of hormones. Any of these treatments may cause an alteration in sexual response or functioning, sometimes requiring people to make changes in their sexual patterns and habits in order to maintain a positive quality of life and healthy interpersonal relationships. As difficult as these changes may be, it is important to remember that the pleasure of sexual closeness can be achieved no matter what treatment has been used. The following suggestions may guide you as you attempt to make adjustments in your sexual functioning.

Get a medical OK
- Check with your health care provider before resuming sexual intercourse. If you have had surgery, it is necessary for any surgical wounds to have healed in order to prevent irritation and infection.
- If your resistance to infection has been lowered by chemotherapy, radiation therapy, or biotherapy, be sure to ask your health care provider's advice on whether sexual activity poses any additional risks.

Ask questions
- Communication plays a big part in helping you cope with sexual changes you may experience or anticipate. Although it may be difficult, you and your partner should discuss sexual issues with your health care provider before you begin your treatment. Here are some questions you may want to ask:
  How will the treatment I am getting affect my sexual desire and/or performance?
  Will the effect of treatment be temporary or permanent?
  Are there any treatments or kinds of therapy (medication, sexual counseling, surgery) that will assist me in adapting to any changes I may experience?
  Do I have any restrictions where sexual activity is concerned?
  Whom should I contact if I am having sexual difficulties?

Set the scene and create the mood.
- Set the stage for sexual contact by choosing a time when both you and your partner are rested and free from distractions.
- A warm shower together allows partners to begin foreplay in a relaxed way. Alternatively, a warm bath, if permitted, may relax muscles and make sexual activity more pleasurable.
- Candlelight, music, and a glass of wine (if permitted) can add to a romantic mood.
- Use of erotic materials, such as books and movies, may help stimulate interest in sexual activity.
- Use of prescribed pain medication or muscle relaxants within the dosing guidelines given by your physician can, if necessary, make sexual activity more comfortable.
- The use of water-soluable lubricants may also help to increase comfort.

Be patient with yourself.
- Many men become anxious about resuming sexual relations with a partner. Sometimes it is helpful to use self-stimulation (masturbation) or partner stimulation as a first step in resuming sexual activity.
- Realize that the first few sexual encounters after cancer treatment may not be as smooth or spontaneous as you might expect or want. This adjustment, like all the

FIGURE 18–4 Regaining Sexual Confidence: For Men with Cancer and Their Partners

others you have made, will probably take a while. Plan sexual encounters for when you and your partner will have sufficient time and privacy.

- Recognize that some patterns may change. Plan to start with gentle touching or massage, so that each partner has a change to enjoy giving and receiving the pleasurable sensations that come from being close.
- Experiment with alternative positions until you find one that is most comfortable for you. If you are feeling fatigued, try positions that require minimal exertion, or just take a rest before proceeding.

Communicate.
- Talk to your partner about what is pleasurable and what you would like done differently. Sometimes it is necessary to experiment with different positions so that both partners can achieve sexual satisfaction.
- Share your feelings with your partner as you go through these adjustments together. It is natural to feel angry, frustrated, or depressed at times. Express those feelings, and let your partner know that it's OK to express them too.

Take appropriate precautions.
- Plan to use appropriate birth control measures, if indicated. Also, unless you are certain that neither you nor your partner has a sexually transmitted disease and that both of you are monogamous, be sure to wear a condom.

Don't hesitate to get help if you need it.
- Pursue the option of sexual rehabilitation or sexual counseling if there are physical or psychological barriers that do not resolve with time.
- If impotence (inability to have or maintain an erection) is an ongoing problem, speak to your health care provider. Impotence can have physical or psychological causes, or a combination of both. Some men may need medication or counseling to control anxiety or depression. Other men may be candidates for surgery that will implant a penile prosthesis, a device that enables men to have an erection.

Learn all you can.
- Obtain a copy of the booklet *Sexuality and Cancer: For the Man Who Has Cancer and His Partner*, a publication available from the American Cancer Society. This booklet offers practical advice on dealing with sexual concerns. You can call 1-800-ACS-2345 to obtain a copy.

- You may want to contact the following organizations for additional information:

  The American Cancer Society. This organization provides educational materials and programs as well as support services to patients with cancer. Contact your local American Cancer Society unit.

  The United Ostomy Association, Inc. This organization provides educational materials, sponsors local Ostomy Association chapters, and published a quarterly newsletter. Write to them at 36 Executive Park, Suite 120, Irvine, CA 92714, or call 1-800-826-0826.

Don't give up.
- Remember that with time, patience, and a little effort by both you and your partner, your sexual relationship can return to what it was . . . or maybe it will be even better.

FIGURE 18–4 Continued

Source: Health Science Communication, Inc. (1993, 1994). *Oncology Patient Care Newsletter*, 3(1) and 4(1). Reprinted with permission.

Having cancer can affect every aspect of your life, including your sexuality. Whether your treatment has entailed surgery, chemotherapy, radiotherapy, biotherapy, or any combination of the four, there will be adjustments to make as you recover. Remember that honest partner-to-partner communication is essential to maintaining a strong, supportive relationship. Be patient, be creative, and ask for advice when needed. The pleasure of sexual closeness enhances quality of life and can be adapted no matter what treatment has been used. After consulting your physician or nurse about specific restrictions, use the following suggestions to promote your sexual recovery.

Before you resume sexual activity . . .
- Focus on your physical recovery first. Emphasize nutrition, rest, and progressive activity.
- Include your partner in all discussions about your care and treatment while you are still in the hospital.
- Be sure that your discharge instructions include advice about resuming sexual activity. If your nurse or doctor doesn't mention it, feel free to ask.
- Obtain a copy of the booklet *Sexuality & Cancer*, a publication available from the American Cancer Society. (Your nurse can tell you how to contact this organization.) Separate booklets are published for men and women.
- Plan to use appropriate birth control measures, if indicated.
- Report any unusual bleeding, discharge, fever, or pain to your doctor or nurse.
- You've been through a lot, and it may take some time before you are interested in sex again. Be patient with yourself.

When you feel ready . . .
- Remember that self-concept and sexuality are linked, so emphasize the positive aspects of your appearance and personality.
- Wear comfortable, attractive lounging clothes and perhaps perfume or cologne, not only to arouse your partner, but also to feel good about yourself.
- Set the stage for sexual contact by choosing a time when both you and your partner are rested and free from distractions.
- A warm shower together allows partners to begin foreplay in a relaxed way.
- A glass of wine, candlelight, and music can add to a romantic mood.
- Mutual massage, not only of the genital area, but also of the neck, chest, buttocks, and thighs, is stimulating to both partners.
- Use of erotic materials, such as books and movies, can help stimulate interest in sexual activity.
- Experiment with alternative positions until you find one that is most comfortable for you. If you are feeling fatigued, try positions that require minimal exertion.
- Use water-soluable lubricant to increase vaginal moisture.
- Use prescribed pain medication or muscle relaxants, if necessary, to make sexual activity more comfortable.
- Conserve energy for sexual activity, perhaps by delegating certain household chores to others.
- Explore alternative ways of expressing physical love.
- Communicate needs and desires so that sexual activity is pleasurable for both partners.
- Consider joining a support group, where you will find couples with concerns similar to yours.

FIGURE 18–5   Regaining Sexual Confidence: For Women with Cancer
and Their Partners

- Pursue the option of sexual rehabilitation or sexual counseling if there are physical or psychological barriers that do not resolve with time.
- Most important of all, remember that, with some effort by both you and your partner, your sexual life may return to what it was . . . or maybe you can discover new and alternative ways to express your feelings for one another.

FIGURE 18–5 Continued

Source: Health Science Communication, Inc. (1993, 1994). *Oncology Patient Care Newsletter, 3*(1) and 4(1). Reprinted with permission.

CONCLUSION

Issues related to sexuality and sexual dysfunction may arise at any time during the disease trajectory, and the nurse is pivotal in offering information and support to the patient and partner. Several resources, such as support groups and printed materials, are available through the American Cancer Society, the National Cancer Institute, and other specialty cancer organizations (e.g., the Leukemia Society of America and the United Ostomy Association) and should be offered to patients as necessary (see Appendix).

BIBLIOGRAPHY

Andersen, B. L., & Lamb, M. A. (1995). Sexuality and cancer. In G. P. Murphy, W. Lawrence, & R. E. Lenhard (Eds.), *American Cancer Society textbook of clinical oncology* (2nd ed.). Atlanta: American Cancer Society.

Annon, J. (1974). *The behavioral treatment of sexual problems. I.* Honolulu: Kapiolani Health Services.

Auchincloss, S. (1991). Sexual dysfunction after cancer treatment. *Journal of Psychosocial Oncology, 9*(1), 23–41.

Halfin, V. P., Morgantaler, A., Barton Burke, M., & Goldstein, I. (1996). Sexuality and cancer. In R. T. Osteen (Ed.), *Cancer manual* (9th ed.). Framingham, MA: Massachusetts Division, American Cancer Society.

Kripke, C. C., Vaias, L., & Elliott, A. (1994). The importance of taking a sensitive sexual history. *Journal of the American Medical Association, 271*(9), 713.

Lamb, M. A., & Woods, N. F. (1981). Sexuality and the cancer patient. *Cancer Nursing, 4*, 137–144.

World Health Organization. (1975). *Education and treatment in human sexuality: The training of health professionals.* Technical Report Series No.572. Geneva: Author.

19

Psychosocial Responses to Disease and Treatment

Ginette G. Ferszt
Ruth C. Waldman

Despite dramatic progress in treatment, **cancer** continues to be one of the most feared of all diseases. Many people still associate cancer with death, suffering, or disfigurement. Some people with cancer fear being ostracized and, therefore, may experience the additional psychological burden of keeping their illness a secret from others.

Cancer may disturb the balance of the entire family system, resulting in increased tension and stress for the person with cancer as well as other members of the extended family. Since family members' responses to the illness will have a significant impact on the patient's adaptation, the nurse needs to incorporate a family-centered approach in assessing and responding to the problems and needs that arise throughout the cancer experience. Children whose parent, sibling, grandparent, or other significant person has cancer are a particularly vulnerable group, and they must be carefully included in the plan of care according to their developmental needs.

In recent years, much oncology nursing research has focused on the quality of life experienced by cancer patients and their families. Quality of life incorporates such concepts as physical health, psychological and spiritual concerns, family relationships, and social and economic issues. Nurses can use this research to develop teaching plans that address all aspects of patient and family needs and contribute to optimal living.

ASSESSMENT OF ISSUES THROUGHOUT
THE CANCER EXPERIENCE

The cancer continuum serves as a useful framework for identifying the complex issues and problems unique to each person who experiences cancer. The nurse who is aware of, and continually assesses for, the concerns of patients and families can do much to improve quality of life through appropriate interventions. Learning to live with cancer involves developing a tolerance for risk and the unknown. Feelings of vulnerability accompany the threat and stress of illness. Sadness and even despair are to be expected, particularly at the time of diagnosis, transitional points of illness, recurrence, and during advanced stages. Grief may be experienced repeatedly as the patient and family cope with the multiple losses associated with the disease and its treatment.

Assessment of patient and family coping should begin with the initial nurse–patient interaction. Early identification of problem areas can prevent a major crisis. The following represent some questions that may be helpful in obtaining a good information baseline from the patient and individual family members as indicated.

- *What types of losses have you experienced in the past?* A person's past history of loss and response to loss may give insight as to how the individual may cope with current losses. An accumulation of losses, particularly over a short period of time, may signal the potential of high risk for psychosocial distress.

- *How did you react or cope with that loss?* Did the person feel afraid, angry, sad, hopeless, or withdrawn? By identifying past coping and grieving styles, the nurse will be better able to understand and respond to present emotional needs.

- *What or who helped you get through that difficult situation?* Some people may focus on creative outlets such as playing music, using guided imagery, or yoga; some may throw pillows; others may reach out to their faith community and/or support groups. By helping the patient and family identify how they dealt with grief or difficult situations in the past, the nurse may be able to assist them in feeling more confident in handling the current situation.

- *What have you been told about your illness and treatment?* This question will help determine whether the patient and family accurately understand the information that has been given. Misunderstandings and knowledge deficits can increase a person's anxiety.

- *How do you think your illness most affects you and your family?* By understanding what impact the illness has on the family system, the nurse can identify and respond to primary concerns. The amount of stress and anxiety the patient and family feel will depend largely on how much their daily life has been disrupted and on their flexibility and adaptability.

- *How does the illness affect your feelings about God, faith or self? What has bothered you most? How do you make sense of the illness?* These questions attempt to discover what meaning the illness has for the individual patient and family. Some persons feel guilty or responsible in some way for the illness; some may question God; others may describe the illness as a natural life event that must be coped with (see Chapter 21).

Even though loss is a universal experience, it is also deeply personal. Patients and families grieve in their own style, for different reasons, and for different periods of time. The response to loss will be largely influenced by the individual's and family's loss history; the way in which previous losses have been dealt with; the presence of concurrent crisis; the availability of support systems; and the person's social, religious, and cultural background. By systematically assessing these critical aspects, the nurse can support the patient and family and assist them in finding the appropriate services that may be helpful in dealing with specific problems and issues.

DIAGNOSIS

The initial reactions of newly diagnosed cancer patients frequently include shock, numbness, fear, and panic. "I can't believe this is really happening to me," "What did I do to deserve this?" and "Am I going to die?" are common themes. Shock reverberates throughout the family system as members try to absorb vast amounts of threatening information. Anxiety, preoccupation, sadness, agitation, fear, and withdrawal are common reactions. The family tries to regain control of an overwhelming situation, often by seeking extensive information.

Emotional and intellectual responses that appear incongruent with the severity of the disease may be mistaken for denial when, in fact, the patient may choose not to deal with the entire situation at this time in order to conserve psychological energy for what lies ahead. The patient and family need time to comprehend fully what has happened, mobilize their psychological resources, and progress past the initial shock.

During the extensive process of diagnosis and staging, patients may undergo myriad radiological, surgical, and physical examinations, and they must hear and attempt to understand extensive amounts of information about their condition, prognosis, and recommended treatment. Patients must make multiple decisions related to their care, and they must now depend on health care providers with whom they have had no previous relationship. Identifying one key professional person to be the primary disseminator of information can decrease anxiety.

During this period, patients and families face issues such as loss of control, changes in body image, and changes in roles and relationships. Patients' lives become focused on the illness and the initial treatment process, and the patient's time may be controlled by external schedules imposed by surgeons, radiologists, physicians, nurses, and hospitals. The nurse must provide structured information about treatment and management of side effects and allow opportunities for patients and families to ask questions and learn what to anticipate. Having at least one family member or friend present during critical times of information giving and discussion of needs will help to facilitate open communication and acknowledgment of the family's needs as well as those of the patient.

TREATMENT

Many people are able to continue active, productive lives during and following cancer treatment. However, the patient and family are challenged to maintain a sense of normalcy in an abnormal situation. Whether treatment involves chemotherapy, radiation therapy, surgery, or a combination of these, cancer patients must concentrate much of their energy on coping with the physical changes and side effects. Conservation of energy is too often learned by trial and error.

As work, family, and social schedules are changed to accommodate the treatments, priorities and goals may also need to be reevaluated. Patients focus on completing the prescribed treatment plan and coping with side effects. It may be necessary for patients to learn new skills associated with the treatments, such as colostomy care or self-injection of medications. These additional stressors may tax the patient's overworked coping strategies, leading to difficulty in concentration and decision making. Suggesting that the patient and family write a list of questions for caregivers to answer may help them focus and use problem-solving skills.

Treatment regimens can place heavy demands on the patient's and family's time and energy. Treatment side effects and distressing symptoms such as nausea, **alopecia** (hair loss), and fatigue often necessitate lifestyle changes, such as buying clothing to accommodate body changes or reassigning responsibilities to conserve physical energy. Innovation, creativity, and supportive resources can make living with these changes easier. Cosmetic and fashion specialists, nutritionists, clinical specialists, social workers, clergy, and support groups can be valuable resources for solutions to difficult problems (see Chapter 20).

SURVIVORSHIP

The meaning of **survivorship** is evolving within oncology nursing. While survivors were originally defined as those who had overcome and been cured of their cancer, recent articles recognize that survivorship is also a journey undertaken by persons who are living with cancer as a chronic illness, and for whom cure is a remote possibility but the prospect of living for an extended period of time is quite probable. Nurses, therefore, must be aware of the issues facing patients and their families and provide needed support and guidance for both those who appear to be disease free and those who have residual disease.

When cancer patients complete the treatment protocol, they feel a great sense of relief at having "beaten the odds" and anticipate resuming their previous lives. At the same time, however, they may be surprised to find themselves frightened at being cast adrift from the close supervision and support of health care professionals and worried about possible disease recurrence. They may recognize that the cancer experience has changed them in fundamental ways and that their lives will never be the same. Anticipatory guidance from nurses can reassure them that these feelings are normal, teach them about signs and symptoms that would indicate the need to seek medical attention, and refer them to individuals or agencies that provide ongoing support and counseling.

One of the problems encountered by those who are cured of their disease is having to confront previously suppressed emotions such as anger at medical personnel who were not helpful, frustration at delays in treatment, and rage at treatment-caused changes in their body image. Individual therapy and support groups can assist the survivor with resolution of these issues. The National Coalition for Cancer Survivorship is a valuable resource and provides information about publications and programs relevant to cancer survivors.

The cancer survivor may encounter barriers when attempting to return to the work force. Employers may be unwilling to allow employees to return to the previous level of responsibility and may demote or refuse to hire them. Health insurance may be impossible, or prohibitively expensive, to obtain. If the patient is continuing with treatment for cancer, the costs of this treatment are an added expense (see Chapter 20 for additional information on workplace discrimination).

An additional challenge faced by cancer survivors is shifting their focus from "one day at a time" to once more being future oriented. The change does not happen overnight, and some people may need help in permitting themselves to plan and dream for the future once again.

Cancer patients often state that only other people who have actually experienced cancer can truly understand their situation. The cancer survivor who wants to help others can serve as a volunteer to talk with people undergoing therapy, demonstrating that positive outcomes do occur and providing hope as well as practical encouragement.

Since there are no guarantees in cancer treatment, the patient will often live with fear of recurrence, especially in the first few months or even years. For some patients, the diagnosis and treatment of cancer may have caused significant physical and emotional changes, necessitating a redefinition of normality. Some patients continue to experience the stigma that can be associated with cancer and find that family, friends, employers, and coworkers continue to treat them as invalids. Many lay people feel awkward talking with people who have cancer and do not know what to say to them or how to act in their presence. This discomfort may cause some people to withdraw from the cancer patient, leaving the patient feeling lonely and isolated.

For the patient surviving with residual disease, there are concerns about ongoing therapy and its impact on physical well-being. Fatigue may interfere greatly with desired activities. Frustration at not being able to engage fully in one's usual roles can lead to depression. The family may also become exhausted by the additional burdens and concerns related to the illness. Patients and their partners may also have difficulty meeting their needs for closeness, intimacy, and sexual expression.

In this phase, patients usually have less contact with their caregivers and may lack knowledge about accessing resources to assist them in their readjustment. It is important for the health care team to establish a follow-up regimen and to provide patients and families with information about psychosocial support services as well as a contact person to call if questions and/or issues arise.

RECURRENCE

Recurrence of cancer is described by many patients as even more difficult than the initial diagnosis. The patient has rebuilt a life at home, at work, and in the community only to have these efforts diminished. The patient must start over again with diagnostic tests to determine the extent of the cancer and receive more treatment to regain control of it. The patient frequently rides a roller coaster of recurrence, treatment, and remission several times before reaching the point of terminal illness.

Advancing disease is usually characterized by increased symptom distress. If symptoms such as pain, nausea, anorexia, stomatitis, or skin excoriation cannot be controlled, patients and families begin to feel helpless and hopeless. Adequate symptom management is crucial during this period. Also, teaching family members to alleviate or manage distressing symptoms can make them feel less helpless. Because the link between physical disease and emotional status is so strong, it is often difficult to separate symptom distress from depression. A referral to psychiatric services should be made if prolonged anxiety, grief, or depression interfere with a normal level of functioning.

The impaired mobility, disfigurement, and loss of energy that accompany difficult prolonged treatment or advancing disease can lead to the patient's social isolation. The physical and emotional toll on the patient and family can manifest as psychological, marital, or family problems. As grief and anxiety strain the patient's and family's ability to cope, continuous and stable relationships with members of the health care team become even more important.

Families in the United States at present are often fairly isolated, functioning without supportive networks. Families coping with prolonged, deteriorating illness must learn to redistribute their workload and change life expectations. Families are often stretched too far, and the unrelenting stress and strain of cancer can cause guilt, anger, and resentment. The patient may feel guilty for being a burden, and family members may be angry because their own needs go unmet. Financial pressures may result from lost income and the burden of health care costs. Nurses need to keep in mind the multiple sources of stress that confront families and assist families in exploring all possible options for assistance and support. Referrals to other members of the health care team, such as social service personnel, the hospice chaplain, the psychiatric nurse specialist, and providers of respite services, may be indicated at this time.

During the advanced phase of illness, the patient and family are challenged to examine their hope system and redefine what they hope for. Maintaining the balance between the energy and motivation necessary to keep going and the physical and emotional losses incurred taxes even the most adaptive family system. Some families may find it difficult to ask for help, but they are often relieved and appreciative of efforts made to provide emotional support.

TERMINAL PHASE

The terminal phase of illness brings a new set of decisions that the patient and family must confront: active treatment or palliation; death at home or in the hospital. As patients and families are faced with impending separation and death, they may experience a wide range of emotions including mood swings, sadness, depression, anger, guilt, powerlessness, withdrawal, and relief. Measures that provide comfort and control pain now have priority.

During this difficult period, patients may question the purpose of their lives. Religious beliefs may be challenged, and existential questions such as the meaning and purpose of suffering are frequently raised. For some patients, this questioning leads to personal transformation and a sense of inner peace; for others, the journey leads to emotional distress and despair.

Patients with terminal cancer must expend increasing amounts of energy fighting progressive symptoms. Their focus shifts from the outside world to their physical comfort. Patients may lose interest in events and experiences that were once important. They are no longer able to participate in many of the activities that were once enjoyable. Their circle of relationships shrinks to close friends and family, and long-term dreams and aspirations may need to be relinquished.

Approaching death sometimes leads to an acute awareness of the significance of the relationship and how deep the loss will be. Patients and families in troubled relationships may grieve because problems may never be resolved. For others, death is a welcome relief or offers the opportunity to experience healing in relationships. The challenge for the nurse lies in accompanying patients and families on their journey, refraining from making judgments or trying to "fix" the situation. The importance of the nurse's support, gentleness, and quiet presence must never be underestimated. The continued commitment to be with the patient and family in one of the most intimate times of life can be the most important gift that is given.

The actual death can be a very stressful time. It may be difficult for families who are not prepared for what they will see and hear to witness the physical dying process. Families may react impulsively, demanding extraordinary measures they have eschewed earlier. If the patient is at home, a specific, written action plan with telephone numbers of people to call can be useful as death approaches.

In some situations, the family struggles to hold on. At times, it may be more difficult for the family to let go than it is for the patient. Families may feel hurt by the patient's emotional withdrawal in the final days. Explaining emotional reactions to families and outlining what they can do for their loved one are important strategies.

Some families will be able to say their last goodbyes and plan for funeral services. In other families, the patient will die without ever having talked about death openly. It is important for the nurse to respect a family's need to grieve and express emotion in a way that is consistent with their own culture, personal style, beliefs, and traditions.

The involvement of children in grief rituals is a concern of families. Many people do not know how to include children and, in an effort to protect them, exclude the children from participation that is important in facilitating their own grief work. Written resources that discuss children's grief and list developmentally appropriate books for children are frequently welcomed by families.

Hospice care can be considered when cure is no longer the treatment goal. Hospice programs address the physical, social, emotional, and spiritual needs of the family with an emphasis on pain and symptom control, volunteer support, and extended care at home. These programs focus on the quality of life that remains, empowering patients and families to make decisions and choices that are consistent with their goals and philosophy. The extensive supportive care that can be provided by hospice programs through their volunteer efforts may give patients and families the necessary support and respite to maximize the final months of life. Most hospice programs also provide bereavement follow-up for a period of time after the patient's death. This can be a valuable service to families who have limited support or who are isolated (see Chapter 21 for more information on hospice and palliative care).

CONCLUSION

Nurses, as well as other members of the health care team, have the opportunity to play a significant role in supporting and empowering patients and families throughout the cancer continuum. Physiological and psychosocial responses to cancer are inseparable from one another. It is often in the context of a helping relationship based on a holistic philosophy that people are able to adapt to and cope with the losses inherent in a life-threatening illness.

BIBLIOGRAPHY

American Cancer Society Resources:
- *Americans with Disabilities Act.* (No. 4571).
- *Caring for the Patient with Cancer at Home: A Guide for Families.* (No.4656).
- *After Diagnosis: Common Questions and Experiences of Cancer Patients and Families.* (No. 0406).
- *Listen with Your Heart. Talking with Cancer Patients.* (No. 4557).

Baird, S., McCorkle, R., & Grant, M. A. (Eds.). (1991). *Cancer nursing.* Philadelphia: W. B. Saunders.

Ferrans, C. E. (1994). Quality of life through the eyes of survivors of breast cancer. *Oncology Nursing Forum, 21*(10), 1645–1651.

Holland, J., & Rowland, J. (Eds.). (1990). *Handbook of Psychooncology.* New York: Oxford University Press.

Rainbow Collection. (1996). *Resources to help people grow through loss and grief.* Burnsville, NC: Author.

Rando, T. A. (1984). *Grief, dying and death: Clinical interventions for caregivers.* Champaign, IL: Research Press.

Schneider, J. (1994). *Finding my way: Healing and transformation through loss and grief.* Colfax, WI: Seasons Press.

Wolfelt, A. (1996). *Helping the bereaved child.* Fort Collins, CO: Companion Press.

20

Rehabilitation

Frances K. Barg

Improved cancer treatment has resulted in more patients living longer than ever before. An important trend in cancer care is a focus on the functional status as well as the quality of life of the person with cancer during and beyond active treatment. As a result, cancer is now frequently considered a chronic illness with episodic physical and emotional effects.

Rehabilitation is a dynamic, ongoing process intended to maximize an individual's capabilities within the limitations of the disease or disability. Cancer has the potential to affect the physical, emotional, and social aspects of a patient's life. The patient's relationships with other family members, coworkers, and employers may be affected by the consequences of the disease and its treatment. However, nurses, in collaboration with the patient, family, and health care team, can help the patient become independent and enable him or her to live a productive, satisfying life whether the cancer is cured, controlled, or palliated. Nurses can assist the patient and family in clarifying goals, values, and needs when planning rehabilitation activities.

THE FAMILY AS THE UNIT OF CARE

A basic tenet of cancer rehabilitation is that the patient and family are treated as a single unit. Most patients do not experience cancer by themselves, but as part of a family, neighborhood, school, work setting, or religious group. It is well established that cancer affects not only the ill person, but family members as well. Studies suggest that cancer leads to altered role relationships and communication patterns. Not only must caregivers assume some roles formerly performed by the ill family member, but they must also assume physical caregiving responsibilities for the ill person.

In recent years there has been an escalating trend toward early discharge of hospital patients. As a result, increasing numbers of patients with cancer are being cared for at home by family members. This demand on family members is not new, but the role of caregiving has dramatically shifted from one of promoting convalescence to one of actively providing care in the home. Because patients are being discharged from acute care settings with fewer days of hospital care and greater health care needs than ever before, family members are being asked to provide more complex care earlier in the patient's recovery.

Caregivers frequently lack the time to develop supportive social relationships. Even though community services might be available, there appear to be barriers that inhibit caregivers from utilizing services to meet their needs. These include (a) a lack of awareness about available services; (b) a lack of knowledge about how to access services; (c) financial constraints; (d) a stigma regarding accepting help; (e) family resistance; (f) a lack of transportation; (g) existing services that are overworked; and (h) health provider goals that are not congruent with patient and family goals.

There is increasing evidence that community-based **support** for caregivers may help to avert some of the adverse consequences of providing care for a family member with cancer. The results of a study involving late-stage lung cancer patients conducted by McCorkle and her colleagues indicated that home health care services assisted patients with forestalling distress from symptoms and maintaining their independence longer in comparison with patients who did not receive such services. In addition, spouses of patients who received home care reported better adaptation for themselves. In a later study, McCorkle demonstrated that cancer patients who are discharged from the hospital with complex problems and who receive home care reported significant improvement in psychosocial distress 3 months after discharge. However, 3 months after discharge their caregivers reported a similar or an increased level of burden. Even as patients' psychological status improved, caregivers reported that they were still required to modify their schedules to assist the patients with their treatment regimens.

Goal Setting

Setting realistic goals is one of the most important factors in cancer rehabilitation. Although cancer can be characterized by significant loss, rehabilitation shifts the focus from what has been lost to what can be done with the remaining strengths and abilities. Goal development can start with an interdisciplinary assessment of deficits, strengths, and potential gains. Rehabilitation goals should be consistent with the specific type and stage of cancer and with goals for cancer treatment. They should also address aspects of prevention, restoration, maintenance, and palliation as appropriate.

BARRIERS TO REHABILITATION

Despite substantial progress, there are significant barriers to successful rehabilitation. Cancer is one of the most feared diseases. Fears of contagion and worker unproductivity, lack of acceptance of the employee by coworkers, and the belief that death is inevitable prevent many from considering cancer rehabilitation possible.

Few cancer treatment centers offer comprehensive rehabilitation services. Rehabilitation care is often fragmented, and emotional support services are frequently lacking. Social support has been identified as an important variable influencing coping and rehabilitation.

Symptom distress can also limit successful rehabilitation. For example, although guidelines for aggressive cancer pain management exist, pain remains a significant problem for many patients. Despite efforts to disseminate accurate information, cancer pain is frequently undertreated, because patients and health professionals lack expertise in managing pain and persist in their fears about addiction and the use of narcotics. (See Chapter 14 for information on pain.)

Patients with cancer frequently experience fatigue and fluctuating endurance. These factors must be considered when planning rehabilitation. Depression is sometimes a result of unrelieved symptom distress, and it also can interfere with energy and motivation.

The fear of disease recurrence also poses a barrier to rehabilitation. Some patients have difficulty believing they are cured. These patients may be less willing to plan long-term intervention based on their current status. Because the disease can recur, many patients may resist rehabilitation activities, thinking, "What's the use?". Nurses can help patients explore their fears about recurrence and set realistic rehabilitation goals. Consistent advocacy of self-care, independence, and self-determination is important regardless of the stage of disease.

Family caregivers who are included in the rehabilitation plan are often overwhelmed by their caregiving role. Frequently, they must juggle their own work schedules, new family roles, or management of their own illnesses with participation in the rehabilitation plan for the person with cancer. While family caregivers often provide significant support to the patient, they do not receive adequate support for themselves.

REHABILITATION AS AN INTERDISCIPLINARY PROCESS

Considering the complex and chronic nature of cancer patient care, the range of potential areas of rehabilitation is vast. Some aspects of care and rehabilitation are short term, such as the management of temporary alopecia from chemotherapy. Other rehabilitation activities address permanent changes, such as those resulting from a laryngectomy or colostomy. An interdisciplinary approach is best for addressing the range of possible patient and family needs. Depending on the needs to be addressed, the team may include nurses, physicians, psychologists, social workers, physical therapists, occupational therapists, speech pathologists, vocational counselors, prosthetists/orthotists, pharmacists, chaplains, enterostomal therapists, dietitians, and of course, the patient and family. By functioning as a team all members can coordinate goals, support and teach each other, enhance communication among the disciplines, and provide a vehicle for accountability. Table 20–1 lists common topics for consideration in the rehabilitation effort.

WORK AND IDENTITY

In general, Americans are bound to the work ethic, so work and productivity issues can pose additional barriers to rehabilitation. Personal identity is intimately linked with occupation. When a person's role changes because of limitations imposed by the disease or its treatment, self-esteem and mood are affected. Rehabilitation embraces the concept that a return to productive function, paid or unpaid, will enhance patients' feelings of mastery, control, and self-esteem.

Workplace discrimination against people with cancer may be overt or covert. Discriminatory employers may be motivated by fears that recovering or recovered cancer patients will be unable to do their jobs, that their turnover and absentee rates will be high, or that their disease will be fatal. Yet anecdotal evidence suggests that turnover and absenteeism are no higher for the employee with cancer than for other employees. The funds employers pay to worker compensation are unaffected, because this program provides insurance for work-related accidents.

The Americans with Disabilities Act (ADA) of 1990 prohibits discrimination in employment on the basis of disability. Since the Rehabilitation Act of 1973, cancer has been deemed a disability for these purposes. State Offices of Vocational Rehabilitation (OVRs) may be valuable resources in helping people with cancer return to work when skill modification or retraining is needed. OVRs can also help employers modify the workplace to accommodate worker disability and educate other employees about cancer. The services available through state vocational rehabilitation and services specific to cancer vary from state to state.

Family caregivers who must modify their work schedules during the treatment or recovery phase of the patient's illness are frequently concerned that time away from the workplace will have a negative impact on their employment status. With passage of the Family Leave Act in 1993, employees with 1 year of employment (in a company with 50 or more employees) are entitled to 12 weeks of unpaid leave to care for a seriously ill family member. Employees retain their health care benefits during the period of leave and are assured of returning to the same or a similar job.

SITE-SPECIFIC REHABILITATION MEASURES

The type of cancer will partly determine the kinds of rehabilitation services a patient needs. For example, a person with a laryngectomy will need information on and assistance with stoma care and communication. A woman who has had a mastectomy will want information about exercises, wound care, prostheses, and possibly reconstruction. Rehabilitation issues associated with common sites of cancer are highlighted in Table 20–2.

TABLE 20–1 Topics for Consideration by the Rehabilitation Team

Areas of Activity	Specific Tasks and Needs
Discharge planning	Follow-up care, community resources, contingency plans
Activities of daily living	Bathing, dressing, feeding, grooming, medication administration, adaptive equipment
	Bed mobility, transfers, ambulation, range of motion, strength, endurance, community access, transportation
Nutrition/swallowing	Enteral and parenteral nutrition, supplements, barriers to swallowing, anorexia
Symptom management	Pain, fatigue, weakness, nausea, sensory alterations, constipation, diarrhea, lymphedema, mucositis, dyspnea, depression, anxiety
Living environment/ home maintenance	Distance from resources, presence of stairs or other architectural barriers, need for help at home, need for special equipment at home
Body functions	Bowel and bladder management, care of skin and mucous membranes
Communication	Speech and language functions
Psychosocial relations	Relations with family members, support systems for patient and family, sexuality, body image, coping skills, role reversal
Financial considerations	Insurance coverage; job security; unreimbursed medical, nutrition, clothing, and custodial care expenses
Vocational	Concerns about return to work, discrimination, adaptation necessary for current job, need for reeducation to obtain a new job, identity issues, family caregiver's job demands
Spirituality	Existential issues

A common problem in cancer rehabilitation is that attention is focused on sites when specific disability is obvious, especially those requiring prostheses or appliances. However, comprehensive rehabilitation plans should include identification of more subtle needs and specific interventions to address them. American Cancer Society offices are prepared to offer information about specific local rehabilitation resources. The chapter bibliographies in this book provide sources of further information on rehabilitation measures that can enhance self-esteem, increase function, and add to productivity.

NURSING'S CONTRIBUTION

Nurses can enhance patient and professional awareness of cancer rehabilitation needs. Dudas and Carlson described five areas in which nurses can have a positive impact:

TABLE 20-2 Rehabilitation Issues Associated with Specific Cancer Sites

Cancer Site	Rehabilitation Issues
Head and neck cancers	Maintenance of optimal nutrition and deglutition Shoulder dysfunction rehabilitation Neck dysfunction rehabilitation Self-care considerations Speech/communication Restoring acceptable appearance and function
Breast cancer	Physical restoration of affected arm Psychosocial rehabilitation regarding loss, body image alterations, and sexuality. Cosmetic rehabilitation with form, prosthesis, or reconstruction for mastectomy patients
Bone and soft tissue malignancies	Restoration of near-normal function through prostheses, appliances, and aids to ambulation Restoration of acceptable appearance Vocational rehabilitation Psychosocial rehabilitation
Lung cancer	Preoperative rehabilitation emphasizes breathing retraining Pulmonary disability prevention after radiation or surgery
Colorectal and bladder malignancies resulting in ostomies	Self-concept adjustment Elimination control and ostomy adjustment Self-care considerations Psychosocial rehabilitation Effective skin care
Central nervous system	Preventing unnecessary loss of function and diminished quality of life Cognitive function evaluation Mobility modifications Retraining for activities of daily living Bowel and bladder management

Source: From DeLisa, J. A., Miller, R. M., Melnick, R. R., Gerber, L. H., & Hillel, A. B. (1989). Rehabilitation of the cancer patient. In V. T. DeVita, S. Hellman, & S. A. Rosenberg (Eds.), *Cancer: Principles and practice* (pp. 2333–2368). Philadelphia: J. B. Lippincott.

1. Promoting a positive attitude toward cancer rehabilitation by emphasizing cancer as a chronic disease.
2. Incorporating potential rehabilitation needs into initial patient assessments.
3. Exposing nursing students to cancer "success" stories.
4. Promoting the independence of people with cancer by referring them to established education and volunteer groups such as I Can Cope or Reach to Recovery and by working with other disciplines.

5. Maximizing functional status by helping patients anticipate potential obstacles and solutions to surmounting them.

Long-term survival has become a reality for an increasing number of people with cancer. The needs of cancer survivors are being articulated by both survivor groups and organizations such as the American Cancer Society. The National Coalition for Cancer Survivors has outlined areas of need specifically concerning work and community. The coalition has also identified a need for health surveillance guidelines and long-term support. Nurses have opportunities through their work or community roles to help survivors return to their usual activities and to educate the public about the positive advances in cancer survival and rehabilitation.

BIBLIOGRAPHY

Anderson, J. L. (1989). The nurse's role in cancer rehabilitation. *Cancer Nursing, 12*(2), 85–94.

DeLisa, J. A., Miller, R. M., Melnick, R. R., Gerber, L. H., & Hillel, A. D. (1989). Rehabilitation of the cancer patient. In V. T. DeVita, S. Hellman, & S. A. Rosenberg (Eds.), *Cancer: Principles and practice* (pp. 2333–2368). Philadelphia: J. B. Lippincott.

Dudas, S., & Carlson, C. E. (1988). Cancer rehabilitation. *Oncology Nursing Forum, 15*(2), 183–188.

Essex-Sorlie, D. (1994). The Americans with Disabilities Act: I. History, summary and key components. *Academic Medicine, 69*(7), 519–524.

Frymark, S. L. (1992). Rehabilitation resources within the team and community. *Seminars in Oncology Nursing, 8*(3), 212–228.

Ganz, P. A. (1990). Current issues in cancer rehabilitation. *Cancer, 65,* 742–751.

Houts, P. S., Yasko, J. M., Harvey, H. A., et al. (1986). Unmet psychological, social, and economic needs of persons with cancer in Pennsylvania. *Cancer, 58,* 2355–2361.

Laizner, A. M., Yost, L. M. S., Barg, F. K., & McCorkle, R. (1993). Needs of family caregivers of persons with cancer: A review. *Seminars in Oncology Nursing, 9*(2), 114–120.

McCorkle, R., Jepson, C., Malone, D., Lusk, E., Braitman, L., Buhler-Wilkerson, K., & Daly, J. (1994). The impact of posthospital home care on patients with cancer. *Research in Nursing and Health, 17*(4), 243–251.

Millette, S. J., & Parker, G. G. (1992). Future directions in cancer rehabilitation. *Seminars in Oncology Nursing, 8*(3), 210–223.

Powell, L. L. (1993). Commentary on life cycle issues affecting cancer rehabilitation. *ONS Nursing Scan in Oncology, 2*(2), 10–11.

Taguiam-Hites, S. G. (1995). The Americans with Disabilities Act of 1990: Implementation and education in rehabilitation nursing. *Rehabilitation Nursing, 20*(1), 43–44.

Watson, P. (1990). Cancer rehabilitation: The evolution of a concept. *Cancer Nursing, 13*(1), 2–8.

Yost, L., McCorkle, R., Buhler-Wilkerson, K., Schultz, D., & Lusk, E. (1993). Determinants of subsequent home health care nursing service use by hospitalized patients with cancer. *Cancer, 72*(11), 3304–3312.

21

Palliative Care

James C. Pace

You matter because you are you. You matter to the last moment of your life, and we will do all we can not only to help you die peacefully, but also to live until you die.

—Dr. Cicely Saunders, Founder
and Director, St. Christopher's Hospice

Palliative care entails providing **support** and caring to persons who are in the final phase of living and their families and significant others. Such support and care enables them to preserve their human dignity and enrich their quality of life. Palliative care usually begins with the awareness that nothing more can be done to effect a cure. Ideally, the patient's physician should be able to acknowledge that the notion that nothing more can be done applies only to treatment aimed at cure, thereby opening the door to palliative care. There is no limit to what can be done to provide as much comfort as possible, enabling the patient to truly live until the very moment of death. This concept of living rather than dying has been influenced most by the modern-day hospice movement. This chapter focuses on the basics of palliative care, concentrating on the concept of hospice and the role of the nurse.

ATTITUDES TOWARD DEATH AND DYING

Death and dying have been taboo topics in Western culture for far too many years. American society has denied death, concentrating instead on youth, beauty, strength, cure of illness, and stamina. In the medical environment, physicians and nurses often have great difficulty sharing a terminal diagnosis with the patient. The effect is a "conspiracy of silence": The patient cannot talk about the subject with health care providers, health care providers do not bring up the subject of dying directly, and the family takes its cues from both groups. The result is that the patient feels isolated and may not have anyone with whom to talk over feelings, fears, frustrations, and plans.

Many Americans fear death because what follows is unknown. And since death has been an unacceptable topic for conversation, its mystery has grown. The fear of death has several component fears: physical pain and suffering, leaving loved ones, being a burden to family members, entering into an unknown realm, losing control, dying alone, and, for a few, the meaninglessness of life. The fears associated with dying provide excellent insight into the needs of dying patients and the approaches caregivers can take in providing support to these patients. It is important to display openness and honesty; provide information; allow participation in care and decision making; understand, value, respect, and listen; provide relief from pain; help promote sleep; give supportive care including peace and quiet when needed; and foster reassurance and hope.

Every culture has its own customs, traditions, and superstitions concerning death and dying. Different ways to prepare the body at the time of death, different beliefs about an afterlife—these customs have been passed on for centuries and continue to be expressed in the way people live their lives. Open communication and the discussion of fears and anxieties often enable the patient and family to better prepare for death. Getting "one's house in order," or getting all the "work of dying" done early allows the patient and family to live better until the moment of death.

HOSPICE CARE

Concept and Goals

Historically, the idea of hospice dates back to medieval times. A hospice offered hospitality—shelter, food, and refuge—to the weary traveler, the sick, the needy, and the poor. Today, the term **hospice** is used to describe an organized institution, either within or outside the hospital setting, designed to provide palliative and supportive care. Hospice care within the hospital can utilize the "scatterbed" approach or be located on a designated unit; outpatient hospices can be home based or freestanding.

The hospice concept began a revolution in the U.S. health care system and in the way Americans regard terminal illness and the care of the dying. The spread of the hospice concept forced the nation to talk about death—to study, plan for, and provide programs to improve long-term care of the chronically and terminally ill. The fundamental goals of any hospice are:

1. To enhance the quality of human life.

2. To provide an alternative to acute care.

3. To provide medical and nursing care by using an interdisciplinary care team (see Figure 21–1)).

4. To provide pain control and symptom management.

To manage and assist with the patient's:

- *Physical symptoms* of pain, nausea, confusion, dyspnea, constipation, lack of mobility, and loss of physical function.
- *Physical signs* of ulceration, decubiti, bowel obstruction, disorientation/dementia, contractures, and labored breathing.
- *Intellectual needs* such as the need to know about one's condition in order to participate in care and the need for the truth, to correct misconceptions about the disease and its prognosis, signs and symptoms to expect, and possible resources for care.
- *Emotional strain* of worry, grief, bereavement, and anxiety.
- *Social disruption* of family, friends, and roles secondary to the disease and its therapy.
- *Financial fears* such as loss of income, cost of treatments, and family future.
- *Spiritual concerns* related to questions of meaning, significance, guilt, and creativity, as well as needs for connection, reconciliation, decreased fear, and controlled anxiety.

FIGURE 21-1   Comprehensive Palliative Plan of Care

5. To lend emotional, spiritual, and social support.

6. To teach basic nursing care to the family.

7. To continuously evaluate and support the patient and family providing 24-hour-a-day, 7-day-a-week coverage.

8. To utilize the gifts and talents of volunteers.

The Unit of Care

The primary unit of care in hospice is the patient, who is viewed as a member of a family and various communities that form his or her environment. Family members have multiple questions and concerns: "What do I tell the kids?" "How can I physically care for my loved one?" "How do I learn to give these treatments?" "I am afraid of death and dying." "What do I do if his breathing becomes worse?" "How can I do all of this alone?" "What will we do for money?" "What if she has horrible pain?" These concerns and many others are the foundation for the hospice treatment plans.

Patient and family hospice care generally begins with a visit by a member of the hospice team, usually a nurse. The hospice professional takes careful note of the family situation: Is the patient the sole source of financial and/or emotional support for the family, or a peripheral member? What are the cultural and behavioral family patterns? What are the long-term conflicts or tensions in the family constellation? The hospice team member attempts to understand the way the family unit functions both in ordinary situations and during stressful times.

Family members caring for a terminally ill patient often deny their own needs and focus solely on the needs of their loved one, leading to feelings of resentment, anger, and neglect. The hospice team attempts to interact with both the family and the patient to provide truly holistic care. Assistance with adjustment to life without the patient begins before death; professional guidance, treatment, and possible referral to other health care disciplines are a part of day-to-day hospice care.

Active participation of the family is part of the process of separation during the dying process. The hospice team soon discovers what a family can and cannot do—who can be relied upon to do what and when. Nursing research has demonstrated that those who are actively involved in the process of care while the patient is alive are less prone to guilt and self-criticism after the patient's death than those who are not involved. The hospice team suggests ways that each family member can be useful, such as providing physical care, taking care of the house or yard, running errands, getting supplies, or sharing cooking responsibilities.

The Interdisciplinary Approach

The terminally ill patient is best served by a team with a holistic approach to patient care. A typical team includes nurse; medical director; social worker; chaplain; volunteers; occupational, physical, and speech therapists; and a variety of consultant services as needed (e.g., psychiatric, radiologic, pediatric). All services are supervised by a physician who is actively involved in the care of the patient at all times.

Most often, however, the major responsibility of day-to-day caregiving falls upon the nurse. The nurse must continuously assess patient and family needs and call upon other members of the team as each situation demands. Interdisciplinary care is a carefully coordinated effort involving professionals, family, close friends, and volunteers.

SPIRITUALITY IN PALLIATIVE AND HOSPICE CARE

The nursing profession has long been an advocate of holistic care incorporating mind, body, and spirit as the object of care and attention. Spiritual well-being is a cornerstone of health and is believed to have an impact on physical well-being. In palliative and hospice care, the patient's spiritual nature is every bit as deserving of care and nurture as the body and mind.

Spirituality and religion have often been confused. Religion is most often defined as an organized, structured system of beliefs, rituals, and values that are expressed through behaviors, creeds, and/or catechisms. Religion can be conceptualized as a map that allows followers to get from the "here" (birth) to the "there" (death/heaven). For many, religion provides the prime opportunity to transcend the physical and come to a greater awareness and knowledge of what lies beyond.

Spirituality may be best described as a journey. A person's ever-evolving experience with life is a spiritual journey. Spirituality denotes a sense of (or lack of) direction. In its healthiest sense, spirituality entails a connectedness to one's self, to other people, and to a supreme being. A person's spirituality is never static: The person continues to grow into and beyond what he or she has been.

Spirituality entails a world view, a paradigm of how things "fit," providing a sense of meaning and purpose to the world and the person's place in it.

Spirituality is a much more comprehensive construct than religion; it captures the life journey of every individual. It may totally subsume the patient's religious beliefs or be totally divorced from religiosity. People who want nothing to do with religion may still be very spiritual. The verbs *becoming, connecting, being,* and *journeying* seem to capture the essence of spirituality. Spirituality is the process of getting from the "here" to the "there" and all that is learned on the journey.

NURSING AND PALLIATIVE CARE

The Role of the Nurse

Palliative care provides a constant challenge to the nurse as well as the other members of the interdisciplinary health care team. A sound working philosophy of nursing care is central to any high-quality palliative care program. It is the practical, mundane, everyday problems that make the most difference to the patient and the family: wet bed sheets, physical discomfort, feelings of isolation, depression, spiritual sadness, insomnia, the loss of physical intimacy. What to do at any given moment to ensure the patient's physical comfort becomes a primary concern for the nurse.

These elements of care delivered from the heart and the soul of the nurse are the core of what constitutes nursing itself. At the bedside of the dying, the nurse is the teacher and the one being taught, the giver and the receiver of care, the healer and the one being healed. These roles are not abstract concepts but realities that require highly skilled, compassionate, and dedicated nurses. High-quality nursing in palliative care entails the following:

- Giving imaginative, unhurried, and attentive care.
- Learning and responding to the patient's mode of communication.
- Learning to sit quietly with those who are dying to keep them in touch with life for as long as possible.
- Knowing one's own limitations.
- Involving family members and interdisciplinary team members to help provide care and do preparatory grief work.
- Knowing and being comfortable with one's own spirituality and growing in the understanding of what gives meaning to life.

Symptom Management

Preventing symptoms related to side effects of drug therapies, inactivity, stresses, and discomfort demands a proactive stance on the part of the nurse. One of the primary goals of palliative care is to maintain or even improve the patient's quality of life. This goal requires that all measures—pharmacologic, psychologic, surgical, medical, and spiritual—be implemented in order to keep the patient at his or her optimal level of functioning.

The use of pharmacologic agents in the palliative control of physical symptoms can both increase the length and improve the quality of life. In the hospice setting, chronic pain is distinguished from acute pain because the meaning of these types of pain is different in the cancer population. Fear of becoming addicted to powerful opioid drugs to control pain is an impediment to the care of the terminally ill. Patients who are dying should never have to wait until pain appears before medication is administered. Pain medication needs to be titrated for each patient's needs and, whenever possible, self-administered to help increase control. Chronic pain can often be controlled with sustained release narcotics or subcutaneously absorbed patches applied to the skin (see Chapter 14).

Symptom control can involve much more than pharmacologic measures. It means providing an environment that is peaceful, safe, and dependable, in which a high quality of care is demonstrated and the family plays a personal role in care and an important role in helping the patient deal with emotional distress.

In summary, the prevention and/or management of pain involves the identification of the pain's etiology (not all pain is caused by the cancer process itself); the prevention of pain *before* it appears, and the administration of medication in as simple a way as possible that allows maximum alertness and normalcy in terms of self-care capabilities and quality of life. Prevention and treatment of other symptoms such as constipation, nausea, fatigue, and insomnia can contribute to increased functional ability, alertness, comfort, and the ability to better enjoy living.

Spiritual Care

Nurses help to identify the spiritual needs of their patients by first listening to the stories of their past journeys. An important part of active listening is commending, congratulating, acknowledging, and giving positive feedback for all the patient's life events that have contributed to his or her well-being. In listening to these accounts, nurses will learn of incidents that may or may not be associated with guilt or shame—for example, past actions, the naming of a diagnosis or surgery, events caused by surgery, hospitalization, or interactions between and among people at various places over time. Shame may be related to such things as the loss of hair or the presence of a newly created stoma. Guilt can occur when a person does not want visitors while feeling unwell. A person may feel ashamed, unclean, or unattractive because of loss of bowel or bladder control, disfiguring surgery, or any type of alteration in appearance. Often there are hurts associated with such events, and it is helpful to have these hurts identified and named. The incident(s) can then be viewed from the perspective of a nonbiased outsider (the nurse) who is willing to reflect on the situation for a few moments and then reach out to the patient.

Often patients feel let down by God or deserted in their time of need. Perhaps they also feel that their faith is not strong enough. Patients who experience doubt and too little faith need encouragement that they are still acceptable to God in spite of their doubts, uncertainties, and questions. The nurse is often the one who first behaves in ways that let patients know they are still loved and accepted for who they have been and currently are.

In addition, patients often believe that others have let them down in some way. Who can they trust? It is important for the nurse to seek to reestablish trust by giving clear and accurate information, following up on promises, providing the reassurance that further treatment or help is available in some form, and providing consistent care that eliminates conflicting signals and information.

Thus, exploring a patient's past journey is the first step to enhancing the patient's spiritual health and well-being. With that accomplished, the nurse then explores the patient's present. Is there anger, suffering, fear, loneliness, helplessness, isolation, lack of functional ability, or fear of the unknown future? Mutually identifying and exploring these possibilities helps the patient and nurse arrive at solutions.

Once the present has been incorporated into the treatment plan, the nurse may then examine how the patient views the possibility for a future. Hope for the future can take many forms, such as hope that a new drug will help, hope of being loved and sharing that love with other people, and hope that a new sense of meaning about life will be discovered and the fear of death will be lessened.

Bereavement Care

The hospice philosophy does not end with the death event. In keeping with the core theme that the unit of care is both the patient and the family, hospice programs provide professional services during the period of mourning and grief for the surviving family members. Grief is the emotion that is involved in the work of mourning. Grief allows individuals to reinvest their emotions in new and productive directions for their future health and welfare. Various patterns of grieving and stages of working through loss have been described in the literature. Patterns and stages, however, are strictly individualized: There is no set or prescribed way to behave in order to mourn successfully. There is also no time limit to "successful" grief work. Eventually, most people learn to cope and get on with their lives, but their love for the one who died is never lost.

Family members often wrestle with feelings of guilt, relief, joy, and/or depression; feelings of being utterly lost; inability to communicate; and inability to get back on track with life. Health care professionals can help these people to feel normal, get on with their day-to-day affairs, and establish short-term goals to guide them through this emotionally labile time. Having someone to communicate with on a regular basis often eases emotional burdens and allows family members the opportunity to work through their feelings. Careful consideration and consultation by the hospice team are required in order to help family members find their own answers.

In summary, the nurse's role in palliative care is to help to integrate the patient's past, present, and future into a meaningful whole that promotes health and well-being. Such growth helps patients become ready to say goodbye and leaves family members feeling that all that could have been done was indeed done. In questioning and analyzing their own beliefs regarding the reassurances, doubts, and answers they provide, nurses can better help patients who are forced to confront their own ultimate truths and the uncertainty of all that comes thereafter. The nurse can be very instrumental in empowering the patient and family to live life more fully; find happiness, a sense of purpose, and well-being; and enjoy the meaning given to life events, including death itself.

ISSUES IN PALLIATIVE AND HOSPICE CARE

Ethical Concerns

To be involved in palliative care is to be in the midst of many ethical issues, including assisted suicide, the role of the primary caregiver in the home, hospice care for the homeless, illegal activities concerning the use of pain medications, substance abuse, physical and/or mental abuse of patients and families, the place of heroic measures in hospice care, aggressive therapy and terminally ill children, and starting or stopping tube feedings. Regular team meetings and discussion among team members can assist with policy formation, procedures, protocols, allowances, and treatment regimens. Team meetings will often require the expertise of ethicists, community leaders, state and local representatives of city/state governments, legal counsel, and religious consultants to more effectively deal with complex issues.

Reimbursement

In 1982, Congress approved benefits for Medicare-eligible individuals who were medically certified as terminally ill—that is, having less than 6 months to live. Hospices (which are certified as Medicare providers) are paid directly by Medicare for services provided. Patients cannot be billed except for a small share of certain outpatient prescriptions and short-term inpatient respite care. There is no limit to the number of days covered as long as the physician certifies that the patient has only 6 months or less of life remaining.

Most major (and many smaller) insurance companies now provide hospice benefits; however, reimbursement is often irregular and inconsistent across states. Many hospices have become proficient at maximizing insurance reimbursement by negotiating modifications or alternative approaches with providers. Providers will agree to this if it saves on expensive hospitalization charges. In addition, hospice leaders have worked hard to encourage private insurance companies to convert from the per-visit, fee-for-service reimbursement model to the per-diem basis, following the Medicare hospice benefit model. The per-diem basis of pay allows for more individualized patient and family services, greater flexibility in provision of care, and a case management approach that leads to better quality of care and more cost-effective management of resources. Hospice care is also reimbursable under Medicaid. Services at most hospices are provided regardless of the patient's ability to pay. Memorial contributions and

United Way funding are always welcomed by the agencies that provide hospice services.

CONCLUSION

To work in the arena of palliative care is to tread on hallowed ground. Nurses journey with those who encounter the veil separating this world from what lies beyond. Nurses both learn from and contribute much to the journey, and it is both an honor and a challenge to be a part of this work.

BIBLIOGRAPHY

Berger, A. S., Badham, P., Kutscher, A. H., Berger, J., Perry, M., & Beloff, J. (Eds.). (1989). *Perspectives on death and dying: Cross cultural and multi-disciplinary views*. Philadelphia: Charles Press.

Corless, I. B., Germino, B. B., & Pittman, M. (Eds.). (1994). *Dying, death, and bereavement: Theoretical perspectives and other ways of knowing*. Sudbury, MA: Jones and Bartlett.

Gonda, T. A., & Ruark, J. E. (Eds.). (1984). *Dying dignified: The health professional's guide to care*. Menlo Park, CA: Addison-Wesley.

Johnson, C. J., & McGee, M. G. (Eds.). (1991). *How different religions view death and afterlife*. Philadelphia: Charles Press.

Morgan, J. D. (1990). *The dying and the bereaved teenager*. Philadelphia: Charles Press.

Petroshino, B. M. (Ed.). (1986). *Nursing in hospice and terminal care: Research and practice*. New York: Haworth.

Rando, T. A. (1984). *Grief, dying, and death*. Champaign, IL: Research Press.

Sherr, L. (Ed.). (1989). *Death, dying and bereavement*. Boston: Blackwell Scientific.

Unit 5

Site-Specific Cancers

22

Cancers of the Head and Neck

Darlene W. Mood

Cancers of the head and neck are malignant **tumors** found in the oral cavity and pharynx, nasal cavity and paranasal sinuses, salivary glands, and larynx. The majority of these tumors are **squamous cell carcinomas;** they account for about 3.2% of all cancer cases and 2.3% of all cancer deaths. Surgery and radiation therapy are the most common primary treatment modalities for head and neck cancers. Treatment regimens that combine modalities (i.e., radiation and surgery, chemotherapy with radiation) are also common in the treatment of some head and neck cancers. Nursing has an important role in both the physical and psychosocial care of persons with head and neck cancer.

Several of the major head and neck cancer sites are subdivided into multiple locations: The oral cavity includes cancers of the lips, tongue, floor of the mouth, buccal mucosa, upper and lower gingivae (gums), retromolar trigone, and hard palate. The pharynx has three major structures: nasopharynx, oropharynx, and hypopharynx (see Figure 22–1). The nasopharynx includes the eustachian tube orifice and the adenoids, as well as the posterosuperior and lateral walls; the oropharynx is composed of the base of the tongue, the tonsils, the soft palate, and the posterior pharyngeal walls; the hypopharyngeal walls, along with the pyriform fossa and postcricoid area, constitute the hypopharynx. The larynx includes three areas: supraglottic, glottic, and subglottic. The other sites in which head and neck cancers occur are the nasal cavity, the paranasal sinuses, and the salivary glands.

INCIDENCE

Cancers of the head and neck account for less than 4% of all cancer cases per year in the United States, although the **incidence** is much higher in other parts

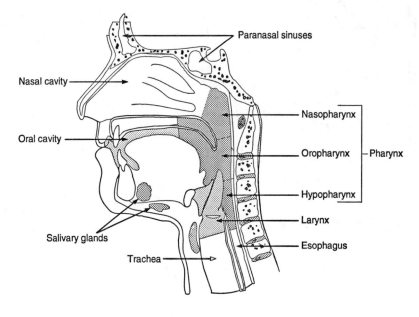

FIGURE 22–1   Oral Cavity and Pharynx

Source: American Cancer Society.

of the world. **Incidence rates** as high as 35% have been seen in Southeast Asia and India. Head and neck cancer represents the sixth most prevalent cancer in the world. In the United States, the annual incidence rate is approximately 10 per 100,000.

The incidence of head and neck cancers is about twice as high in men (4.1% of all cases; 13.5 cases per 100,000) as it is in women (2.1% of all cases; 5.3 cases per 100,000). Similarly, death rates for men (3%) are twice that for women (1.5%). However, both incidence and death rates are decreasing for men while increasing for women, presumably due to women's increased use of tobacco products and alcohol. More than 90% of head and neck cancer patients are over the age of 40, with more than 50% older than 65 years. Furthermore, the incidence of head and neck cancers, especially pharyngeal tumors, is rising in African Americans of all ages.

The 5-year **survival rate** from all head and neck cancers is poor: 55% for whites and 34% for African Americans. However, survival rates are strongly correlated with the stage of disease at diagnosis. Patients who present with Stage I disease have an 85% probability of surviving for 5 years. In contrast, patients who present with Stage IV tumors have 5-year survival rates of 34%. The annual incidence-to-death ratio for head and neck cancers is about 3:1.

RISK FACTORS

Researchers have established a strong relationship between tobacco use (i.e., cigarettes, cigars, pipes, and smokeless chewing tobacco) or alcohol intake and the development of cancers of the head and neck. In fact, the use of tobacco and/or alcohol has been associated with more than 95% of the squamous cell carcinomas of the head and neck. In addition, tobacco and alcohol are thought to have a synergistic effect in increasing the **risk** of developing these tumors, with data indicating a relative risk about five times higher for heavy-smoking drinkers than for heavy smokers who do not drink or heavy drinkers who do not smoke.

Poor nutrition and poor oral hygiene also have been identified as **risk factors** for head and neck cancer. While trauma has been suggested as a possible risk factor, research fails to confirm this. The oral sites that have the lowest incidence of tumors (i.e., tip of the tongue, gums, cheeks, and hard palate) are also the sites receiving the most trauma. Unlike some other cancers, cancer of the head and neck is, in itself, a risk factor for the appearance of another primary head and neck cancer. Exposure to noxious substances appears to be a risk factor, with a higher-than-expected incidence of various head and neck cancers observed among workers in leather, chemicals, cotton, wool, and asphalt. Exposure to sunlight has been implicated in some lip carcinomas, while the Epstein-Barr virus has been associated with nasopharyngeal carcinomas. While poverty and race have a positive association with the incidence of head and neck cancer, these correlations are probably a function of the combinations of risk factors that are more prevalent among poor people and among African Americans than in the general population.

DETECTION

Early **detection** of head and neck cancer is associated with excellent chances for long-term survival and minimal dysfunction. Health professionals, especially dentists and oral hygienists, as well as physicians and nurse practitioners, may discover asymptomatic lesions during a routine oral examination. Easy visualization of structures within the oral cavity makes identification of many precancerous or early malignant lesions possible. Although **leukoplakia** (thickened whitish patches on the tongue or mucous membranes) has been regarded as the most common premalignant lesion, in fact, only about 30% of these are associated with a later diagnosis of a malignancy. **Mucosal erythroplasia** (red inflammatory lesions) is actually the earliest visual sign of oral and pharyngeal squamous cell carcinomas.

Unfortunately, most head and neck cancers are detected only after patients become symptomatic. Attention should be given to individuals showing any of the warning signs of head and neck cancer: sores that do not heal, chronic changes in the appearance of oral mucous membranes, persistent hoarseness or changes in voice quality, and lumps or swelling in the mouth or neck. In particular, health professionals should have a high index of suspicion about such signs and symptoms in patients who are more than 45 years old, especially those who use tobacco products or drink heavily, or who are employed in occupations that expose them to toxic substances. Patients may also present complaining of pain in the face, jaw, or ear; bleeding; stuffy noses; headaches; sore throat; loss of sensation in the tongue; difficulty chewing or swallowing; and/or feeling a mass. Depending on the duration and severity of the symptoms, detection may occur after the disease has advanced.

DIAGNOSIS

The diagnostic examination may include direct, indirect, and fiberoptic laryngoscopy, esophagoscopy, bronchoscopy, radiographic and computerized tomography (CT) scans, and a biopsy of suspicious tissue. The procedures of choice depend on the suspected location of the tumor. Needle and simple open biopsies are typical approaches to determining the **histology** of the tumor. A staining substance, toluidine blue, can be used in suspected oral cancer to differentiate malignant lesions from normal tissue. It is also essential that the regional lymph nodes be examined carefully.

STAGING

Head and neck cancers are typically staged by the **tumor-node-metastasis (TNM) system** proposed by the American Joint Committee on Cancer. The T-component of the TNM system consists of four stages, T1 through T4, which differ according to the tumor size and extent of invasion into deep muscle or bone. The exact definition of the T-component differs for the various tumor sites, with oral cavity and oropharynx determined by their surface dimensions, in contrast to tumors in the nasopharynx, hypopharynx, and larynx, which are staged by their extent into adjacent anatomic areas. The nodal stage, or N-component of the TNM system, is applied consistently across these tumor sites and is determined by size, location, and number of affected lymph nodes. Variations in the type, severity, location, and duration of presenting signs and symptoms are associated with differences in the stage of the disease.

TREATMENT

The precise location of the tumor is essential to accurate **staging** of the head and neck cancer, which in turn determines the most effective treatment plan. In addition to tumor location, volume, and patterns of spread, consideration must be given to the likely effects of treatment on functional status, appearance, and potential for rehabilitation. While the major goal of cancer treatment is cure of the cancer, there are important conditions unique to head and neck cancer that must be considered: for example, for tumors of the oral cavity, hypopharynx, and larynx, restoration or retention of patients' ability to chew and swallow, as well as their ability to speak; for tumors of the nasal cavity and paranasal sinuses, the patients' appearance. Other factors upon which treatment decisions may depend are patients' age, general state of health, prior treatment, and ability to comply with treatment demands, as well as cost, convenience, and availability of support systems.

Surgery and radiation have been shown to be about equally effective in early stage disease. With advanced disease, however, combinations of modalities have been found to yield superior results compared to single-modality therapy regimens. Protocols combining surgery with radiation therapy appear to be most effective. The data from **chemotherapy** trials in head and neck cancer have not been encouraging, although there is some recent evidence that the combination of chemotherapy with radiation may be an effective treatment plan for some head and neck cancers.

Ideally, every patient preparing to be treated, especially for cancers in the oral cavity and salivary glands, should be given a careful dental evaluation. This is particularly critical for patients receiving radiation therapy. Dental caries should be repaired or teeth extracted. Fluoride treatments should be provided for patients who are scheduled for radiation therapy, and pretreatment assessments made in anticipation of posttreatment dental prostheses.

Surgery

Large tumors or those that extend into adjacent structures may necessitate surgical resection of portions of bone, muscle, and soft tissue. Common surgical procedures are outlined in Table 22–1. Surgery for cancers of the head and neck may result in impaired chewing, swallowing, speech articulation, or control of saliva, as well as cosmetic defects. Every effort is made to conserve chewing and swallowing functions, voice and speech quality, and appearance without sacrificing patients' chances for survival. Nonetheless, despite its cost in function and appearance, radical neck dissection is the treatment of choice in many advanced head and neck cancers. Through advanced surgical techniques, some defects can be reconstructed using grafts and myocutaneous flaps. Reconstruction may be performed during the initial surgery or delayed until posttreatment status can be evaluated. Often, maxillofacial prosthetic devices are used to correct intraoral defects, particularly those involving the hard palate and nasal fossa. Closure of a hard palate with an obturator can prevent passage of food into the nasal fossa and improve the quality of speech.

Because of refined surgical procedures, total laryngectomy may not be necessary for some patients with laryngeal cancers. Depending on the size and location of the lesion, a less radical surgical procedure that permits preservation of parts of the laryngeal tissue and partial conservation of the natural voice may be possible. Similarly, better understanding of the patterns of tumor invasion of the mandible has led to the development of mandible-sparing approaches such as marginal mandibulectomy and mandibulotomy. Cryosurgery and laser excision may also be used to help to control tumor growth. Cryosurgery is often useful in

TABLE 22–1   Common Surgical Procedures for Cancers of the Head and Neck

Procedure	Structures Involved
Neck dissection (simple, radical)	Removal of cervical lymph nodes and surrounding tissue
Composite resection	May include radical neck dissection, resection of part of floor of mouth, tongue, cheek, or tonsillar area, and mandibulectomy
Glossectomy (total hemi-)	Removal of all or part of the tongue
Laryngectomy (total supraglottic)	Removal of all or part of the larynx
Maxillectomy, mandibulectomy	Removal of some portion of the upper or lower jawbone

treating recurrent tumors in patients who have already had radiation. Laser excision is useful in treating small lesions.

Radiation

In radiation therapy for head and neck cancers, the principle of shrinking fields is used to minimize the toxic effects of radiation to large volumes of tissue. With this approach, the maximal dose is delivered to the tumor site, while smaller doses are given to the surrounding tissue and lymph nodes. External beam radiation therapy or combinations of external beam and interstitial radiotherapy (**brachytherapy**) are increasingly selected as a first line of defense in many early stage head and neck cancers. Good results with this combination of radiotherapy treatments have been observed in patients with tumors of the oropharynx, resulting in the preservation of the swallowing function. Also, for some early stage laryngeal tumors, it has been found that the quality of the voice is better preserved with radiation therapy. Where adjacent lymph nodes are involved, a simple or radical neck dissection is frequently performed to prevent distant metastases, followed by radiation therapy to the involved nodes. Radiation therapy to the contralateral side, known to be a common site of recurrence, is also recommended if **metastasis** is suspected.

Chemotherapy

Because chemotherapy is not considered curative in head and neck cancers, its use is generally reserved for patients with advanced disease or those who have failed other forms of treatment. Researchers are currently exploring the role of chemotherapy as an adjunct to either surgery or radiation. When combined with surgery, chemotherapy is given preoperatively to reduce tumor size, thus permitting less extensive surgical resection and minimizing subsequent functional impairment and deformity. Good results have been seen in patients with advanced laryngeal cancers treated with **induction chemotherapy** followed by radiation, preserving the larynx in these patients who otherwise would have received a total laryngectomy. Nonetheless, at this point the use of chemotherapy in the treatment of head and neck cancer is still limited, and considerable research is needed to establish its effectiveness for these carcinomas.

REHABILITATION

The treatment of cancers of the head and neck can result in long-term sequelae that interfere with function and appearance and, in turn, can negatively affect patients' quality of life. Thus, a comprehensive program of rehabilitation, which includes psychosocial and behavioral functions as well as physical functions, is essential to the proper care of the head and neck cancer patient. This may require the involvement of many other health professionals in addition to the otolaryngologist-surgeon, medical and radiation oncologists, and nurses. Among the other specialists who may be called upon to participate in the rehabilitation programs of head and neck cancer patients are dentists, diagnostic radiologists, speech pathologists and speech therapists, audiologists, physical therapists, occupational therapists, social workers, and dietitians. When the number of technical specialists (e.g., radiation technologists, dental technicians, physician assistants) in these fields is added to the list, plus other persons such as a chaplain and volunteers, the number of different individuals advising, teaching, and otherwise providing care to the head and neck patient can be overwhelming—and it is often the nurse who serves the triage function of coordinating the complex care program that provides for the effective interface of all of these members of the care team.

NURSING CONSIDERATIONS

Nursing has an important role to play in every aspect of the prevention, detection, treatment, and rehabilitation of patients with head and neck cancer. In the area of prevention, knowing the clear relationship that exists between smoking and/or drinking and the risk of head and neck cancer, nurses in many settings are in a position to provide information and support for avoidance of these toxic chemicals and for the discontinuation of their use by those already smoking or drinking heavily. Referral to groups that have shown success in assisting individuals to quit drinking or stop smoking is something nurses can do to help prevent this disease. Public health education often is nursing's responsibility, and modification of lifestyle to healthier choices is part of the important message to be shared. The holistic model that guides much of nursing practice requires the inclusion of assessment for health-threatening lifestyle behaviors in their evaluation of patients and the use of every opportunity to reinforce healthy choices.

With regard to detection, nurses who are aware of the risk factors for head and neck cancer, including age, race, and occupation as well as use of tobacco and excessive alcohol, can be more vigilant—especially with patients at risk—and monitor for signs and symptoms of the disease in their physical assessment of these patients. Of particular importance is the examination of the oral cavity, watching for evidence of erythroplasia. Potential problems related to uncontrolled tumor growth include airway obstruction, difficulty with chewing and swallowing, impaired speaking ability, hoarseness and pain, and unexplained weight loss. Recognizing these as potential symptoms of head and neck cancer can help prevent, among other things, death through starvation, airway obstruction, or massive hemorrhage following carotid artery rupture.

During treatment for head and neck cancer, nurses are critical members of the health care team from the time of diagnosis through rehabilitation and follow-up care. As suggested earlier, it is often the nurse's responsibility to coordinate patients' complex treatment plans. In their role as patient educators, nurses assist in the preparation of patients for their treatment regimens by providing information regarding the treatment itself, the potential side effects and management strategies to deal with those side effects, the importance of completing the full treatment program even if the symptoms subside, and the roles the various health professionals will have in the comprehensive program that is planned uniquely for that patient. Preoperatively, patients need to be prepared for what they can expect: that is, pain and pain management strategies in the immediate postoperative period; difficulties that may be experienced in breathing, speaking, and eating; changes in appearance; and others. Postoperatively, nurses have major responsibilities in assisting patients in their wound and pain management and other aspects of physical care, as well as alterations in communication, nutritional maintenance, and psychosocial adjustment. In addition to the effects of surgery, radiation and chemotherapy can result in problems that ultimately affect the patient's ability to eat or communicate, and they pose a major threat to an individual's self-esteem, body image, and **sexuality**. With the current trend toward shortened hospital stays, patients with head and neck cancer are being discharged sooner and are receiving more of their medical and rehabilitative care on an outpatient basis. Many leave the hospital with artificial airways or feeding tubes, or after having only a short time to learn the new skills required to handle changes caused by the disease and its treatment. Communication with nurses in community-based nursing agencies who will provide ongoing care is essential if these patients and their caregivers are to manage at home. Some of the most important areas of nursing care are in response to the conditions described in the following sections.

Alterations in Airway

Surgery to remove large tumors often results in edema of the upper airway with the need for a temporary tracheostomy. In cases where total laryngectomy is required, the patient must learn to care for a permanent tracheostomy. Nurses should assess respiratory status, manage the tracheostomy, and assist with the use of an alternative means of communication while the tracheostomy is in place. When the tracheostomy is used for long-term airway management, home care teaching and follow-up referral to community agencies is required. These patients frequently experience strange sensations associated with the tube, fear of suffocation or drowning while taking a bath, and anxiety about not being able to talk. Nurses can increase these patients' confidence by involving them in self-care as early as possible and allowing sufficient time for learning new skills.

Altered Nutrition

Head and neck patients with advanced tumors and those with intraoral defects or swallowing problems following tumor resection may have difficulty maintaining adequate oral intake. Nutritional failure is a significant morbidity factor in head and neck cancer patients, stemming from both poor eating habits that are common among heavy drinkers and a high incidence of **cachexia** (the inability to absorb the nutritional value of the food eaten). Difficulties in chewing and swallowing are common, exacerbating the difficulties in maintaining adequate nutrition. Postoperatively, patients are frequently fed **enterally** (nutrition administered directly to the stomach or small intestine) to prevent stress on intraoral or pharyngeal suture lines, to reduce the risk of aspiration, or to bypass an interruption in the alimentary canal. While a nasogastric tube is most commonly employed, esophagostomy or gastrostomy/jejunostomy tubes also are used. Patients are given high-protein liquid feedings and must be monitored for complications such as tube blockage or dislodgment, aspiration, intolerance of the feedings, and fluid and electrolyte imbalance. Many patients can be taught to administer their own feedings. If the individual is to be discharged with a feeding tube in place, commercially prepared liquid diets or blenderized foods may be administered at home. **Enteral feeding** is continued until the patient is able to safely resume oral feedings.

After the need for enteral feeding has passed, it is important for the nurse to continue to assess patients' nutritional status, taking their eating habits and preferences into account. Careful monitoring of patients' weight is important, as is consultation with a dietitian for assistance in planning meals that will increase calories and proteins. Research is currently being done to identify surgical strategies that will better preserve the chewing and swallowing functions, but rehabilitation with a speech pathologist or occupational therapist may be required after treatment. Pretreatment dental evaluation with follow-up dental care is essential because of the threat of radiation-induced dental disease and **xerostomia,** an abnormal dryness of the mouth due to insufficient secretions. Patients may need to devote considerably more attention to their oral hygiene than has been their habit, and the specialized techniques to preserve their teeth and the health of the oral cavity need to be taught (see Chapter 16).

Wound and Pain Management

Head and neck surgery often results in swelling of the face and neck and extensive highly visible suture lines. To decrease swelling and promote healing, nurses can help the patient elevate the head, avoid constricting clothing or ties around the neck, and maintain adequate oxygen exchange and optimal nutritional status. Large wounds require suction drainage systems to prevent hematoma formation under skin flaps. If vascular flaps and grafts have been used in reconstruction, special care must be taken to avoid pressure on the flap beds and pedicles, and the neck should not be hyperextended or twisted. Health care professionals should check these wounds frequently for evidence of impaired healing. If the patient received radiation prior to surgery, the risk of delayed healing is increased. Unusual drainage may indicate the development of a fistula. Once formed, fistulae are difficult to heal and may require additional surgery. Requirements for special wound care vary. Stress on suture lines within the oral cavity should be reduced by avoiding undue trauma from oral care, suctioning, or eating until healing has progressed. Following consultation with the surgeon, a program of oral care should be initiated with the patient. Wound management also may involve teaching a patient to use and care for an intraoral prosthesis.

Pain can be a major rehabilitation problem for head and neck cancer patients. Pain anywhere in the head and neck area tends to be amplified in the patient's experience and is therefore considered both severe and inescapable. Pain management is difficult, especially in light of the personal histories of substance abuse in some head and neck cancer patients. Noninvasive pain management strategies (e.g., biofeedback, relaxation) can be used alone by the nurse or in combination with medication in the effort to produce maximum relief (see Chapter 14).

Altered Communication

Loss of the ability to speak, even temporarily, is one of the most frightening aspects of head and neck cancer treatment. It is vital that an alternate method of communication be devised before surgery. Magic slates, writing tablets, picture boards, or hand signals can be used. Since it will take the patient longer to communicate, nurses must be sure to allocate adequate time when giving care. Careful listening is another essential nursing care action. The tracheostomy patient will eventually be able to speak again; the patient with more radical surgery frequently has problems with speech articulation and may require referral to a speech therapist.

A patient undergoing total laryngectomy has lost the natural organ of speech and will have to establish another form of communication. Alternative forms of speech include esophageal speech, the use of a voice prosthesis, or the use of an external mechanical device such as the electrolarynx. The alternative of choice is a function of the patient's capabilities, resources, and preference. The use of such devices is not only difficult for some patients, but also contributes to the development of negative attitudes that can lower self-esteem. The appearance of the stoma is also a concern for some patients, and there are some options available for covering the stoma (e.g., bibs, scarves, high-neck shirts, or shirts with ties) to improve appearance. Nurses can provide information regarding common behaviors that the patient with a laryngectomy will have to alter (e.g., coughing or blowing one's nose) and other restrictions that will apply (e.g., no swimming). Examination by an audiologist may also be necessary if there is any reason to suspect that hearing has been impaired as a result of the disease or its treatment. Additional sources of support and information are available through the Lost

Chord Club, an organization of laryngectomy survivors, which will send a member to visit the patient and provide support, encouragement, and practical advice (see Appendix).

Psychosocial Adjustment

The disfigurement and dysfunction resulting from head and neck cancer and its treatment carry psychological and social costs in addition to the physical sequelae. Head and neck cancer patients with visible scars and distorted features may feel stigmatized, and they are often reluctant to participate in such "public" functions as eating and speaking. Nurses must address concerns related to body image in order to decrease patients' isolation and promote their reintegration into the community. Depression must also be considered in the patient who shows evidence of nutritional failure, unresponsiveness to self-care recommendations, or other signs of poor coping and adjustment. Consultation with mental health professionals may be required. **Support** groups and peer counseling (i.e., developing a working relationship with a survivor of a similar type of cancer) are effective rehabilitation strategies.

A note of caution: Nurses and other health professionals must not impose their own expectations and values on patients whose expectations and values may be different. For example, nurses sometimes behave as if denial or uncertainty are "bad" and interfere with the patient's ability to care for himself or herself. Nursing research, in fact, suggests that both denial and uncertainty can be positive for some patients and under some conditions, leaving room for a level of optimism when certainty would remove all hope. Nurses must be sensitive to the potentially positive values of these behaviors, adjusting their desire to have a fully informed patient to take the patient's immediate needs into account.

In addition to patient education programs, nurses have used a variety of behavioral strategies to help patients cope more effectively with the demands of their cancer experience. Contingency contracting is one technique that is easily used by nurses to promote positive health and coping behaviors. Based on social learning theory, contingency contracting involves the identification of mutually agreeable health goals, criteria for goal attainment, a time line, and a reward. The goals are set so that the patient has some challenge to meet, but within a readily attainable range, since the objective of the technique is to be able to reward the patient as often as possible. Research has shown that the size of the reward is relatively unimportant to the effectiveness of the strategy. A popular reward option is lottery tickets. Paperback books, magazines, small plants, and coupons for food or sporting events are among some of the relatively inexpensive reward options that can be used.

Sensitivity to cultural and social class differences is another way in which nurses can assist patients and their families in their adjustment to head and neck cancer. For example, in some cultures, the concept of self-care is unknown for a very ill person. The responsibility for care falls to the spouse or other family members. In such a case, teaching the patient alone is unlikely to result in adequate maintenance or adherence to the care plan. Rather, including a critical family member in the teaching sessions is essential. Similarly, dietary recommendations need to consider cultural food preferences and resources. In an effort to increase protein and calories, suggesting daily inclusion of a milkshake to an individual for whom milkshakes are foreign to the diet, or who has no blender or resources to purchase ice cream, is probably useless. Rather, learning about the food preferences of the patient and/or the patient's access to foods is necessary to make recommendations that are likely to be implemented.

It is also important to assess patients' role functions. What is the patient's usual work? Is the patient a parent of a dependent child? A spouse? A community leader? A churchgoer? A bowler? Patients feel more like themselves when they can fulfill the roles they had prior to their diagnosis. Patients need assistance to evaluate their abilities and limitations and to regain as much of their functional ability as possible. Occupational and social rehabilitation may be required. Returning to work is encouraged if it is within the individual's capability. Engaging in social activities with family and friends is also encouraged. Encouraging patients to resume their normal activities to whatever extent they are capable is an essential element of nursing care. Referral to community resources, counseling opportunities, alcohol or smoking cessation programs, or other support groups can be helpful to enhance patients' adjustment.

Caring for the head and neck patient in the context of his or her family is critical to the patient's psychosocial adjustment. While patients with histories of excessive drinking may have poor or unstable relationships in which the nurse is not prepared to intervene, those patients whose families want to assist in their care and provide support need to be assisted to do so. Communication barriers that often arise among patients and their family members or friends (sometimes called "the conspiracy of silence") need to be broken. Role playing with patients can be a useful technique to help them communicate more directly about their needs and their feelings. Including family members in patient education programs or support groups also promotes improved family functioning. The local chapter of the American Cancer Society may offer programs such as the We Can Weekend or I Can Cope, which assist patients and their families in meeting the challenges of the diagnosis and treatment of head and neck cancer (see Appendix).

CONCLUSION

Nursing care of the head and neck cancer patient includes the provision of support and encouragement as patients adjust to the demands of their rehabilitation program. Patients are usually willing to keep appointments and remain active in their care program as long as they are involved in activities that relieve symptoms and improve function. The importance of follow-up, however, is sometimes overlooked. The relative risk of recurrent disease in head and neck cancer is high, and it tends to occur within the first 2 to 3 years following treatment. Thus, patients should be examined at regular intervals (e.g., bimonthly) during that time. Since the risk of a second primary tumor continues to rise with time to as high as 40% in long-term survivors, patients' follow-up care should continue indefinitely, but with longer times between visits. As is the case with every other aspect of the complex care program experienced by most head and neck cancer patients, nurses can assist patients to understand both the expectations and the value of this final aspect of care.

BIBLIOGRAPHY

Baker, K. H., & Feldman, J. E. (1987). Cancers of the head and neck. *Cancer Nursing, 10*, 293–299.

Burke, J. (1989). Maintaining adequate nutrition in the head and neck patient undergoing radiation therapy. *The Journal of the Society of Otorhinolaryngology and Head-Neck Nurses, 7*(11), 8–11.

Dropkin, M. J. (1989). Coping with disfigurement and dysfunction after head and neck cancer surgery: A conceptual framework. *Seminars in Oncology Nursing, 5*, 213–219.

Flanders, W. D., & Rothman, K. J. (1982). Interaction of alcohol and tobacco in laryngeal cancer. *American Journal of Epidemiology, 115*, 371–379.

Logemann, J. A. (1989). Swallowing and communication rehabilitation. *Seminars in Oncology Nursing, 5*, 205–212.

Mashberg, A., & Samit, A. (1995). Early diagnosis of asymptomatic oral and oropharyngeal squamous cancers. *CA—A Cancer Journal for Clinicians, 45*, 328–351.

Mathog, R. H. (1991). Rehabilitation of head and neck cancer patients: Consensus on recommendations from the International Conference on Rehabilitation of the Head and Neck Cancer Patient. *Head and Neck, 13*, 1–15.

Mood, D. W., Parzuchowski, J., Grant, M. M., & Ensley, J. (1991). Psychosocial care needs of patients with head and neck cancers. *Head and Neck, 13*, 3–4.

Reese, J. L. (1991). Head and neck cancer. In S. Baird, R. McCorkle, & Grant, M. (Eds.), *Cancer nursing: A comprehensive textbook* (pp. 567–583). Philadelphia: W. B. Saunders.

Schleper, J. R. (1989). Prevention, detection, and diagnosis of head and neck cancers. *Seminars in Oncology Nursing, 5*, 139–149.

Shah, J. P., & Lydiatt, W. (1995). Treatment of cancer of the head and neck. *CA—A Cancer Journal for Clinicians, 45*, 352–368.

Sigler, B. (1988). Nursing care of the head and neck cancer patient. *Oncology, 2*(12), 49–53.

Steckel, S. (1982). *Patient contracting.* Norwalk, CT: Appleton Century Crofts.

23

Lung Cancer

Elizabeth J. White

Primary lung cancers account for 25% of all cancer deaths in the United States. Lung cancer is the leading cause of cancer deaths in both men and women, accounting for 158,700 deaths per year. Although the incidence of lung cancer is almost two times greater for men than for women, the incidence for women continues to increase.

RISK FACTORS

An estimated 80% to 90% of lung cancer cases are attributed to the **carcinogens** in tobacco smoke. The **risk** of developing lung cancer is related to how long a person has smoked and the number of packs of cigarettes smoked per day and is commonly referred to as pack years (packs per day × number of years). The risk of developing lung cancer increases significantly at 10 pack years. Fortunately, the risk declines after 5 years of smoking cessation, but it is not equal to the risk of the nonsmoker until 10 to 15 years after cessation. There is evidence that exposure to secondary or passive smoke in the environment increases the **incidence** of lung disease in nonsmokers and accounts for approximately 3,000 cases of lung cancer per year.

Other factors associated with the development of lung cancer include exposure to industrial and environmental carcinogens: asbestos, coal tar, nickel, silver, radon, chloromethyl ethers, chromate, and vinyl chlorides. Research continues on the impact of genetics on lung cancer.

PREVENTION

Smoking deterrence, smoking cessation strategies, and avoidance of exposure to secondhand smoke could prevent the vast majority of lung cancer cases.

Cough	Dyspnea
Hemoptysis	Pneumonia
Chest, shoulder, or arm pain	Weight loss
Bone pain	Hoarseness
Headaches or seizures	Swelling of the face or neck

FIGURE 23–1   Common Signs and Symptoms of Lung Cancer

Source: E. W. Humphrey, H. B. Ward, & R. T. Perri, "Lung Cancer." In *American Cancer Society Textbook of Clinical Oncology* 1996:223. Reprinted with permission.

Adherence to industrial safety standards and control of environmental radon, asbestos, and other carcinogens could assist in the prevention of additional lung cancer cases. See Chapter 3 for further information on prevention.

EARLY DETECTION

Early **detection** of lung cancers is uncommon because these tumors do not produce symptoms at the outset. In many cases, patients seek medical attention after months have passed and when multiple symptoms are present. The prognosis for lung cancer is poor, with only 13% of patients surviving 5 years. The poor prognosis results from the regional or distant **metastases** identified at **diagnosis** in 80% of patients with lung cancer and from lack of effective treatment.

Screening programs of the general population and high-risk populations have not been cost effective in detecting early lung cancers and have failed to decrease **mortality.**

DIAGNOSTIC EVALUATION AND STAGING

Lung cancer treatment depends on accurate diagnosis and confirmation by cytology, histology, and stage. Two discrete subgroups of lung cancer exist: **non-small-cell lung cancer (NSCLC)** and **small-cell lung cancer (SCLC).** Treatment for these subgroups differs greatly. Diagnostic work-up and **staging** are designed to differentiate between the two subgroups of lung cancers (and noncancer diagnoses), the extent and **histology** of the disease, and the ability of the patient to tolerate treatment. All patients receive a thorough history and physical examination, including pulmonary function and cardiac status, x-rays, general blood work, and **computerized tomography (CT)** scans.

The most frequent reasons people seek medical attention include the signs and symptoms listed in Figure 23–1. Vague symptoms of cough, **dyspnea,** wheezes, and hemoptysis are associated with smoking, emphysema, and infectious diseases, as well as cancer, and they may persist for long periods of time before treatment is sought. Pain, weight loss, pleural effusion, neurological changes, swelling of the face and neck **(superior vena cava syndrome),** paraneoplastic syndromes, and jaundice herald advanced disease.

TABLE 23–1   Diagnositic and Staging Work-Up for Small-Cell
and Non-Small-Cell Lung Cancer

Procedure & Purpose	SCLC	NSCLC
History: Determine risk factors, family history of lung cancer and lung cancer symptoms.	X	X
Physical Exam: Determine signs of lung cancer.	X	X
Lab Work (CBC, chemistry, LFT, AST, & CA): Provide information regarding general health and signs of paraneoplastic syndromes.	X	X
Chest x-ray: Determine lesion location.	X	X
Sputum Cytology: Confirm pathologic diagnosis.	X	X
Fiberoptic Exam (brochoscopy with biopsy, brushing, needle aspiration): Confirm pathologic diagnosis.	X	X
Percutaneous Fine-Needle Aspiration: Obtain sample for cytology or histology.		X
Video-Assisted Thorascopy (VAT) (wedge excision, needle apiration): Confirm pathologic diagnosis.		X
Thorocotomy: Tumor biopsy.		X
Mediastinoscopy: Biopsy		X
Metastatic Disease Identification		
CT scan of liver and brain	X	X
Radionuclide scanning	X	X
Bone x-rays	X	X
Bilateral bone marrow aspirates	X	
Monoclonal antibodies studies	X	

* Diagnostic studies will vary according to individual patient signs and symptoms.

Non-small-cell lung cancers include three main histologic groupings: **squamous-cell** or epidermoid carcinoma, **adenocarcinoma,** and large-cell or **undifferentiated** carcinoma. They represent 75% of all lung cancers. Most adenocarcinomas, a dominant histology for women, and large-cell undifferentiated carcinomas will present in the peripheral zone on x-ray. Fiberoptic bronchoscopy of these **tumors** is not possible. Sixty-five percent of squamous-cell carcinomas, the histology most frequently associated with cigarette smoke, are found in the central zone of the lung on x-ray, thus making fiberoptic bronchoscopy feasible. The diagnostic work-up for NSCLC involves many of the same procedures as SCLC. A more involved surgical work-up determines whether or not surgery will be used to treat local disease. Table 23–1 lists components of the diagnostic work-up. Many of the procedures are overlapping for both NSCLC and SCLC. Table 23–2

TABLE 23–2   TNM Staging System for Lung Cancer

Stage	Descriptors	5-Year Survival (%)
I	T1-2N0M0	60–80
II	T1-2N1M0	25–50
IIIA	T3N0-1M0	25–40
	T1-3N2M0	10–30
IIIB	Any T4 or any N3M0	< 5
IV	Any M1	< 5

T Descriptor	Definition
TX	Positive malignant cell; no lesion seen
T1	< 3 cm diameter
T2	> 3 cm diameter
	Distal atelectasis
T3	Extension to pleura, chest wall diaphragm or pericardium
	< 2 cm from carina or total atelectasis
T4	Invasion of mediastinal organs
	Malignant pleural effusion

N Descriptor	Node Involvement
N0	No involvement
N1	Ipsilateral bronchopulmonary or hilar
N2	Ipsilateral or subcarinal mediastinal
	Ipsilateral supraclavicular nodes
N3	Contralateral mediastinal hilum or supraclavicular

M Descriptor	Metastatic Involvement
M0	None
M1	Metastases present

Source: Mina, J., Pass, H., Gladstein, E., & Pass, D. (1993). Lung cancer. In V. DeVita, S. Hellman, & S. Rosenberg (Eds.), *Cancer principles and practice of oncology*. Philadelphia: J. B. Lippincott Co., p. 682. Reprinted with permission.

shows the internationally accepted TNM staging system for lung cancer, which is used in staging NSCLC.

Small-cell lung cancers include oat cell, intermediate, and mixed (small-cell combined with other cell types of lung carcinoma) and account for 25% of all lung cancers. SCLC is often treated as a systemic disease. Lesions occur centrally but are difficult to biopsy by bronchoscopy. They grow rapidly, most having spread at the time of diagnosis. Distant sites include the brain, liver, bone, bone marrow, lymph nodes, and subcutaneous lesions. Although applicable to SCLC, the TNM staging system is not useful for a disease treated primarily by **chemotherapy** and therefore is rarely used.

Clinicians stage SCLC using a simple two-step staging system developed by the Veterans Administration Lung Cancer Study Group. Limited disease includes tumors confined to the hemithorax of origin, the mediastinum, and the supraclavicular nodes, which can be captured within a tolerable radiotherapy port. The definition is loose and varies among study groups. Extensive disease includes all disease excluded by the definition of limited disease.

Cellular characteristics of SCLC include two subgroups: the radiosensitive classic cell line, with high levels of neuroendocrine markers, and less radiosensitive variant cell lines, with reduced marker levels. The **paraneoplastic syndromes** (ectopic Cushing syndrome, inappropriate antidiuretic hormone secretion, Lamber-Eaton myasthenic syndrome, and carcinoid syndrome) summarized in Table 23–3, are associated with the neuroendocrine nature of SCLC cells. SCLC cells undergo multiple genetic changes. Three myc-oncogenes have been associated with SCLC. Development of various monoclonal antibodies against SCLC-associated antigens continues to provide research fronts in diagnosis and targeted treatment.

TREATMENT

Non-Small-Cell Lung Cancer

Early discovery of NSCLC, before metastasis to the lymph system, gives the best chance of cure. In Stage I and Stage II NSCLC, surgery is the treatment of choice. Radiotherapy is recommended for Stage I and Stage II individuals who are poor surgical risks, including those having poor pulmonary function, cardiac disease, or other debilitating conditions. Clinical trials of postsurgical chemotherapy, chemoprevention following other therapy, and internal photodynamics continue.

In Stage II NSCLC, combinations of surgery with or without radiation and with or without chemotherapy are also implemented.

Surgery is recommended for Stage IIIA NSCLC but not for Stage IIIB NSCLC. Radiation with or without chemotherapy is used for both Stage III groups, while chemotherapy alone and chemotherapy plus radiation have been studied for Stage IIIB disease. A few trials have also tested preoperative (**neoadjuvant**) chemotherapy and surgery. The 13% 5-year **survival rate** has not changed with the use of chemotherapy; however, some authors have reported an increase in the mean survival time between those treated with best supportive care and with chemotherapy and radiation. They cite a reduction in cough, hemoptysis, bone pain, malaise, and weight loss as good reasons for implementing therapy. New antiemetic agents and **colony-stimulating factors** make chemotherapy more tolerable. Cisplatin, doxorubicin, and cyclophosphamide are standard agents for NSCLC, while paclitaxel, docetaxel, toptecan irinotecan, and vinorelbine are investigational.

The treatment for Stage IV NSLC is palliative; it can include radiation and chemotherapy as single agents or in combination. Other types of care are used to promote comfort.

TABLE 23-3 Paraneoplastic Syndromes Associated with Small-Cell Lung Cancer

Syndrome	Prevalence	Mechanism	Signs/Symptoms
Ectopic corticotrophin syndrome (Cushing's syndrome)	5% of all small-cell lung cancer (SCLC)	Increased secretion of adrenocorticotrophin hormone from the SCLC	Edema, proximal myopathy, elevated plasma and urinary-free cortisol levels, hypokalemic alkalosis, and hyperglycemia
Syndrome of inappropriate antidiuretic hormone secretion (SIADH)	5%–10% of all SCLC	Increased secretion of antidiuretic hormone from the SCLC	Confusion, lethargy, high urine osmolality, low serum sodium, and plasma osmolality reflecting a retention of fluid
Lambert-Eaton myasthenic syndrome (LEMS)	Rare	Caused by down-regulation of presynaptic voltage-grated calcium channels (VGCC) following cross-linking by divalent anti-VGCC IgG antibodies	Myasthenia-like symptoms (e.g., weakness of legs and arms, ptosis, diplopia, difficulty chewing, dysphagia) usually affects the limbs but ocular and bulbar muscles are spared
Carcinoid syndrome	Rare	Associated with carcinoid tumors Caused by serotonin, prostaglandin, and other active substances secreted by the SCLC	Attacks of severe cyanotic flushing (bluish discoloration) of the skin lasting from minutes to days, diarrheal watery stools, broncho-constrictive attacks, sudden drops in blood pressure, edema, and ascites

Source: Glover, J., & Miaskowski, C. (1994). Small cell lung cancer: Pathophysiologic mechanisms and nursing implications. *Oncology Nursing Forum, 21,* 88. Reprinted with permission.

Standard Chemotherapy Regimens
EP or EC: etoposide + cisplatin or caboplatin
CAV: cyclophosphamide + doxorubicin + vincristine
CAE: cyclophosphamide + doxorubicin + etoposide
ICE: ifosfamide + carboplatin + etoposide

Other Regimens with Similar Outcomes,
Studied Less Extensively or Not as Frequently Used
CCMV: cyclophosphamide + methotrexate + lomustine + vincristine
cyclophosphamide + methotrexate + lomustine
cyclophosphamide + doxorubicin + etoposide + vincristine
CEV: cyclophosphomide + etoposide + vincristine
oral etoposide

FIGURE 23–2　Standard Chemotherapy Regimens for Small-Cell Lung Cancer

---

Source: PDQ® (Physician Data Query). [Database online]. Bethesda, MD: National Cancer Institute; 1995—updated Dec. 1995]. *Small cell lung cancer treatment statement for health care professionals*.

Small-Cell Lung Cancer

Treatment for limited-stage SCLC involves chemotherapy with two to four drug regimens. In a select number of cases (5%), the treatment is surgery followed by chemotherapy with or without prophylactic cranial irradiation (PCI). Survival time, although four times better than with previous treatments, is dismal; the median is 10 to 16 months for limited-stage disease and 6 to 12 months for extensive-stage disease. Increased survival time has not been gained by exceeding six cycles of treatment. Radiotherapy improves survival when used in combination with chemotherapy. PCI is considered when complete response to therapy occurs. Limitations of PCI relate to neurotoxicity. Clinical trials continue on variation in dose schedules, timing of radiation, and changes in the quality of life during treatment. Commonly used chemotherapy combinations are listed in Figure 23–2.

Treatment for extensive-stage SCLC consists of multidrug chemotherapy. Poor performance status associated with advanced disease necessitates less intensive treatment. Single-agent IV etoposide or oral etoposide in combination with other active drugs provides symptomatic relief. Investigational use of teniposide and paclitaxel continue in patients with extensive disease. Palliative radiotherapy is used on brain, epidural, and bone metastases.

LONG-TERM SEQUELAE

For patients who have a limited surgical excision there is always the possibility of a second primary lesion or of other lesions not seen at the time of surgery. Pulmonary and esophageal fibrosis, carditis, and pneumonitis are long-term sequelae of radiation therapy to the chest. Reduced pulmonary function can be attributed to surgical removal of lung tissue, the cancer itself, or coexisting chronic obstructive pulmonary disease (COPD) and emphysema. The increased toxicities of combined modality treatment increase the risk of these long-term side effects. Patients with smoking histories have a greater risk for second tobacco-related cancers.

NURSING CONSIDERATIONS

Nurses care for people with lung cancers across the continuum of the disease and in vastly different practice settings. The importance of patient teaching increases as a greater percentage of care is delivered in outpatient settings. Patients need to be aware of side effect management techniques and when and whom to call for help as effects of therapy occur at home after discharge.

Surgical patients must learn what is expected in the hours following surgery, including turning, coughing and deep breathing, and incentive spirometry. Nurses can assist patients with smoking cessation preoperatively as well as postoperatively. The effects of anesthesia and the loss of lung tissue when resection is performed place patients at an increased risk for postoperative complications. Pain limits mobility as well as the patient's ability to perform coughing and deep breathing exercises. Effective pain management is essential after surgery. If pain increases or changes locations, the possibility of other complications, such as infection, pulmonary embolism, and thrombophlebitis, should be considered. Nurses need to assess and monitor the patient's healing, laboratory work, response to treatment, and coping. (See Chapter 7.)

Patients receiving chemotherapy need to have nausea and vomiting prevented or managed. They need to know when their blood counts are expected to fall. They must know how to prevent infection as well as what to do if and when they become sick. Additional information on chemotherapy and symptom management can be found in Chapters 9, 13, and 14.

In addition, radiation patients can be expected to need assistance with skin care, weight loss, and fatigue. Patients undergoing radiotherapy need to know how to treat the skin within the radiation portal. They need to know what products exist to combat the **dysphasia** and pain resulting from esophagitis. Dyclonine hydrochloride or viscous lidocaine can be administered before mealtime to provide comfort and improve food and liquid intake. Weight loss, **anorexia,** and **cachexia** are problems associated with lung cancer and its treatments. Soft foods and liquid dietary supplements help provide the calories and protein needed during treatment. Since fatigue accompanies radiation, patients may find it helpful to scale back activities and add rest and exercise periods to their daily schedule.

Acute radiation pneumonitis is characterized by dyspnea, hacking cough, and mild chest pain. Symptoms usually subside after 3 to 4 weeks, although larger doses of radiation can result in permanent fibrotic changes. If pulmonary fibrosis occurs, symptoms develop several weeks to months after treatment. Since there is no cure for this complication, patients must learn to deal with diminished pulmonary function. The nurse should work with the health care team to implement an appropriate pulmonary rehabilitation program including pursed-lip breathing, abdominal-diaphragmatic breathing, and positioning for comfort. Planning should include prioritizing activities and utilization of community and personal resources to assist patients with personal care and housework. See Chapter 8 for further information on radiation therapy.

NURSING MANAGEMENT OF ADVANCED LUNG CANCER

Nursing interventions for patients with advanced lung cancers are aimed at decreasing the respiratory problems they experience, including dyspnea, hemoptysis (blood-tinged sputum from the lungs), and cough. Since length of survival is short, there is a great urgency for nurses to move quickly in helping patients address issues related to advanced disease.

Obstructed airways or restriction of lung expansion most frequently lead to dyspnea for lung cancer patients, many of whom have preexisting chronic obstructive lung disease or emphysema. Postobstructive pneumonitis, atelectasis, pleural effusion, and treatment-related problems may also contribute to this problem. Immediate coping strategies include positioning, moving slower, use of inhalers, administration of medications, and pursed-lip breathing. Distraction, meditation, guided imagery, and relaxation techniques may also be helpful in combating pain and anxiety. Long-term adaptive strategies such as changing or decreasing the activities of daily living, transferring them to others, or scheduling them at different times of day are useful methods of conserving energy.

Other general nursing measures include increasing the patient's fluid intake to thin out secretions and educating the patient about the appropriate purpose, dose, and side effects of medication used to treat dyspnea. Anxiolitics used during acute episodes of dyspnea can decrease the associated anxiety. Beta antagonists provide symptomatic relief for patients with underlying chronic obstructive pulmonary disease (COPD). Although metered-dose inhalers provide good relief, they are frequently misused and thus considered ineffective by patients. Teaching patients appropriate use of inhalers and spacers enhances their effectiveness. Low-dose opioids reduce the respiratory drive and provide comfort without producing significant respiratory depression. Oral or inhaled adrenal glucocorticosteroids reduce edema and bronchospasm. Antibiotics are used to treat infections. Chlorpromazine, diazepam, and metoclopramide are useful in treating hiccups, which can become exhausting and painful. Humidified air, cough suppressants, and codeine can reduce cough. Atropine or scopolamine can be used to dry up secretions distal to an obstruction or terminal airway obstruction (death rattle).

Low-flow home oxygen is indicated for patients with significant hypoxia. However, if the patient's blood gases are normal, supplemental oxygen will not help. The patient and family members need assistance in understanding why oxygen will not be useful and opioids and anxiolytics can be used instead.

Hemoptysis is not uncommon with lung cancer patients. It results from capillary trauma, tumor sloughing, or pulmonary infection. Radiation therapy or laser surgery may be used to stop moderate hemoptysis. Major, life-threatening hemorrhage may occur in advanced lung cancer. Whether a family decides on hospitalization or chooses to care for the patient at home, it is important that nurses help the family in developing an emergency plan to reduce anxiety and increase feelings of security in the event of hemorrhage. Hemorrhage is a rare occurrence but a common fear for patients and their families when hemoptysis is present.

Cough, which frequently accompanies lung cancer, can be caused by infection, inflammation, or the tumor pressing against the bronchi or trachea. Persistent coughing disrupts sleep; increases musculoskeletal chest pain and hemoptysis; and aggravates nausea, vomiting, and anxiety. A cough may lead to pathologic rib fractures, which are an additional risk for patients with metastatic lesions to the bone or those using steroids on a long-term basis. Coughing is one indicator of pulmonary infection, and antibiotics are appropriate for acute respiratory tract infection. Antipyretics, cough suppressants, hydration, and humidification of secretions may also reduce cough.

Psychosocial and spiritual issues are important for those with life-threatening illnesses. Nurses attend to these issues through active listening and appropriate referral. (See Chapters 19, 20, and 21.)

CONCLUSION

Lung cancer is a frequently occurring and deadly form of cancer. Nurses play a significant role in maintaining a patient's quality of life through symptom management; disease and treatment education; and attention to the spiritual, social, and psychological sequelae of the disease. Nursing leadership, by example, community eduation, and political activism—to discourage smoking and encourage smoking cessation—continues to be more effective in saving lives than any treatment currently available.

BIBLIOGRAPHY

Mina, J., Pass, H., Gladstein, E., & Pass, D. (1993). Lung cancer. In V. DeVita, S. Hellman, & S. Rosenberg (Eds.), Cancer principles and practice of oncology. Philadelphia: J. B. Lippincott.

Evans, W. K. (1993). Management of metastatic non-small-cell lung cancer. Chest, 103, 68s–71s.

Glover, J., & Miaskowski, C. (1994). Small cell lung cancer: Pathophysiologic mechanisms and nursing implications. Oncology Nursing Forum, 21, 87–95.

Humphrey, E., Ward, H. B., & Perri, R. T. (1995). Lung cancer. In G. H. Murphy, W. Lawrence, & R. E. Lenhard Jr. (Eds.), American Cancer Society textbook of clinical oncology. Atlanta: American Cancer Society.

PDQ (Physician Data Query). [Database online] Bethesda, MD: National Cancer Institute; 1984-updated Dec 12; cited 1995 Dec 31]. *Small cell lung cancer health professional summary.* Available from National Cancer Institute; National Library of Medicine, Bethesda, MD; OVID Technologies, Inc., New York, NY; Lexis-Nexis, Miamisburg, OH.

PDQ (Physician Data Query). [Database online] Bethesda, MD: National Cancer Institute; 1984-updated Jan 1996; cited 1995 Feb 2]. *Nonsmall cell lung cancer health professional summary.* Available from National Cancer Institute; National Library of Medicine, Bethesda, MD; OVID Technologies, Inc., New York, NY; Lexis-Nexis, Miamisburg, OH.

Rose, M. A., Shrader-Bogen, C. L., Korlath, G., Priem, J., & Larson, L. R. (1996). Identifying patient symptoms after radiation using a nurse managed telephone interview. *Oncology Nursing Forum, 23,* 99–102.

Seale, D. D., & Beaver, B. M. (1992). Pathophysiology of lung cancer. *Nursing Clinics of North America, 27,* 603–613.

Turrisi, A. T. III. (1993). Innovations in multimodality therapy for lung cancer. *Chest, 103,* 56s–59s.

24

Breast Cancer

Karen Hassey Dow

INCIDENCE

Breast cancer is a major health problem in the United States and represents the most common malignancy among women. In 1996, the American Cancer Society (ACS) estimated 184,300 new cases of invasive breast cancer in women. The **incidence** of breast cancer has increased steadily at the rate of 2% each year since 1980. This increased **incidence** is most often attributed to the corresponding increase in mammographic screening.

The ACS estimated 44,300 deaths in 1996, making breast cancer the second leading cause of cancer death in women. While the incidence of breast cancer has increased, **mortality rates** have remained steady for the past 40 years, suggesting that current available treatment (surgery, radiation therapy, and chemotherapy) have achieved moderate gains toward improving survival. Ethnic differences have been noted in mortality. For example, in the period from 1973 to 1988, mortality rates among white women increased 1.1% compared to a 19.4% increase among African-American women. Racial differences are thought to be related to several factors. Research suggests that breast cancer in African-American women may be diagnosed at later stages, may be more likely to be estrogen negative, and may be more likely to be related to socioeconomic factors. Age differences in survival have also been noted, with younger women surviving longer than older women.

RISK FACTORS

By the year 2000, nearly 2 million women in the United States are projected to have a breast cancer diagnosis. Currently, there is no known cure, nor is there one known cause of breast cancer. It is believed that breast cancer may result from a series of genetic, hormonal, and possibly environmental events that contribute to its etiology and development. Genetic alterations, such as changes or mutations in normal genes, and the expression of proteins that either suppress or promote the development of tumors are increasingly implicated in breast cancer. Steroid hormones produced by the ovaries—estradiol and progesterone—have a focal role in breast cancer. They are altered in the cellular environment, which can affect growth factors for breast cancer.

While there are several identified **risk factors** for breast cancer, roughly 60% of women diagnosed do not have any factors placing them at high **risk.** Thus, all women should be considered at risk for developing breast cancer during their lifetime. Risk factors help to provide a means for identifying women who may benefit from increased surveillance and early treatment. In addition, further research into risk factors will help develop effective strategies to prevent or modify breast cancer in the future.

The major risk factors for breast cancer are (a) increasing age; (b) first-degree relative with breast cancer (mother, daughter, sister); and (c) a personal history of breast cancer. *Lifetime risk* refers to the probability that an individual, over the course of her life, will be diagnosed with or die from cancer. A woman in the United States has a 1 in 8 risk of developing breast cancer. This risk varies among age groups. For example, the risk of developing breast cancer by age 30 is 1 in 233, while the risk by age 60 is 1 in 29. Thus, women over the age of 60 years have a higher risk of developing breast cancer than younger women.

Women with a family history of breast cancer in a first-degree relative have a relative risk of 1.5 to 2.0. **Relative risk** is a measure of the strength of the relationship between a risk factor, such as family history, and cancer. The relative risk may increase two times if the mother was affected with the malignancy before the age of 60; the risk dramatically increases four to six times if two first-degree relatives were affected. Women with a personal history of breast cancer have a relative risk of developing contralateral breast cancer that increases by approximately 1% per year.

Reproductive risk factors include early age at menarche (before age 12); nulliparity or later age at first birth; late age of menopause (after age 55); and lengthy exposure to cyclic estrogens.

Dietary risk factors include a slightly increased risk in women who consume even one alcoholic drink per day. A high-fat diet was initially thought to increase the risk of breast cancer because of international variations that showed differences in breast cancer related to fat intake. However, recent cohort studies have shown only weak or inconclusive associations between a high-fat diet and increased risk of breast cancer.

PREVENTION

Strategies to prevent breast cancer have focused on hereditary factors, dietary changes, and chemoprevention. Several ongoing studies are evaluating these prevention strategies. For example, hereditary factors include the newly identified breast cancer genes (BRCA1, BRCA2) located on chromosome 17. BRCA1 and BRCA2 are thought to be related to approximately 5% to 10% of all breast cancers. Women who have mutations of these genes seem to have a higher risk of developing breast cancer at a younger age. The identification of these genes has led to developing screening tests for women who have high breast cancer rates in their families.

Dietary intervention using reduced fat intake has also been evaluated in the prevention of breast cancer. However, some researchers argue that it will take a lifetime of dietary change to decrease risk. In addition, these changes in breast cancer incidence will not be evident for at least one generation. Limited data also suggest a potentially protective effect of vitamin A intake against breast cancer, and clinical trials are evaluating this hypothesis.

Chemopreventive agents are drugs used in the prevention of cancer. In breast cancer, the antiestrogen tamoxifen is used as adjuvant therapy to control growth of tumors or prevent tumors from recurring. The major problem with the use of tamoxifen as a chemopreventive agent is the inability to determine with certainty who will develop breast cancer. Until the findings of ongoing clinical trials of tamoxifen as a chemopreventive agent are available, it should not be provided to the general population. Proponents of tamoxifen argue for its protective effect against osteoporosis and heart disease in addition to the potential benefit of reducing risk of breast cancer.

SCREENING AND EARLY DETECTION

Since we do not know what causes breast cancer, the best way to improve survival is through screening and early detection of the disease. Currently, the best combination of screening for breast cancer is mammography with physical examination of the breast and breast self-examination.

Mammography

Screening mammography has reduced mortality from breast cancer by 30% in women aged 50 to 69 years. Its effectiveness in reducing mortality among younger women has not yet been determined. The American Cancer Society recommends beginning mammography by the age of 40. Recommendations for screening mammography are listed in Table 24–1. Younger women with a high risk profile, in consultation with their health care provider, may consider beginning mammography earlier and/or having it more frequently.

The mammographic procedure takes about 20 minutes and is usually performed in the radiology department of a hospital or freestanding center. Two views are taken of each breast, à craniocaudad view and a mediolateral view, with the breast compressed from top to bottom and side to side. Women experience some discomfort because maximum breast compression is needed to visualize breast tissue.

TABLE 24–1   American Cancer Society Screening Recommendations

Test	Age	Frequency
Breast self-examination	20 and over	Monthly
Clinical breast examination	20–40	Every 3 years
	40 and over	Annually
Mammography	Begin by age 40	Once
	40–49	Every 1–2 years
	50 and over	Annually

Several barriers exist to obtaining mammograms in this country. First is the lack of adherence to recommended guidelines by physicians. The poor, women of color, and those without health insurance face significant barriers to obtaining a mammogram (see Chapter 5). Second, the quality of mammography and technologists' skills vary widely across the country. The Mammography Quality Standards Act of 1992 was enacted to ensure the use of high-quality machines and experienced personnel. Nurses can make great strides in the fight to improve breast cancer survival by educating women about the benefits of mammographic screening, helping to overcome barriers to screening mammography, especially among the poor and underserved, and working to develop low-literacy and educational materials targeted to specific ethnic groups.

Clinical Breast Examination and Breast Self-Examination

A clinical breast examination (CBE) is recommended at least every 3 years for women aged 20 to 40, and then annually thereafter. CBE and **breast self-examination (BSE)** are considered complementary to mammography. BSE proponents argue that most lesions are self-detected, making BSE the first-line defense for early detection of breast cancer. Others believe that lumps detected by BSE are an incidental finding and that no conclusive studies have demonstrated that BSE decreases overall mortality from breast cancer. Studies have also revealed that only a minority of women (25%–30%) perform BSE proficiently and regularly each month. Younger women, in particular those who may have normal lumps in their breasts, have found it particularly difficult to perform BSE. Studies have documented that increased anxiety, difficulties in performing BSE, fear of the results, psychologic factors, modesty, ethnic and cultural influences, and older age are barriers to BSE. Yet, BSE has many benefits. Women can learn to find breast changes. Studies have demonstrated that women who examine their breasts regularly can find breast changes earlier than women who do not examine regularly. It continues to be an important part of health promotion. Nurses in any setting can educate women about the benefits of regular BSE and urge them to seek prompt attention when lumps are found. Several BSE teaching programs, pamphlets, and videos may be obtained from the American Cancer Society.

DIAGNOSIS

Several techniques are available for diagnosing breast masses, and the techniques used will depend on whether the breast mass is palpable or nonpalpable. Techniques commonly used for palpable masses include fine-needle aspiration biopsy (FNAB), core-cutting needle biopsy, excisional biopsy, and incisional biopsy.

The FNAB is done on an outpatient basis and can be performed with either a local or no anesthetic. Advantages of this procedure are accuracy, low morbidity, lower cost, and faster results for ease of communication with the patient.

The core-cutting needle biopsy uses a special needle (Tru-Cut) with a large lumen to remove a core of tissue. This procedure is used when a **tumor** is relatively large and is located close to the surface of the skin.

The excisional biopsy is generally performed on an outpatient basis under local anesthesia. This procedure is used for any palpable breast mass. The entire lesion is removed with a margin of surrounding tissue. When a cancer **diagnosis** is suspected, proper handling of the biopsy specimen is needed so that prognostic indicators such as estrogen and progesterone hormone receptors can be assessed accurately.

The incisional biopsy is used to remove a portion of a mass for definitive pathologic examination. It is used when complete removal of a mass is not planned or when a mastectomy will be indicated.

With the increase in nonpalpable breast lesions detected by mammography, several newer techniques have been developed to evaluate these breast lesions. These include needle localization, stereotactic core breast biopsy, and ultrasound-guided percutaneous needle biopsy.

In summary, any palpable or nonpalpable breast lesion should be thoroughly evaluated. It is not unusual for women to be anxious, fearful, and uncomfortable during evaluation of a breast mass. Nurses can best prepare patients by providing accurate written and verbal instruction, delineating differences between benign and malignant breast conditions, discussing sensations women may likely experience during diagnostic procedures, and ensuring prompt follow-up of results.

STAGING

Staging helps to determine the best choice of treatment available, estimate prognosis, and compare results of alternative treatments. The most widely used staging system for breast cancer is the **TNM system** developed by the American Joint Committee on Cancer (See Table 24–2). In this system, the stage is based on size of tumor, number of involved nodes, and evidence of distant **metastasis.**

TYPES OF BREAST CANCER

There are several different **histologies** or types of breast cancer. Knowledge of the types of breast cancer provides an indication of tumor growth and prognosis. The various types are described in the following list.

TABLE 24–2　AJCC Staging System for Breast Cancer

Stage	Description
Tx	Primary tumor cannot be assessed
T0	No evidence of primary tumor
Tis	Carcinoma in situ: intraductal, lobular carcinoma in situ; Paget disease
T1	Tumors 2 cm or less in greatest dimension
T2	Tumors more than 2 cm but no more than 5 cm in greatest dimension
T3	Tumors more than 5 cm in greatest dimension
T4	Tumors of any size with direct extension to chest wall or skin
Nx	Regional lymph nodes cannot be assessed
N0	No regional lymph node metastasis
N1	Metastasis to one or more movable ipsilateral axillary nodes
N2	Metastasis to one or more movable ipsilateral axillary nodes fixed to one or another or to other structures
N3	Metastases to ipsilateral internal mammary lymph nodes
Mx	Presence of distant metastases cannot be assessed
M0	No distant metastasis
M1	Distant metastasis (including metastases to one or more ipsilateral supraclavicular nodes)

Source: Adapted from American Joint Committee on Cancer. (1992). *Manual for staging of cancer* (4th ed., pp. 151–152). Philadelphia: J. B. Lippincott.

- Infiltrating ductal carcinomas are the most common histologic type and account for 75% of all breast cancers.

- Infiltrating lobular carcinoma accounts for 5% to 10% of breast cancers. These tumors are most often multicentric, either in the same breast or in the opposite breast.

- Medullary carcinoma comprise 6% of breast cancers and grows in a capsule inside a duct. These tumors can become larger but are slow to expand.

- Mucinous cancer accounts for 3% of breast cancers. The cancers are mucus producers that are also slow growing and have a good prognosis.

- Tubular ductal cancer is rare, accounting for only 2% of cancers, and has good prognosis.

- Inflammatory carcinoma is a rare type of breast cancer (1%–2%) associated with unusual symptoms. The tumor is tender and painful; the breast is abnormally firm, enlarged with edema, and has nipple retraction. Symptoms rapidly increase in severity.

- Paget's disease of the breast is a less common type of breast cancer. Burning and itching are frequent symptoms. A tumor mass cannot be palpated underneath the nipple, where this disease arises.

- **In situ carcinoma** of the breast is characterized by the proliferation of malignant cells within the ducts and lobules, without invasion into the surrounding tissue. Types of in situ carcinoma are ductal (DCIS) and lobular (LCIS).

PROGNOSTIC FACTORS

Knowledge of prognostic factors helps to determine the best possible treatment and the potential for success with the selected treatment regimen. In addition to the TNM classification and histologic type, other prognostic factors include estrogen and progesterone receptor status and measures of cellular proliferation.

The presence of estrogen and progesterone receptor proteins indicates that the regulatory controls of the mammary epithelium are functioning. Presence of both receptor proteins is associated with an improved prognosis; their absence is indicative of poorer prognosis.

A tumor with a high degree of **differentiation** is associated with a better prognosis than a poorly differentiated, anaplastic tumor. Assessment of a tumor's proliferative rate (S-phase fraction) and DNA content (ploidy) by flow cytometry may also be a useful prognostic indicator. Tumors classified as diploid (normal DNA content) are associated with a better prognosis than tumors classified as aneuploid (abnormal DNA content).

TREATMENT

Treatment of breast cancer consists of both local management and systemic treatment. Today, most women are treated with combination therapy using both local and systemic treatment. The selection of local management (surgery and/or radiation therapy) and/or systemic treatment (chemotherapy or hormonal therapy) is based on the individual characteristics of the patient and the disease.

Local Therapy

The main goal of local therapy is eradication of local disease. The procedures most often used in local management of breast cancer are mastectomy, with or without reconstruction, and breast-conserving surgery combined with radiation therapy.

Modified Radical Mastectomy   This procedure involves excision of the tumor, entire breast, and axillary lymph nodes, leaving the pectoralis major and pectoralis minor muscles intact. Since the major drawbacks to modified radical mastectomy are cosmetic deformity and altered body image and self-concept, efforts are made to avoid a visible and restrictive mastectomy scar. Another objective is to maintain or restore normal function to the hand, arm, and shoulder girdle on the affected side. After mastectomy, a temporary breast prosthesis may be worn. In 4 to 6 weeks, a woman can be fitted for a permanent prosthesis. A wide choice of materials, shapes, sizes, and colors of prosthesis are available.

Side Effects/Complications   Even though women may be prepared for and knowledgeable about mastectomy, the actual experience may be physically hard and emotionally difficult to accept. Thus, side effects are numerous and include physical, psychological, and emotional sequelae. Infection, seroma, and hematoma may occur at the incision site. In addition, lymphedema and nerve trauma with resultant phantom breast sensations have been noted in the postoperative recovery period and for several years after mastectomy. Impaired arm and shoulder mobility and chest wall tightness can occur due to the disruption in lymphatic and venous drainage. Women should be encouraged to do hand and arm exercises to increase range of motion and decrease tightness in the affected arm.

Approximately 15% to 20% of women develop lymphedema after treatment. The incidence of lymphedema is related to the extent of surgical dissection, infection after surgery, radiation to the axilla, and older age. Lymphedema is a troublesome and traumatic effect of therapy. Several interventions ranging from nothing to aggressive surgical procedures have been used with limited success. The most common interventions include elevation, compression sleeves, exercises, and pneumatic compression.

All women should be instructed in arm and hand care after treatment. Since lymphedema may occur many years after treatment, women should follow good hand and arm care for the rest of their lives. They should be taught to use meticulous skin, nail, and cuticle care; avoid constricting sleeves or jewelry on the affected side; avoid heat, sunburns, tanning, baths, and hot saunas to the affected extremity; and avoid violent and strenuous exertion of the affected limb.

Psychologically, the loss of a breast is related to altered body image and self-concept (see Chapter 19). Women may experience difficulties in adjusting to their new bodies, they may not want to look at the mastectomy site for several weeks, and they may have up and down emotional periods relating to the loss of their breast. Several programs are available, specifically Reach to Recovery, which provides specific assistance in prosthesis, and Look Good . . . Feel Better, which provides help with cosmetics and support (see Appendix II).

Breast Reconstruction   Women may elect to have reconstructive surgery after mastectomy. This offers considerable psychologic benefit. Some concerns that women may have about reconstructive surgery are cost, safety, and whether to have immediate (done at the time of mastectomy) or delayed (done 6 months or up to a year after surgery) reconstruction. Cost to the patient may vary depending on the insurer, but it is considered rehabilitative surgery and therefore is often reimbursed. Side effects with reconstruction include infection and potential for an unsatisfactory reconstructive result.

If a woman decides to have reconstructive surgery at the time of the mastectomy, she avoids future surgery, although the total operative time is lengthened. Some women have found that immediate reconstruction lessens the feelings of loss and disfigurement. Occasionally, reconstruction cannot be done because skin and muscles are too tight. Other women benefit by a waiting period before another surgical procedure. Not all women desire reconstruction, and not all are candidates for reconstructive surgery. Reconstructive surgery is contraindicated if a woman has locally advanced, metastatic, or inflammatory breast cancer.

Primary Radiation Therapy When radiation therapy is the primary treatment of choice, a wide local excision that removes the entire tumor is followed by a course of radiation therapy to remove residual microscopic disease. The objectives of this treatment are to conserve the breast, decrease the chance of recurrence, and eradicate residual cancer. External beam radiation using a linear accelerator delivering photons is given daily over a 4½-week period to the entire breast region. In addition, a concentrated radiation dose or "boost" is given to the primary tumor site via electrons. Prior to the delivery of radiation, patients undergo a radiation treatment planning session that will serve as the template for daily treatments. Small permanent ink markings are used to delineate the breast tissue to be irradiated. Patients need reassurance about the procedure and specific self-care instructions about side effects and their management (see Chapter 8).

Side Effects Radiation therapy is generally well tolerated, and women may continue working during treatment. Side effects (see Chapter 14) are temporary and usually consist of a mild to moderate skin reaction and fatigue. Fatigue usually begins about 2 weeks after treatment and may last for several weeks after treatment is completed. Fatigue can be discouraging, and the patient needs reassurance that it is normal. She should also be given specific instructions on how to manage and cope with fatigue. Rare complications of radiation therapy to the breast include pneumonitis, rib fracture, and breast fibrosis.

Patient self-care instructions are based on maintaining skin integrity. They include (a) use of mild soap with minimal rubbing; (b) avoidance of perfumed soaps or deodorants; (c) use of hydrophilic lotions (Lubriderm®, Aquaphor®, Eucerin®) for dryness; (d) use of Aveeno® soap if pruritus occurs; and (e) avoidance of tight clothes, underwire bras, and excessive temperatures or ultraviolet light. After treatment ends, patients should minimize exposure of the treated area to the sun for 1 year. They also need reassurance that minor twinges and shooting pain in the breast are normal reactions after radiation treatment.

Systemic Therapy

Chemotherapy Chemotherapy is given to eradicate micrometastatic spread of the disease. An overview of chemotherapy is presented in Chapter 9. Chemotherapy regimens for breast cancer combine several chemotherapeutic agents to increase tumor cell kill and to minimize drug resistance. Chemotherapeutic agents used most often in combination are cyclophosphamide (C), methotrexate (M), fluorouracil (F), and Adriamycin® (A). A CMF or CAF regimen is the most commonly used treatment protocol. Less commonly used are CMFVP (V = Vincristine, P = prednisone) or AC. Decisions regarding the chemotherapy protocol are based on the individual patient's age, physical status, disease status, and whether she is participating in a clinical trial.

Anticipatory anxiety is a common response among patients facing chemotherapy. Today, however, side effects can be managed well, with women continuing their daily work and routine schedules. This is due in large measure to the meticulous educational and psychological preparation provided to patients and their families by their oncology nurses, oncologists, social workers, and other members of the health care team.

Common physical side effects of chemotherapy for breast cancer include nausea, vomiting, taste changes, **alopecia, mucositis,** dermatitis, fatigue, weight gain, and bone marrow depression (see Chapters 13 and 14). Less commonly occurring side effects include hemorrhagic cystitis and conjunctivitis. In addition, younger women receiving chemotherapy may experience temporary or permanent amenorrhea leading to sterility. Side effects vary depending on the chemotherapeutic agent used. Nausea is generally well controlled with the administration of combination antiemetics. Adriamycin® may cause alopecia. Obtaining a wig prior to hair loss and using stylish hats or scarves may be helpful. Reassurance that new growth will occur when treatment is completed is helpful, although the color and texture of the hair may differ. The ACS Look Good . . . Feel Better program provides useful tips for applying make-up during chemotherapy. Taking time to explain side effects and possible solutions may alleviate some of the anxiety of women who are uncomfortable asking questions.

Emotional responses to chemotherapy may have a negative effect on self-esteem, **sexuality,** and well-being. Certainly, these side effects, when combined with having to deal with a potentially life-threatening diagnosis, can be overwhelming in some instances. However, the majority of women with breast cancer today are treated in an environment where a multidisciplinary approach to holistic care is used. In addition, numerous **support** and advocacy groups in the community are available for patients and their families. Important aspects of care include communication, support groups, encouragement to ask questions, and promoting trust and faith in care providers.

Hormonal Therapy   Decisions about hormonal therapy for breast cancer are based on the index of estrogen and progesterone receptors provided by the **hormone receptor assay.** Normal breast tissue contains receptor sites for estrogen. However, only about one third of breast malignancies are estrogen dependent or ER-positive (ER+). An ER+ assay indicates that tumor growth depends on estrogen supply. Thus, measures to reduce hormone production may limit disease progression. ER+ tumors may grow more slowly than ER-negative tumors. Less than 3 fmol/mg is considered negative. Values of 3 to 10 are questionable, and values greater than 10 are considered positive. The greater the value, the more a beneficial effect from hormone suppression can be expected.

Hormonal therapy can be ablative or additive. *Ablative therapy* includes removal of endocrine glands that produce hormones (i.e., ovary, pituitary, or adrenal glands). Oophorectomy is a treatment option for premenopausal women with estrogen-dependent tumors. *Additive therapy* usually consists of tamoxifen treatment followed by progestins, aminoglutethimide, estrogens, or androgens for second- and third-line therapy. Tamoxifen has few side effects, but some patients may experience nausea, vomiting, hot flashes, fluid retention, and depression.

TABLE 24–3 Late Sequelae Associated with Breast Cancer

Physical	*Surgery:* Lymphedema
	Radiation therapy: Shooting pains in the breast; rib fracture, pneumonitis
	Chemotherapy: Infertility, early menopause
	Other: fatigue
Psychological	Fear of recurrence, uncertainty over the future
Social	Barriers to insurance; work-related problems
Emotional	Anxiety, depression, hopelessness

Bone Marrow Transplantation

Since the doses of chemotherapy and radiation therapy are limited by the degree of marrow toxicity, **autologous bone marrow transplantation (ABMT)** (see Chapter 11) has been used in women who are at high risk for recurrence. Recent studies indicate that ABMT induces a response in 50% to 80% of women, 30% of whom have a complete response for several years. Initially, mortality rates were high with ABMT due to sepsis. However, the use of growth factors (see Chapter 10) to stimulate the bone marrow have led to an overall decline in mortality from BMT. The procedure involves the removal of bone marrow from the patient, after which high doses of chemotherapy are given. The patient's bone marrow, spared from the effects of chemotherapy, is then reinfused intravenously and engrafts to "rescue" the marrow from the toxic effects of chemotherapy. This highly specialized procedure requires intensive patient preparation, education, and support.

Treatment Summary

Several local and systemic treatments are used for breast cancer depending on the particular woman and her specific disease characteristics. Treatment for breast cancer has changed dramatically and is often given in some combination of local treatment and systemic therapy. Side effects may be specific to each treatment. In addition, women experience significant emotional and psychological side effects, which may linger long after treatment ends.

LONG-TERM SEQUELAE

Since women are living longer with breast cancer, they may experience a number of sequelae that may be related to treatment, disease, or social issues. Some of the major concerns in long-term sequelae are listed on Table 24–3. These factors must be weighed against the overall improvements in treatment allowing longer periods of survival. Efforts are in progress to improve survival and minimize late effects.

NURSING CONSIDERATIONS

Nurses have a tremendous role in the care of women with breast cancer and their families. Opportunities exist in teaching and support with regard to prevention, screening, and early detection of the disease. In addition, nurses have made tremendous strides in decreasing symptoms associated with treatment. Efforts continue in the care of women with recurrent, advanced, or end-stage disease, and nurses are working to improve the overall quality of survival. Nurses have used their talents and skills in all areas of nursing practice, education, administration, and research to reduce the burden of breast cancer in the United States and will continue to do so in the future.

BIBLIOGRAPHY

Dow, K. H. (Ed.). (1996). *Contemporary issues in breast cancer*. Sudbury, MA: Jones and Bartlett.

Gross, J. (Ed). (1991). Breast cancer. *Seminars in Oncology Nursing, 7*(3), entire issue.

Harris, J., Lippman, M., Veronesi, U., & Willett, W. (1992). Review article: breast cancer. *New England Journal of Medicine, 327*, 319–327; 390–397; 473–480.

Hughes, K. (1993). Decision making by patients with breast cancer: The role of information in treatment selection. *Oncology Nursing Forum, 20*, 623–628.

LaTour, K. (1993). *The breast cancer companion*. New York: Morrow.

Long, E. (1993). Breast cancer in African-American women. *Cancer Nursing, 16*, 1–24.

Knobf, M. (1990). Symptoms and rehabilitation needs of patients with early stage breast cancer during primary therapy. *Cancer, 66*, 1392–1401.

Knobf, M., & Stahl, R. Reconstructive surgery in primary breast cancer treatment. *Seminars in Oncology Nursing, 7*, 200–206.

Schover L. (1991). The impact of breast cancer on sexuality, body image and intimate relationships. *CA—A Cancer Journal for Clinicians, 41*, 112–120.

Varricchio, C., & Johnson, K. (1993). The use of tamoxifen in the prevention and treatment of breast cancer. In S. Hubbard, P. Green, & M. Knobf (Eds.), *Current issues in cancer nursing practice*. Philadelphia: J. B. Lippincott.

25

Colorectal Cancer

Marlyn D. Boyd

INCIDENCE

Cancers of the colon and rectum (colorectal cancer) occur in the lower portion of the gastrointestinal tract. These are the third most commonly diagnosed cancers in both men and women. Colorectal cancer is also the second leading cause of cancer-related **mortality** within the United States. Approximately 7% of Americans will develop colorectal cancer in their lifetimes. It is typically a disease associated with increasing age. Over 90% of patients diagnosed with colorectal cancer are over the age of 50. The average age at the time of **diagnosis** is 60. Fewer than 6% of all colorectal cancers are found in persons younger than 50. It is estimated that in 1996 there will be 133,500 new cases of colorectal cancer and approximately 54,900 deaths. The **incidence** of colorectal cancer is slightly higher in men, and African Americans have a higher incidence than whites.

RISK FACTORS

The two primary **risk factors** for colorectal cancer are being male and increasing age. The risk of developing these cancers begins to increase after the age of 40, rises sharply between the ages of 50 and 55, then continues to increase with age. Other risk factors include a history of inflammatory bowel disease, a family history of large bowel cancer, familial polyposis syndromes (genetic predisposition to developing **polyps**), a personal history of colorectal polyps and/or colorectal cancer or other cancers, exposure to certain chemicals, anal intercourse and genital warts (for rectal cancer), cigarette smoking, sedentary lifestyle, high-fat and/or low-fiber diets, high calorie intake/obesity, and alcohol consumption.

Approximately 70% of those who develop colorectal cancers are not members of identified high **risk** groups. About 1% of colorectal cancers are due to a history of inflammatory bowel disease; 1% are due to familial adeno-polyposis; 5% are due to **hereditary nonpolyposis colorectal cancers** (HNPCC); and 15% to 20% are due to a family history of having one or two first-degree relatives (mother, father, siblings) with colorectal cancer.

PREVENTION

Modifying lifestyle factors and, in the cases of familial polyposis syndromes, preemptive surgery, are the only methods at present to prevent or decrease the likelihood of developing colorectal cancer. Recommended lifestyle changes include eating a diet high in insoluble fiber and low in animal fats, alcohol use in moderation, maintaining an optimal weight, and being physically active. Some evidence suggests that daily aspirin therapy, as well as increasing calcium intake through a supplement or in the diet, may decrease the incidence of colorectal cancer.

EARLY DETECTION

Early **detection** is the most crucial factor in increasing **survival rates.** Survival rates vary greatly depending upon the stage of colorectal cancer at the time of diagnosis. Persons diagnosed at a localized stage (the cancer is confined to the colon or rectal mucosa) have a 5-year survival rate of 91% compared to 60% at the regional stage (the cancer has moved through the colon or rectal wall) and a 6% survival rate when the diagnosis is made with the cancer in the advanced stage (cancer has metastasized to other parts of the body). Unfortunately, only 37% of colorectal cancers are diagnosed while the cancer is localized.

The American Cancer Society recommends that both men and women have a yearly digital rectal examination beginning at age 40; a fecal occult blood test every year beginning at the age of 50; and preferably a flexible sigmoidoscopy every 3 to 5 years beginning at the age of 50. Persons with identifiable risk factors should have a **screening** schedule as recommended by their physician.

DIAGNOSTIC EVALUATION

Diagnosis of colorectal cancer involves one or more of the following procedures.

A *physical examination* is done to identify any physical signs of colorectal cancer, and a careful *history* is taken to determine whether there are any genetic predispositions, identifiable risk factors, or symptoms of colorectal cancer. Typically, there are no symptoms when colorectal cancer is in the localized stage. Symptoms begin as the colon or rectal structures are compromised by the invasion and growth of the cancer. Common symptoms include cramping or gnawing abdominal pain; a change in bowel habits such as diarrhea, constipation, or narrowing of the stool; blood in the stool; an urgent, painful need to defecate; unexplained weight loss; **anemia;** unusual paleness; and fatigue.

A **digital rectal examination (DRE)** involves the physician's feeling the interior walls of the rectum. Although it is beneficial as a screening tool, only those growths within the reach of the finger, which is usually only about 10 cm, can be detected.

Fecal occult blood testing (FOBT) is a chemical test used to identify blood in the stool. FOBT is not a test for cancer, but a test for blood in the stool; therefore, it may result in false negative or false positive results for cancer. Certain medications such as aspirin and other nonsteroidal anti-inflammatory drugs, eating red meat or raw vegetables, or bleeding hemorrhoids may cause a false positive result for cancer. False negatives may occur because polyps and some cancers may not bleed or may bleed only occasionally. However, FOBT is accurate in identifying 25% to 40% of colorectal cancers. It is most effective in identifying cancers in the sigmoid colon and less effective for identifying cancers of the right colon. FOBT is not an effective test for identifying polyps. Annual screening with FOBT can decrease colorectal cancer mortality by 33% to 57%.

Flexible sigmoidoscopy is an invasive procedure. The physician uses a hollow, lighted tube to visually inspect the wall of the rectum and the distal colon. With the 60 cm scope, the physician can detect 65% to 75% of polyps and 49% to 60% of colorectal cancers. Screening by sigmoidoscopy can result in a 65% to 95% reduction in mortality for individuals with cancers that are within reach of the scope. Flexible sigmoidoscopy is used both as a screening tool for persons at risk and as a diagnostic tool if the person has a positive FOBT or symptoms of colorectal cancer.

Barium enema with air contrast examination involves x-rays of the colon after the patient drinks a contrast medium. This test is almost 100% effective in identifying growths throughout the colon; however, it is not an effective method for identifying growths in the rectum.

Carcinoembryonic antigen (CEA) assay is a test used to measure the peripheral blood level of the **tumor** marker CEA. Many patients with colorectal cancer have elevated blood levels of CEA. The CEA, like the FOBT, is an imperfect test. It is not always elevated in people with colorectal cancer, and some persons who do not have colorectal cancer can have abnormally high levels of CEA.

Biopsies, which entail taking small tissue samples of polyps or "washing" cells off the colon or rectal wall, are performed to make the diagnosis of cancer. Biopsies are usually collected during endoscopic procedures.

STAGING

Once the diagnosis of cancer has been made, then the extent of the cancer is determined and identified through a series of stages. Various **staging** schemes have been proposed over the years; however, two are most commonly used, the **Duke's staging system** and the **TNM staging system** (see Table 25–1).

TABLE 25-1   Staging for Colorectal Carcinoma

Stage	Primary Tumor	Nodes	Metastasis	Stage
Stage O	Tis	NO	MO	
Stage I	T1	NO	MO	DUKES A
	T2	NO	MO	
Stage II	T3	NO	MO	Dukes B
	T4	NO	MO	
Stage III	Any T	N1	MO	Dukes C
	Any T	N2, N3	MO	
Stage IV	Any T	Any N	M1	

T = Primary Tumor; N = Regional Lymph Node; M = Distant Metastasis

Primary Tumor (T)

TX	Primary tumor cannot be assessed
TO	No evidence of primary tumor
Tis	Carcinoma in situ
T1	Tumor invades submucosa
T2	Tumor invades muscularis propria
T3	Tumor invades through the muscularis propria into the subserosa or into nonperitonealized tissue or perirectal tissues
T4	Tumor perforates the visceral peritoneum or directly invades other organs or structures

Regional Lymph Nodes (N)

NX	Regional lymph nodes cannot be assessed
NO	No regional lymph node metastasis
N1	Metastasis in 1 to 3 pericolic or perirectal lymph nodes
N2	Metastasis in 3 to 4 pericolic or perirectal lymph nodes
N3	Metastasis in any lymph node along the course of named vascular trunk

Distant Metastasis (M)

MX	Presence of distant metastasis cannot be assessed
MO	No distant metastasis
M1	Distant metastasis

Source: Adapted from American Joint Committee on Cancer, American Cancer Society, Pub. No. 89-25M-No.3485.02

PATHOPHYSIOLOGY

Colorectal cancers progress from normal mucosal cell division to mutation of the cell, causing overproliferation. This proliferation of cells causes an adenomatosis polyp to form on the mucosal walls of the colon. These cells are benign because they cannot invade or metastasize. They do not produce tumor-associated

antigens. This mutative process may be reversed with a nonsteroidal anti-inflammatory agent. However, unless the person is in an identified high-risk group that warrants earlier and more frequent screening, polyps at this reversible stage may not be detected. Next, the cells undergo further mutation and produce cancerous cells. Once these cells reach a critical mass, they begin to invade the colonic wall and eventually metastasize. **Metastasis** usually occurs first to the liver and then to the lungs. The typical time period from polyp formation to cancer development is about 10 years.

TREATMENTS

Surgery

Surgery provides the most promise of a cure in colorectal cancers. However, its effectiveness is primarily dependent upon the stage and extent of the disease at the time of surgery. About 85% of persons diagnosed with colorectal cancer in the localized stage can have surgery leading to a cure. Surgical goals for every patient are to remove the cancerous tissue and preserve as much functional capacity as possible. Because of recent advances in surgical techniques, only one out of every eight patients undergoing surgery will require a permanent colostomy to provide for elimination when the anus is nonfunctional. Temporary or loop colostomies are performed to divert fecal materials away from an inflamed area or a surgical site. Often, temporary colostomies are avoided as well, and when they are necessary, they are usually closed within 2 to 3 months. If the colorectal cancer is diagnosed in the early stages, a colostomy rarely is necessary.

Radiation

Radiation therapy can be used as an adjunct to surgery. Preoperative radiation therapy is often used for borderline operable rectal cancers. Because rectal cancers are located away from other sensitive structures, radiation therapy is used more frequently as an adjunct to surgery than with cancers located higher in the colon.

Although colon cancer is responsive to radiation therapy, it can cause damage to the adjacent small intestine. Special procedures are necessary to move or shield the small intestine and kidneys from the radiation treatment area.

Radiation therapy has proven to be effective in helping prevent recurrence and metastasis of tumors and in relieving pain. In addition, radiation therapy can be useful in treating bowel obstruction and bleeding often associated with colorectal cancer.

Chemotherapy

Chemotherapy is often used as an adjunct to surgery in colorectal cancer. Until recently, chemotherapy was used predominately to help control pain in persons with advanced stage disease. However, recent studies have shown that chemotherapy has a broader role in the treatment of colorectal cancer.

Chemotherapy using a combination of drugs such as 5-flurouracil (5-FU) with methyl-CCNU, leukovorin, methotrexate, cisplatin, or others has been shown to be of benefit in decreasing the recurrence of rectal cancer following early stage surgical removal.

In colon cancer, recent data have shown that, by using 5-FU and levamisole, recurrence of early stage disease has been significantly reduced, leading to a reduction in cancer-related deaths. The chemotherapy agent 5-FU is used to shrink tumors and provide pain relief for those who are in the late stages of the disease.

The liver represents the most frequent site for colon cancer metastasis. Liver metastasis from colon cancer is also responsive to chemotherapeutic agents. An arterial hepatic pump delivers a constant infusion of chemotherapy into the liver via a small catheter. This method has been shown to cause significant regression of liver disease. Other methods of delivering chemotherapeutic agents include **intraperitoneal implanted ports** that deliver chemotherapeutic agents such as 5-FU into the peritoneal cavity.

Other Treatments

Advances in surgical techniques continue to improve the success and outcomes of colorectal cancer surgeries. More work is being done in the use of chemotherapy agents. Promising new adjuncts to surgery—**biological response modifiers** (immunotherapy) such as **interferon** and **interleukin**—are undergoing study and may add new weapons to the treatment arsenal for colorectal cancer.

PROGNOSIS

The pivotal factors in determining the prognosis of colorectal cancer are its location and the stage of the disease at the time of diagnosis. Other factors that play an important role in determining the prognosis include the pathology of the cells and the person's age and general health. The 5-year **survival rate** for colon cancer detected in the early, localized stage is 93%; for rectal cancer it is 87%. If the cancer is diagnosed after it has spread regionally to surrounding organs or lymph nodes, the 5-year survival rate drops to 63% for colon cancer and 53% for rectal cancer. Once the cancer has metastasized, the 5-year survival rate drops to 7%. Survival rates continue to decline after 5 years; however, 51% of persons diagnosed with colorectal cancers survive 10 years or more. Unfortunately only 37% of colorectal cancers are diagnosed while in the early stage.

TREATMENT SIDE EFFECTS AND COMPLICATIONS

The possible side effects and complications from procedures, surgery, radiation, and pharmacologic agents used in colorectal cancer treatments depend on a host of factors, including the stage and location of the disease at the time of treatment, the patient's response to treatment, and the patient's general health.

Surgery

The most common complication of bowel surgery is infection due to opening the bowel. To curtail this possibility, preoperative cleansing of the bowel is done and prophylactic antibiotics are given pre- and postoperatively. Other potential complications from bowel surgery are obstructions and perforation of the bowel. These can occur due to adhesions or recurrence of the cancer.

Sexual dysfunction is not uncommon in males following abdominal perineal resection. This extensive procedure involves the nerves responsible for sexual functioning. As a consequence of the loss of nerve function, retrograde ejaculation occurs. In women, sexual dysfunction is less common but may occur due to scarring or contracture of the vagina and surrounding structures.

Radiation

Common side effects of radiation include surface tissue irritation causing sensitivity, pain and diarrhea, nausea and vomiting, loss of appetite, weight loss, and fatigue. Possible complications include radiation damage to surrounding tissues and organs, leading to dysfunction of those particular structures, such as bladder irritation, or scarring, leading to urinary problems or ovarian dysfunction.

Chemotherapy

Depending upon the method used to deliver the chemotherapeutic agent(s), the type of therapeutic agent(s) used, the doses and frequency of dosage, side effects and possible complications of chemotherapy can include nausea, vomiting, hair loss, loss of appetite, change in bowel habits, and fatigue. For example, diarrhea and **mucositis** are not uncommon side effects of treatment with 5-FU.

LONG-TERM SEQUELAE

Colorectal cancers can reoccur at the initial site or in new areas due to metastasis. Persons with large bowel disease have a 2% to 10% chance of developing a new cancer in the colon or rectum. These new cancers are not a recurrence of the original tumor. Because of the possibility of recurrence and the potential for adhesions or perforation of the bowel, regular checkups are necessary.

Follow-up studies include a physical examination, history, fecal occult blood test, sigmoidoscopy, double-contrast barium enema, blood tests including CEA assay, and x-rays. If a new polyp formation or a new tumor is found, then the treatment regimen of surgery, radiation, and/or chemotherapy will be started once again.

NURSING CONSIDERATIONS

In the preoperative stage of the care of patients with colorectal cancer, the nurse serves primarily as a patient educator and advocate and assesses for psychological readiness for the treatment. Helping the patient identify his or her emotions and validating them as normal is beneficial. Helping the patient grieve over the loss of health, changes in body image, and possible changes in sexual functioning is essential.

Showing pictures of stomas to patients who will have an ostomy, to prepare them to see their own, is necessary to promote postoperative readiness for learning stoma care. Likewise, helping patients identify resources for coping with cancer, possible sexual dysfunction, and having a stoma may empower them and help them adapt to lifestyle changes, thereby increasing their quality of life.

Nurses must help patients acknowledge their fears, clarify misconceptions, and plan for treatment. Patients often have informational and emotional needs that nurses may not be aware of, therefore, the nurse needs to assess what those needs are before planning teaching content. A "one size fits all" approach will seldom meet all of a patient's needs. Once the patient's needs are addressed, then the nurse can cover necessary content to prepare and support the patient as he or she undergoes staging, treatment, and follow-up.

Nurses must remember that the patient is expending a great deal of emotional and physical energy on coping with the diagnosis and treatment. The amount of concentration and energy that the patient can devote to learning may initially be limited. Therefore, teaching must be ongoing, not a one-time affair.

Teaching content must be appropriate to the patient's literacy level, culturally sensitive, and pertinent to the particular learner. Written, audiovisual, and oral material must be presented in such a way that patients are cued to important content. Expectations for learning should be presented before teaching begins so that the patient knows what are the essential information and skills that he or she will need.

Learning and retention of information and skills will be greater if multiple methods are used, such as print, audiovisual, discussion, demonstration, and return demonstration. Reviewing essential information as often as possible will help the patient remember key points and decrease the possibility of misunderstandings or incomplete information. Likewise, print materials can be used at home to reinforce content and to provide information that is "nice to know" or nonessential.

During the immediate postoperative stage, the nurse needs to monitor for postsurgery complications, particularly elimination patterns, abdominal cramping or pain, and fatigue. As the immediate postoperative period passes, the nurse will need to devote time to helping patients adjust to their change in body image, particularly if they have a stoma. Instruction of colostomy care should progress in an orderly fashion from organizing supplies to eventually completing the care independently. Having a visit from a person who has successfully integrated living with a colostomy with a full and satisfying lifestyle can provide encouragement to the patient and promote a more positive attitude.

During radiation and chemotherapy, nurses must prepare patients to expect changes in appetite and instruct them in necessary dietary changes, how to handle nausea and vomiting, changes in elimination patterns, and the need to conserve energy.

Throughout the patient's experience of colorectal cancer, from diagnosis to ongoing follow-up, the nurse should include significant others in teaching and provide emotional support as they cope with their loved one's diagnosis, treatment, and follow-up.

CONCLUSION

Research is ongoing into the causes of colorectal cancer and effective screening and treatment options. These efforts offer hope to thousands of Americans who are at risk of developing colorectal cancer. As health professionals strive to improve screening and treatment outcomes, it is becoming increasingly clear that for the majority of Americans, changing their lifestyle choices may be their greatest opportunity to reduce their risk and provide for early detection.

BIBLIOGRAPHY

American Cancer Society. (1991). *American Cancer Society textbook of clinical oncology.* Atlanta, GA: Author.

Barsevick, A. M., Pasacreta, J., & Orsi, A. (1995). Psychological distress and functional dependency in colorectal cancer patients. *Cancer Practice, 3*(2), 105–110.

Burris, J., & McGovern, P. (1993). Mass colorectal cancer screening: Choosing an effective strategy. *AAOHN Journal, 41*(4), 186–191.

DeCosse, J. J., & Cennerazzo, W. (1992). Treatment options for the patient with colorectal cancer. Proceedings of the American Cancer Society National Conference on Colorectal Cancer. *Cancer, 70*(5), 1342–1345.

Hoebler, L., & Irwin, M. M. (1992). Gastrointestinal tract cancer: Current knowledge, medical treatment, and nursing management. *Oncology Nursing Forum, 19*(9), 1403–1415.

Martin, W. L. (1992). Colorectal cancer: Recent developments and continuing controversies. *Post Graduate Medicine, 91*(1), 153–160.

Weinrich, S. P., Boyd, M. D., Johnson, E., & Frank-Stromberg, M. (1992). Knowledge of colorectal cancer among older persons. *Cancer Nursing, 15*(5), 322–330.

Weinrich, S. P., Weinrich, M. C., & Boyd, M. D. (1994). Teaching older adults by adaptations for aging changes. *Cancer Nursing, 17*(6), 494–500.

26

Urinary Tract Cancers

Julena Lind

BLADDER CANCER

Incidence and Risk Factors

Bladder cancer accounts for approximately 4% to 5% of all cancers in the United States. The **incidence** of bladder cancer in men is three times that in women, and the age-adjusted bladder cancer rate in white men is almost twice that in African-American men.

Possible etiologic factors include exposure to chemicals called *arylamines* (used in the textile and rubber industries), cigarette smoking, dietary nitrosamines, and exposure to *Schistosoma haematobium*, a parasite commonly encountered in Asia, Africa, and South America.

Most bladder cancers are **carcinomas** of the transitional epithelium of the bladder's mucosal lining. Although 90% of the cases are localized at **diagnosis,** up to 80% will recur.

Prevention and Early Detection

There are no generally accepted guidelines for prevention or early **detection** of bladder cancer in the United States.

Diagnostic Evaluation and Staging

Patients with bladder cancer usually present with gross hematuria. Other manifestations include bladder irritability (dysuria, frequency, or urgency) and symptoms of urethral obstruction. Obstruction of the ureters causes flank pain and results in hydronephrosis. Advanced **tumors** may compress the pelvic lymph nodes, resulting in rectal obstruction, pelvic pain, and lower extremity edema.

TABLE 26–1 Jewett/Marshall Bladder Staging System

Stage	Description
Stage O	Carcinoma in situ (CIS) or superficial papillary tumor confined to the mucosa without invasion
Stage A	Papillary tumor invading the lamina propria
Stage B1	Tumor with superficial muscle invasion
Stage B2	Tumor with deep muscle invasion
Stage C	Invasion of the perivesical fat
Stage D1	Involvement of adjacent viscera and/or pelvic nodes
Stage D2	Involvement of nodes above the aortic bifurcation or distant spread

To identify the cause of clinical symptoms an excretory urogram (also known as intravenous pyelogram, IVP, or intravenous urogram, IVU) is initially performed, preferably before cystoscopy. The diagnosis is then confirmed by cystoscopy and biopsy of the suspicious lesion, and a staging work-up is performed.

Staging of this cancer is based on the depth of invasion into the bladder muscle and surrounding structures. The most common bladder staging systems used in the United States are the Jewett-Strong system (modified by Marshall) and the **TNM system** (Tables 26–1, 26–2, 26–3). In addition to anatomical staging, it is also important in this cancer to assess the tumor grade. Tumors are graded according to degree of cellular abnormality, with the most atypical cells designated as high-grade tumors. Approximately 25% to 33% of bladder cancers present with a high-grade, muscle-invasive tumor. The majority present with low-grade, superficial disease.

The staging work-up includes a **computerized tomography (CT)** scan to identify intra-abdominal and pelvic node enlargements greater than 1.5 cm. CT primarily has a role in staging large or bulky tumors. **Flow cytometry,** which is a technique that examines urine cells for the relative amount of DNA content per cell, may also be used as part of staging to help detect the presence of muscle-invasive tumors. Unfortunately, flow cytometry is not widely available clinically.

Treatment

Superficial Bladder Cancer Tumors that are limited to the inner layer of the bladder (i.e., the mucosa and the submucosa) are classified as *superficial*. The term includes carcinoma in situ (CIS), tumors that are limited to the mucosa (0,Ta), and the more invasive forms that penetrate into the lamina propria (A,T1).

Superficial bladder cancer is generally treated by transurethral resection (TUR) and intravesical chemotherapy. **Intravesical chemotherapy** describes the procedure in which chemotherapy is given directly into the bladder to concentrate the drug at the tumor site and eliminate any residual tumor mass after resection. The literature strongly indicates that coupling of TUR with intravesical therapy achieves better results than either alone. The most common drugs used

TABLE 26–2   TNM Bladder Classification

Primary Tumor (T)
TX = Primary tumor cannot be assessed
TO = No evidence of primary tumor
Tis = Carcinoma in situ
Ta = Noninvasive papillary carcinoma
T1 = Tumor invades submucosa/lamina propria
T2 = Tumor invades superficial muscle
T3a = Tumor invades deep muscle
T3b = Tumor invades perivesical fat
T4 = Tumor invades adjacent organs

Regional Lymph Nodes (below aortic bifurcation) (N)
NX = Regional lymph nodes cannot be assessed
NO = No regional lymph node metastasis
NI = Metastasis in single node < 2 cm
N2 = Metastasis in single node > 2 cm but < 5 cm, or multiple nodes < 5 cm
N3 = Metastasis in nodes > 5 cm

Distant Metastases (M)
MX = Presence of distant metastasis cannot be assessed
MO = No distant metastasis
M1 = Distant metastases present

T = tumor; M = node; M = metastases.

are thiotepa, mitomycin C, doxorubicin, or the immunotherapeutic agent BCG (bacillus Calmette Guerin). To date there is no consensus on the choice of drug, the timing for the start, the duration of treatment, or the schedule. Superficial recurrences are managed by repeated transurethral resections and intravesical chemotherapy.

Side effects associated with TUR include initial bladder irritability and frequency. Nursing considerations include patient education on the use of bladder antispasmodics and on adequate hydration, up to 2 liters per day.

TABLE 26–3   Bladder Stage Groupings

Jewett/ Marshall Stage	TNM Stage	TNM Classification
CIS, O	O	Tis NO MO; Ta NO MO
A	I	T1 NO MO
B1	II	T2 NO MO
B2, C	III	T3a NO MO; T3b NO MO
D1, D2	IV Any N, M1	T4 NO MO; Any T, N1, N2, N3 MO; Any T

The side effects of intravesical chemotherapy depend on the drug used and are correlated with transvesical absorption of the drug, which depends mostly on molecular weight. The principal systemic effect of thiotepa is **myelosuppression,** which is directly related to the monthly cumulative dose (over 80–90 mg increases the risk of myelosuppression). Mitomycin absorption is low due to its high molecular weight, but allergic reactions are somewhat more common (3%–20%). Absorption of doxorubicin is negligible. BCG adverse effects may be severe, even though less than 5% of patients manifest general reactions. These effects include fever, granulomatous prostatitis in men, systemic infection, sepsis, allergic reactions, and arthralgia. (See Chapter 9 on chemotherapy for nursing considerations associated with these side effects.)

Although superficial tumors are generally treated with TUR, in some centers, patients with high-grade T1 tumors associated with CIS, or invasion of the lymphatics, receive a radical cystectomy with pelvic **lymphadenectomy.**

Muscle-Invasive Bladder Cancer Radical cystectomy with urinary diversion has reemerged in the United States as the treatment of choice in invasive bladder cancer. However, when there are only solitary lesions in the dome of the bladder and random mucosal biopsies of distant bladder sites are normal, a partial cystectomy may be performed. About 50% of patients with high-stage, high-grade tumors will eventually relapse following cystectomy. Surgery is seldom performed to palliate symptoms in these patients.

In men, radical cystectomy is usually synonymous with prostatocystectomy. The procedure includes excision of the bladder with the pericystic fat, the attached peritoneum, and the entire prostate and seminal vesicles. In women, radical cystectomy includes removal of the bladder and entire urethra, uterus, ovaries, fallopian tubes, and anterior wall of the vagina. Pelvic lymph node dissection is frequently performed during the cystectomy to stage the disease and to attempt to prevent local pelvic recurrence and **metastasis.**

In both men and women the removal of the bladder necessitates a urinary diversion. An experienced enterostomal therapist should assist in preoperative teaching and in marking for stomal placement of the anticipated urinary diversion.

The urinary diversion associated with radical cystectomy may be an intestinal conduit such as an ileal conduit, or a **continent urinary reservoir.** Figure 26–1 shows an ileal conduit; Figure 26–2 depicts one type of continent urinary reservoir called a *Kock pouch,* which is constructed with a piece of ileum.

Side effects associated with an ileal conduit include wound infections, enteric fistulae, urine leaks, ureteral obstruction, bowel obstruction, and pelvic abscesses, which may occur for the first month after surgery. Later complications include stomal stenosis, peristomal hernias, chronic pyelonephritis, ureteroileal obstruction, intestinal obstruction, calculi, and hyperchloremic acidosis.

Postoperative nursing care includes monitoring the urinary diversion for urine secretion immediately following surgery. The urinary stoma, which protrudes approximately one-half inch above the skin, should be fitted with a urinary appliance. The color of the stoma should be checked frequently for several days

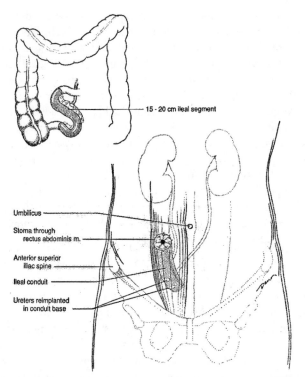

FIGURE 26–1   Urinary Diversion Using a Segment of Ileum

As short a segment as possible is used, and it is usually positioned in the right lower quadrant of the abdomen in an isoperistaltic direction.

Source: From Carroll, P. R. & Barbour, S. (1992). Urinary diversion & bladder substitution. In E. Tanagho & J. McAninch (Eds.), *Smith's general urology* (13th ed., p. 427). Norwalk, CT: Appleton & Lange.

after surgery. Normal color is deep pink to dark red. A dusky appearance could indicate stomal necrosis.

Mucous will be present in all urinary diversions constructed from bowel segments because the intestine normally produces mucus. Excessive mucous can clog the urinary appliance. This problem can be minimized by increasing the patient's fluid intake to 3 liters per day. Nurses should teach patients adequate skin care and pouching of the stoma. Other topics include handling equipment, early identification of kidney infections, community- and hospital-based resources, and body image issues. Generally, the nurse should not begin teaching these procedures until patients' physical discomfort has subsided and their physiologic state has returned more or less to normal.

With a continent ileal reservoir, there is no need for an external appliance, and catheterization of the pouch duplicates normal bladder function. These patients will need to learn self-catheterization techniques. Many stomal complications associated with an ileal conduit can be prevented by good stomal care

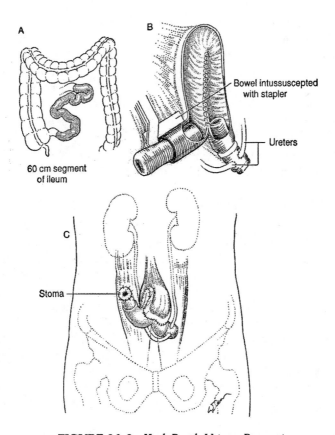

FIGURE 26–2   Kock Pouch Urinary Reservoir

(A) Shaded area indicates section of small intestine selected for reservoir construction. (B) Ureters implanted on afferent (nonrefluxing) limb and efferent limb (with nipple valve) for stoma created by using stapling devices. (C) Completed reservoir with the efferent limb drawn through the abdominal wall and stoma created.

Source: From Carroll, P. R. & Barbour, S. (1992). Urinary diversion & bladder substitution. In E. Tanagho & J. McAninch (Eds.), *Smith's general urology* (13th ed., p. 432). Norwalk, CT: Appleton & Lange.

and appropriate teaching by an enterostomal therapist trained in the recognition of peristomal skin complications and in urinary diversion management.

In cystectomy, operative damage to nerves responsible for erectile function renders most male patients physiologically unable to have or maintain an erection, but some patients are still able to achieve orgasm. Because the prostate and seminal vesicles are removed, men experience dry orgasms without emission of semen. Penile implants may be useful for some patients. Women who undergo cystectomy may experience some physiologic problems during intercourse as a result of a shortened vagina.

Radiation therapy has been the chosen modality of treatment for invasive bladder cancer in many other countries, notably England. Complications of radiotherapy include radiation enteritis or colitis and skin reactions.

Half of all patients, independent of treatment with surgery and/or radiation, will have disseminated disease. Systemic chemotherapy may be used to manage advanced bladder cancer or as an adjuvant to surgery and/or radiation therapy. Complete response rates of 40–67% have been reported using a combination protocol called MVAC, which consists of methotrexate, vinblastine, adriamycin (doxorubicin), and cisplatin. Single-agent chemotherapy has demonstrated limited success, with cisplatin proving the most effective agent.

CANCER OF THE KIDNEY

Incidence and Risk Factors

Renal cell carcinoma (also called hypernephroma and adenocarcinoma), which occurs in the parenchyma of the kidney, is the most common type of renal cancer, accounting for 90% of all kidney cancers and approximately 3% of all adult malignancies. Renal cell carcinoma (RCC) is more common in males than in females (2:1) and is rare in people under age 35.

Although the etiology of RCC is unclear, cigarette smoking is the most definitive **risk factor,** with approximately 25% to 30% of cases directly attributable to smoking. Other risk factors for renal cell carcinoma are the use of phenacetin-containing analgesics and exposure to asbestos, cadmium, or gasoline. Patients who develop cystic disease while on chronic hemodialysis may also be at a greater risk for renal cell cancer.

There is also a genetic link. Like many cancers, RCC occurs in both familial and nonfamilial (sporadic) forms. Rare family constellations have been described in which multiple family members develop RCC, and predisposition to the disease is inherited in an autosomal dominant fashion. The patients with familial RCC have a translocation of the short arm of chromosome 3, and unaffected family members do not carry these translocations. A second form of hereditary RCC is seen as part of von Hippel-Lindau (VHL) disease. This rare disease is a cancer syndrome in which affected patients are predisposed to develop multiple, bilateral renal cysts and carcinomas, bilateral pheochromocytomas, retinal angiomas, hemangioblastomas of the central nervous system (CNS), pancreatic cysts and tumors, and/or epididymal cysts. Recent studies have found that the same gene is involved in both the sporadic and familial forms of RCC.

Prevention and Early Detection

Aside from smoking cessation and avoidance of asbestos, there are no guidelines or procedures for the prevention or early detection of RCC.

Diagnostic Evaluation and Staging

Over 40% of patients with renal cell cancer exhibit gross hematuria. Patients may also present with a dull, aching flank pain or a palpable abdominal mass.

TABLE 26-4 Robson's Renal Cell Cancer Classification

Stage	Description
Stage I/A	Tumor within renal capsule
Stage II/B	Tumor outside capsule but within Gerota's fascia
Stage III/C	Involvement of regional lymph nodes, renal vein, or vena cava
Stage IV/D	Adjacent organs or distant metastases

Other presenting symptoms include fever, weight loss, **anemia,** and **hypercalcemia.** More and more tumors are presenting as incidental findings on IVP, abdominal ultrasound, or CT scans.

One-third of RCC patients present with metastatic disease, and 30% to 40% of the remainder will develop distant metastasis. The median survival time for patients with metastasis is less than 1 year. Renal cell carcinoma spreads locally to the medullary portion of the kidney, to the renal vein, and sometimes into the vena cava. The most common sites of distant metastasis are the lungs, bones, brain, and liver.

The first step in diagnosis of RCC is to differentiate it from the more common benign renal cysts. **Ultrasound** can effectively define the solid or cystic nature of the mass. If a cystic mass is at all suspicious, then fine-needle cyst puncture should be performed to rule out malignancy.

Diagnostic and staging tests for renal cell cancer include kidney/ureters/bladder radiograph (KUB), excretory urogram (IVP), renal ultrasound, CT, and renal angiography. One of the unique features of RCC is its pattern of growth intraluminally into the renal vein, the inferior vena cava (IVC), and occasionally the right atrium. **Magnetic resonance imaging (MRI)** is an accurate noninvasive method for delineating the full extent of an IVC thrombus and is now the preferred caval imaging modality. The staging system used for kidney cancer can be seen in Tables 26-4 and 26-5.

TREATMENT

Surgery Radical nephrectomy is the mainstay of curative treatment for localized renal cell cancer. Recently the role of surgery has been changing for localized RCC, with nephron-sparing surgery being accepted more often in situations where radical nephrectomy would leave a patient anephric, and palliative nephrectomy being done for selected patients with metastatic disease who are experiencing severe disability from associated local symptoms.

Pain can be a severe side effect after nephrectomy. Patients may experience incisional pain and, as a result of the position on the operating table, muscular discomfort as well. Before the operation, it may be useful to explain the surgical positioning and resulting discomfort. Postoperatively, in addition to medication,

TABLE 26–5   TNM Renal Cell Classification

Primary Tumor (T)
T0 = No evidence of tumor
T1 = Tumor < 2.5 cm and confined to kidney
T2 = Tumor > 2.5 cm and confined to kidney
T3a = Extends to perinephric tissues
T3b = Involves renal vein
T3c = Involves renal vein and IVC
T4 = Invades adjacent tissues beyond Gerota's fascia

Regional Lymph Nodes (N)
N0 = No lymph node metastases
N1 = A single node 2 cm or less
N2 = One or more nodes 2–5 cm
N3 = One or more nodes > 5 cm

Distant Metastases (M)
M0 = No distant metastases
M1 = Distant metastases present

T = Tumor; N = Node; M = Metastases

relief can be provided with moist heat, massage, and pillows to support the patient's back while he or she is lying on one side.

Other nursing considerations include teaching about the procedure, postoperative care, and care and education at home. Individuals who are undergoing diagnostic procedures or treatment of a kidney malignancy are naturally anxious about the procedure and the outcome. The nurse can help by providing information and reassurance that life with only one kidney can be normal.

Postoperative nursing interventions include pain relief and prevention of atelectasis, pneumonia, and infection at the incision site; assessment of the remaining kidney function; and monitoring for bleeding and paralytic ileus.

At home, patients and their families should be taught the importance of liberal fluid intake (at least 2.5 liters/day). Patients should be advised to have an annual follow-up to monitor for metastasis or contralateral tumors. The nurse should also teach the patient and family to report any signs of respiratory distress, hemoptysis, pain, or fracture of an extremity, which could indicate metastasis.

Radiation   The use of radiotherapy for renal cell tumors is controversial, but pre- and postoperative radiotherapy have been combined with nephrectomy. The role of radiation in managing disseminated RCC is usually limited to palliation of metastases, especially bony lesions. An objective shrinkage of tumor is often noted following 4,000 to 5,000 rads of palliative external-beam radiation.

Chemotherapy   Renal cell cancer remains resistant to chemotherapy.

Immunotherapy It was first found in 1984 that RCC is particularly responsive to adoptive **immunotherapy** using **interleukin-2** (IL-2) with or without **lymphokine-activated killer (LAK) cells.** However, this treatment is complicated, toxic, and expensive. While LAK cell infusions alone are well tolerated, high-dose IL-2 has caused many complications, including malaise; fever; hepatic dysfunction; **thrombocytopenia;** somnolence; disorientation; pulmonary edema; and, rarely, respiratory distress, coma, and myocardial infarctions. Nursing interventions include extensive patient education and support and intensive monitoring of the severe side effects.

Alpha **interferon** has also been evaluated for the treatment of advanced renal cell carcinoma. It shows modest activity, with overall response rates of 15% to 20%.

There is considerable interest today in using a combination of alpha interferon with low-dose IL-2. Trials have shown improved response rates and much lower toxicity, allowing the treatment to be given on an outpatient basis. Side effects of alpha interferon include flu-like symptoms, myelosuppression, fatigue, and depression. (See Chapter 10 for further information on biotherapy.)

CONCLUSION

The two urinary tract cancers discussed in this chapter are relatively rare, together accounting for only about 6% of all cancers. Smoking is an etiologic factor for both types of cancers, although there are individual risk factors for each cancer as well. Surgery is the usual treatment of choice for cure in the United States for most bladder and kidney cancers; however, radiation therapy is the mainstay of treatment for bladder cancer in many other countries. Advances in the treatment of bladder cancer have been made in the improved surgical procedures for continent urinary diversion. Late-stage kidney cancer has recently shown improved response rates and lower toxicity to treatment with a combination of alpha interferon with interleukin-2.

BIBLIOGRAPHY

Bono, A. V. (1994). Superficial bladder cancer: State of the art. *Cancer Chemotherapy and Pharmacology, 35* (suppl.), S101–S109.

Esrig, D., Freeman, J., Stein, J., & Skinner, D. (1995). Surgery in the management of bladder cancer. *Comprehensive Therapy, 21,* 20–24.

Gnarra, J., Lerman, M., Zbar, B., & Linehan, W. M. (1995). Genetics of renal-cell carcinoma and evidence for a critical role for von Hippel-Lindau in renal tumorigenesis. *Seminars in Oncology, 22,* 3–8.

Lind, J., Kravitz, K. & Grieg, B. (1993). Urologic and male genital malignancies. In S. L. Groenwald, M. H. Frogge, M. Goodman, & C. H. Yarbro (Eds.), *Cancer nursing: Principles and practice* (3rd ed., pp. 1258–1315). Sudbury, MA: Jones and Bartlett.

McFarlane, M., deKernion, J., & Figlin, R. (1993). Neoplasms of the bladder. In J. F. Holland, & E. Frei (Eds.), *Cancer medicine* (3rd ed., p. 1546). Philadelphia: Lea & Febiger.

Novick, A. C. (1995). Current surgical approaches, nephron-sparing surgery, and the role of surgery in the integrated immunologic approach to renal-cell carcinoma. *Seminars in Oncology, 22,* 29–33.

Richie, J. (1993). Renal cell carcinoma. In J. F. Holland, & E. Frei (Eds.), *Cancer medicine* (3rd ed., p. 1529). Philadelphia: Lea & Febiger.

Taneja, S. S., Pierce, W., Figlin, R., & Belldegrun, A. (1994). Management of disseminated kidney cancer. *Urologic Clinics of North America, 21,* 625–637.

27

Male Genital Cancers

Debra L. Brock

The most common cancers of the male genital tract are those of the prostate, testis, and penis. Prostate and penile cancers usually affect men over age 50, but testicular cancer is most common in adolescent and young adult males.

PROSTATE CANCER

Prostate cancer is the most common cancer in men in the United States. The **incidence** is increasing in part due to an increase in awareness and improved detection, but also due to the aging of the U.S. population. The American Cancer Society (ACS) estimated that there would be 317,100 new cases and 41,400 prostate cancer deaths in 1996. The overall 5-year **survival rate** for men with localized prostate cancer is 95%. Currently, approximately 60% of men have localized disease at the time of diagnosis.

African-American men have the highest incidence of prostate cancer in the United States. They also tend to develop it at an earlier age than Caucasian men, and **mortality** is higher. Japanese men have the lowest incidence, although among second-generation immigrants to the United States the incidence of this cancer is similar to that of American men in general.

Risk Factors and Etiology

Because the exact causes of prostate cancer are unknown, there are no known measures to prevent it. The most important **risk factor** is age. It is a rare cancer in young men, with 80% of cases found in men over the age of 65. Of autopsied men over age 80, more than 60% are found to have microscopic prostate cancer. The median age at diagnosis is 70 years. Studies have found no consistent relationship of prostate cancer to infections, dietary habits, smoking, sexual habits, or occupational exposure, and there is no known relationship between benign prostatic hypertrophy (BPH) and prostate cancer.

There is some familial association, but it is unknown whether this is due to genetic or environmental factors. Men with a family history of prostate cancer are three times more likely to develop the disease. If a man has a father or brother who has had prostate cancer before age 65, his chances for developing it increase fourfold. Some chromosomal studies have reported abnormalities found in chromosomes 1, 7, and 10 in men with prostate cancer.

There appears to be some hormonal relationship associated with a greater risk of prostate cancer. The exact role of hormones in the development of prostate cancer needs further investigation.

Clinical Manifestations

Prostate cancer can grow for years without symptoms. The primary symptoms are similar to those of benign prostatic hypertrophy and/or urinary tract infections. These include a weak or interrupted urine flow; difficulty starting or stopping the stream; the need to urinate frequently, especially at night; blood in the urine; pain or burning with urination; and pain in the low back, pelvis, or upper thighs. Bone pain is the most frequent complaint of patients who present with metastatic disease.

Detection

The American Cancer Society recommends that every male over age 40 have a yearly **digital rectal exam (DRE)** during a regular annual physical and that a **prostate-specific antigen (PSA)** blood level be measured annually on all males age 50 and over. There is controversy regarding the use of the PSA as a **screening** tool. The PSA is prostate specific but not cancer specific. Benign prostatic hypertrophy can also cause mild elevations in the PSA level. Prostate-specific antigen levels increase with age and prostate volume. A PSA test is usually recommended if there is a family history of prostate cancer, especially in immediate family members. If either a DRE or a PSA is abnormal, a transrectal **ultrasound** of the prostate (TRUS) with possible biopsy will most likely be performed.

Treatment

Treatment depends upon the stage of the cancer at **diagnosis** (Table 27–1). Treatment may consist of surgery such as a prostatectomy or hormonal manipulation with bilateral **orchiectomy.** Radiation therapy may also be used as a treatment option if the cancer is confined to the prostate or surrounding tissues. Radiotherapy may be an option for some men who are elderly and are poor surgical candidates. In some asymptomatic men with very slow-growing **tumors** who are elderly or have other medical conditions, close observation and follow-up may be the best choice.

Hormonal therapy is another possible treatment option for prostate cancer. Newer pharmacological agents such as the **leutinizing hormone-releasing hor-**

TABLE 27-1   American Urological Staging System for Prostate Cancer

Stage	Description
Stage A	No palpable lesion
A1	Single focal area of well-differentiated tumor
A2	Multiple areas of cancer in the gland, or cancer is poorly differentiated
Stage B	Tumor palpable but confined to the prostate
B1	Small single nodule < 2 cm
B2	Multiple nodules or single nodule > 2 cm
Stage C	Tumor is localized to periprostatic area
C1	No involvement of seminal vesicles, tumor < 70 gm
C2	Involvement of seminal vesicles, tumor > 70 gm
Stage D	Advanced Disease
D1	Pelvic lymph node metastases or ureteral obstruction
D2	Bone or distant lymph node organ or soft tissue metastases

mone **(LHRH)** agonists stimulate the pituitary to increase leutinizing hormone (LH), thereby stimulating testosterone production. After a few weeks with continued treatment, the pituitary no longer initiates the production of LH or testosterone. A LHRH agonist may also be combined with an antiandrogen to produce total androgen blockade in the treatment of prostate cancer.

Chemotherapy is not widely used in the treatment of prostate cancer due to its questionable benefit in this malignancy. Chemotherapy is occasionally used when a man is refractory to hormone treatment. As newer drugs become available and research continues, the possibility of using chemotherapy as a single modality or in combination therapy may become a more viable option.

Nursing Considerations

Nursing care of men with prostate cancer may occur at any point along the course of the disease. Besides coping with a diagnosis of cancer, many men are concerned about the effect of treatment on their sexual function and urinary continence. These concerns should be discussed before treatment begins. When a prostatectomy is planned men should be told that while newer surgical techniques have decreased the incidence of incontinence and impotence, both of these problems can occur. Techniques for management of incontinence and exercises to strengthen perineal muscles can be taught preoperatively. Patients should be given ample opportunity to discuss concerns about sexual function with a nurse or other health professional (see Chapter 18).

Men undergoing surgical resection of the prostate need particular attention to prevention of bleeding and infection in the early postoperative period. The nurse should ensure catheter patency and be prepared to administer antispasmodics to decrease bladder spasms, a common and painful occurrence after prostatectomy.

Patients undergoing radiation therapy to the prostate are likely to experience diarrhea and possibly bladder spasms or cystitis at some point during treatment. If diarrhea occurs, they should be instructed to decrease dietary fiber and may need antidiarrheal medications. Antispasmodics may be needed for relief of bladder spasms. It is also important to instruct the patient to drink plenty of fluids to decrease the risk and discomfort of cystitis.

The nurse should understand the action, side effects, and management of any chemotherapeutic or hormonal agents being administered and should teach the patient and family about these agents (see Chapter 9).

With advanced prostate cancer, bone **metastasis** is common, resulting in chronic and often severe pain. Palliative radiation, analgesics, and noninvasive pain management techniques should be considered in achieving the goal of freedom from pain (see Chapter 14).

TESTICULAR CANCER

While testicular cancer is an uncommon malignancy, representing approximately 1% of all male cancers, it is the most common malignancy among young adult men between the ages of 15 and 35 years. The ACS has estimated that there would be 7,400 new cases and 370 deaths in 1996 due to testicular cancer. The incidence of testicular cancer is low among nonwhites. The greatest incidence is in North America and Europe, with Denmark having the highest rate. The lowest incidence is in Asia and Africa. Testicular cancer is potentially curable, even when found in advanced stages. The 5-year survival rate for all stages of testicular cancer is approximately 90%. Approximately 15% of men with testicular cancer are diagnosed in advanced stages. More than half are diagnosed with Stage 1 disease, in which the cancer is confined to the testis. Monthly testicular self-examination (TSE) is the best screening tool for testicular cancer. Because testicular cancer is rare, it is neither cost effective nor practical to screen for the disease.

Risk Factors and Etiology

A history of cryptorchidism (an undescended testicle) is the most significant known risk factor for developing testicular cancer. Approximately 25% of men with a history of unilateral undescended testicle will develop testicular cancer in the contralateral testicle. A successful orchiopexy performed before the age of 6 is thought to decrease the risk for tumor development. In general, males who have been diagnosed with testicular cancer have about a 1% to 2% chance of developing testicular cancer in the contralateral testicle either occurring simultaneously or at a later date. Men with Klinefelter's syndrome are also at an increased risk for developing germ cell tumors.

Many theories concerning a possible etiology of testicular cancer have been studied, such as age, trauma, hormonal drugs, genetic abnormality diseases, and socioeconomic factors. Recently it has been recognized that an abnormality located on chromosome 12 is associated with testicular cancer and extragonadal tumors. Approximately 80% of patients with germ cell tumors have been found to have the abnormality. It is especially important to stress the performance of testicular self-examination to men who have previously been diagnosed with testicular cancer.

Clinical Manifestations

A scrotal mass that is accidentally discovered by the male is usually the presenting symptom. The most common sign of testicular cancer is a small, painless lump in the scrotum. A male may also complain of a dragging sensation, dull aching or pain in the scrotal area, or swelling of the scrotum. Low back pain is sometimes the presenting symptom, indicating that the cancer has spread into the retroperitoneal lymph nodes. **Gynecomastia** may also be a symptom due to an elevation of beta **human chorionic gonadotropin** (BhCG). If pulmonary metastasis is present, the male may present with a chronic cough, **dyspnea,** chest pain, or hemoptysis.

Testicular cancer is an aggressive cancer and spreads rather quickly. It also spreads in an orderly fashion. Usual spread is from the testis to the retroperitoneal lymph nodes and to the lung. Although advanced-stage disease at diagnosis is rare, it would involve metastasis to the liver, brain, or bone. Early diagnosis and treatment are of utmost importance in achieving favorable outcomes.

Detection

As previously mentioned, TSE is the best available tool for the detection of testicular cancer. A male should be taught how to perform monthly TSE by the time he is 15 years old. Some states now require that TSE be taught to males in high school. There are testicular models, pamphlets, and videos available to assist in teaching TSE.

Treatment

Testicular tumors are classified into two major histologic categories: **seminoma** and **nonseminomatous germ cell tumors.** Treatment depends upon the classification and **staging** of the testis tumor (Table 27–2). Treatment should consist of an inguinal orchiectomy for pathologic confirmation and histologic diagnosis. A transcrotal fine-needle biopsy or other surgical violation of the scrotum can result in metastasis to the inguinal lymph nodes and an increase in the risk of recurrence of the cancer. Treatment for testicular cancer may consist of a retroperitoneal lymph node dissection (RPLND), radiation therapy, chemotherapy, or bone marrow transplant, or a combination of these.

Sterility due to surgery, chemotherapy, or radiation therapy, is of concern to most males who are facing treatment for testicular cancer. Often, questions arise concerning sperm banking prior to initiation of treatment. Although there is no known cause, up to 80% of males are found to be oligospermic at diagnosis before initiation of any treatment. Due to the aggressiveness of germ cell tumors and the finding that most males are oligospermic before treatment initiation, the treatment should not be delayed for sperm banking. Studies have found that approx-

TABLE 27-2   Indiana Staging System for Testicular Cancer

Stage	Description
Minimal	1. Elevated markers only 2. Cervical lymph nodes (+ or – nonpalpable retroperitoneal nodes) 3. Unresectable, nonpalpable retroperitoneal disease 4. Fewer than 5 pulmonary metastases per lung field and largest < 2 cm (+ or – nonpalpable retroperitoneal nodes)
Moderate	1. Palpable abdominal mass only (no supradiaphragmatic disease) 2. Moderate pulmonary metastasis: 5–10 metastasis per lung field and largest < 3 cm or solitary pulmonary metastasis of any size > 2 cm (+ or – nonpalpable retroperitoneal disease)
Advanced	1. Advanced pulmonary metastasis—primary mediastinal nonseminomatous germ cell tumor or > 10 pulmonary metastases per lung field or multiple pulmonary metastasis with largest > 3 cm (+ or – nonpalpable retroperitoneal disease) 2. Palpable abdominal mass + supradiaphragmatic disease 3. Liver, bone, or central nervous system metastasis

imately 50% of males treated with chemotherapy will regain both spermatogenesis and Leydig cell function within 2 years after treatment. If a male is more than 30 years old, received treatment for longer than 6 months, or received prior abdominal radiation therapy and **autologous bone marrow transplantation** with high-dose chemotherapy, his chances for return of spermatogenesis decrease greatly. The Indiana University Cancer Center found in one study that the rate of pregnancy and incidence of congenital anomalies among offspring of testicular cancer survivors treated with chemotherapy alone were no different from those among a control group in the study and were similar to the national average. They reported one congenital anomaly and one spontaneous abortion in 60 pregnancies.

Nursing Considerations

Because testicular cancer usually affects adolescent and young adult men, concerns about future fertility are often expressed. Counseling concerning the potential for permanent sterility should be given by someone with up-to-date knowledge and expertise in fertility and sexual counseling. Patients should be instructed to use a reliable method of birth control during and for at least 6 months after treatment.

Testicular cancer treatment often includes aggressive chemotherapy, and patients will need to be taught about the side effects and self-care management related to each chemotherapeutic agent they receive. (See Chapter 9.)

PENILE CANCER

Etiology

Penile cancer is rare in the United States, especially in men under the age of 40. It has been attributed to poor hygienic practices in males who have not been circumcised. Smegma is thought to be the primary cause of penile cancer. A history of sexually transmitted disease also increases the risk of developing cancer of the penis.

Clinical Manifestations

Symptoms of penile cancer include a painless ulcer or nodule on the penis. Penile discharge may or may not be present, and pain or bleeding are late symptoms. The male with penile cancer may also have experienced phimosis, a constriction of the foreskin in uncircumcised males.

Treatment

Treatment is usually surgical. The extent of the surgery depends on the extent of the disease at diagnosis. More extensive disease may require a partial or complete penectomy. If regional lymph nodes are involved, a **lymphadenectomy** may also be performed. Radiation and or chemotherapy may also be utilized in the treatment of penile cancer, especially for those with metastatic disease.

Nursing Considerations

Body image changes are understandably severe for most men with penile cancer, and sensitive counseling and guidance by the nurse or other health professional are required. Cancer of the penis usually results in severe sexual dysfunction. These patients and their partners may need extensive counseling about techniques and alternative ways of maintaining a mutually satisfying sexual relationship.

CONCLUSION

Cancers of the male genital tract each have unique etiologies, manifestations, and treatment approaches. All of them potentially threaten a male's self-image and sexuality. Nurses should be especially sensitive to these concerns when caring for patients with male genital cancers. For additional information on sexuality, see Chapter 18.

BIBLIOGRAPHY

Brock, D. L., Fox, S., Hossan, E., & Maxwell, M. (1993). Genitourinary malignancies. In C. Henke Yarbro (Ed.), *Seminars in oncology nursing* (9)4, 217–292. Philadelphia: W. B. Saunders.

Einhorn, L. H., Richie, J. P., & Shipley, W. U. (1993). Cancer of the testis. In V. T. Devita, S. Hellman, & S. A. Rosenberg (Eds.), *Cancer: Principles and practice of oncology*. Philadelphia: J. B. Lippincott.

Gittes, R. F. (1991). Carcinoma of the prostate. *New England Journal of Medicine, 324,* 236–245.

Heinrich-Renning, T. (1987). Prostate cancer treatments and their effects on sexual functioning. *Oncology Nursing Forum, 14,* 37–41.

Kassabian, V. S., & Graham, S. D. (1995). Urologic and male genital cancers. In G. P. Murphy, W. Lawrence, Jr., & R. E. Lenhard (Eds.), *American Cancer Society textbook of clinical oncology* (2nd Ed.). Atlanta, GA: American Cancer Society.

Mahon, S. M., Casperson, D., & Wozniak-Petrofsky, J. (1990). Prostate cancer: Screening through treatment and nursing implications. *Urological Nursing, 10,* 5–11.

Moon, T. (1992). Prostate cancer. *Journal of the American Geriatric Society, 40,* 622–627.

Roth, B. J., Griest, A., & Kublis, P. S. (1988). Cisplatin-based chemotherapy for disseminated germ cell tumors: Long-term follow-up. *Journal of Clinical Oncology, 6,* 1239–1247.

Senturia, Y. D., Peckham, C. S., & Peckham, M. J. (1985). Children fathered by men treated for testicular cancer. *Lancet, 2,* 766–769.

28
Gynecologic Malignancies

Virginia R. Martin

Gynecologic cancers account for 13% of all cancers in women. **Screening** is particularly effective for many of these cancers, because it is possible to identify preinvasive and in-situ cancers, which are curable. However, there are still several gynecologic cancers for which we do not have valid and reliable screening and that continue to be diagnosed at an advanced stage. The multifaceted care of women with gynecologic cancer at either end of this spectrum is both rewarding and challenging to nurses.

ENDOMETRIAL CANCER

Incidence, Etiology, and Risk Factors

Endometrial cancer is the most common cancer of the female genital tract. In the United States, it was estimated that 34,000 new cases would be diagnosed in 1996 and 6,000 women would die from this disease. Endometrial cancer is predominantly a disease of postmenopausal women, with the average age at presentation being 59. It is suggested that the disease is hormonally related and may be associated with either endogenous or exogenous estrogen. **Adenocarcinoma** of the endometrium originates in the endometrial epithelium of the body of the uterus.

The following conditions have been identified as possible **risk factors** for endometrial cancer: obesity, nulliparity, history of infertility or failure to ovulate, dysfunctional uterine bleeding during menopause, late menopause, diabetes mellitus, hypertension, unopposed estrogen, and complex atypical hyperplasia.

Prevention and Early Detection

An annual pelvic examination and **Papanicolaou (Pap) smear** are recommended for women age 40 and over as a part of routine health maintenance. Unfortu-

TABLE 28–1   FIGO Staging for Endometrial Carcinoma (1988)

Stage	Findings
IA GI23	No myometrial invasion
Ib G123	< ½ Myometrial invasion
Ic G123	> ½ Myometrial invasion
IIa G123	Extension to endocervical glands
IIb G123	Cervical stromal invasion
IIIa G123	Positive serosa, adnexae, or cytology
IIIb G123	Vaginal metastasis
IIIc G123	Positive pelvic or periaortic lymph nodes
IVa G123	Bladder or bower mucosal metastasis
IVb	Distant intraabdominal or inguinal lymph node metastasis

Source: International Federation of Gynecology and Obstetrics.

nately, the Pap test, highly effective for screening in cervical cancer, is not an adequate screening test for endometrial cancer. Mass screening with an endometrial sampling is not practical or cost effective for all women, but screening is important for women identified as high risk.

Since diet and estrogen have been identified as possible risk factors, women should aim to maintain a desirable weight and health providers need to evaluate each woman's personal risks and benefits before prescribing estrogen for menopausal symptom management. Including progesterone in estrogen replacement therapy helps to minimize the risk of endometrial cancer.

Evaluation and Staging

Often the only significant clinical signs of this disease are vaginal bleeding, unusually heavy menses, and intermenstrual, postmenopausal, or postcoital bleeding. All warrant further diagnostic studies. An aspiration currettage or endometrial biopsy is usually the preliminary step in diagnosis of endometrial cancer. A fractional dilatation and currettage (D & C), is performed to confirm the diagnosis. After the **diagnosis** is made, a thorough evaluation is performed to complete the work-up for the patient. Prior to 1988 endometrial cancer **staging** was done clinically, but because of the discrepancy between clinical and actual stage the International Federation of Gynecology and Obstetrics (FIGO) adopted a pathological staging classification system outlined in Table 28–1. The surgical staging classification of endometrial cancers is based on uterine size, cervical involvement, and **tumor** cell **differentiation.** Seventy-five percent of patients are diagnosed in the early stages.

Treatment

The treatment plan must be individualized and take into account prognostic factors determined by surgical staging. The mainstay of treatment is surgery. Surgical intervention consists of a total abdominal hysterectomy bilateral salpingo-oophorectomy (TAH-BSO), a sampling of the peritoneal fluid, biopsy of any extrauterine lesions, and sampling or excision of suspicious lymph nodes. Further treatment after surgical staging depends on the stage, and usually surgery is combined with radiation therapy. Radiation can also be used in the **adjuvant** setting so that initial treatment consists of a combination of radiation first and then surgery. Advanced endometrial cancer (Stage IV) is treated with hormonal agents. Recurrent endometrial cancer may be treated with radiation if the patient has not received it before; more radical surgical intervention may be considered; and, most often, hormonal therapy and/or chemotherapy is given. **Chemotherapy** may be single agent or a combination of agents. Some of the most common chemotherapy agents used in endometrial cancer include adriamycin®, cisplatin, and, most recently, paclitaxel.

Side Effects, Complications, and Nursing Considerations

Postoperative wound care, the possibility of bladder irritation or infection or bowel irritability from radiation, and the side effects associated with chemotherapy must all be included in the individualized teaching plan of the patient with endometrial cancer. Psychosocial assessment of needs must be included, because these women will need **support** when confronted with a new cancer diagnosis, including alleviation of fears related to treatment and concern about their **sexuality.** (See Chapter 19.)

CERVICAL CANCER

Incidence, Etiology, and Risk Factors

Cervical cancer **incidence** was estimated to reach 15,700 new cases for 1996, with 4,700 projected deaths. The death rate from cervical cancer has dropped from number one among all cancers in women to number eight because of the development of an effective screening test, the Pap smear. Cases of **carcinoma in situ** of the cervix were estimated to reach 65,000 for 1996, significantly higher than the number of cases of invasive cancer.

The cause of cervical cancer is unknown, but its development seems to be related to multiple insults and injuries sustained by the cervix. A number of risk factors have been identified, including early age of first intercourse, multiple sex partners, cigarette smoking, and infection with certain types of human papillomavirus (HPV). Cervical intraepithelial neoplasia (CIN) and carcinoma in situ are points on a spectrum of disease that begins with mild dysplasia and concludes with invasive cancer of the cervix. Carcinoma in situ and preinvasive forms of this disease are highly curable. At the onset of the disease, cellular growth is slow; once invasive, it grows rapidly.

Prevention and Early Detection

Screening is both simple and cost effective. The Pap test is a simple procedure that can be performed at appropriate intervals by health care professionals as part of a pelvic examination. The test must be performed accurately. The recommended procedure is to take a sample of cells from the endothelium of the cervix using a wooden spatula and a sample of cells from the epithelium of the endocervix using a cervical brush. The cells are swabbed on a slide and then examined under a microscope. Abnormal smears must be fully evaluated with **colposcopy** and/or biopsy. The most important requirement of the Pap smear is that the specimen be adequate for accurate evaluation. Using the technique described here will ensure that this is accomplished. If the cytology report indicates an inadequate specimen, the Pap smear must be repeated.

The American Cancer Society recommends that all women who are or have been sexually active, or who have reached the age of 18, undergo an annual Pap test and pelvic examination. After a women has had three or more consecutive annual examinations with normal findings, the Pap test may be performed less frequently at the discretion of the physician.

Nurses have a role in educating youth today to understand the risks associated with being sexually active at an early age and educate them about the importance of seeing a health care professional if they are sexually active. Additionally, education must be provided about the correlation of smoking with cervical cancer.

Evaluation and Staging

A thin, watery, blood-tinged vaginal discharge may be noted intermittently in cervical cancer's early stages. Painless spotting postcoitally or after douching is another sign. Vaginal bleeding increases as the cancer grows, and a late symptom may be pain, either in the flank or in the leg.

Initial evaluation of this disease takes place in the office with a clinical appraisal and may include a colposcopy, biopsy, and/or endocervical currettage. The diagnosis is confirmed with an examination under anesthesia that often includes a cystoscopy and proctosigmoidoscopy. The clinical staging (Table 28–2) is based on FIGO, taking into account the clinical extent of the disease, the class of cytologic interpretation, and the histologic grade.

Treatment

The choice of therapy is dictated by the stage of the disease. The decision should be made with both a gynecologic oncologist and a radiation therapist, since surgery and radiation are often utilized together.

Patients with preinvasive cervical cancer or Stage 0 may be treated with various conservative treatment options including local excision, electrocautery, cryosurgery, laser surgery, **conization,** loop electrosurgical excision procedure (LEEP), or hysterectomy. Close follow-up is mandated with many of these treatment options.

For Stage I through Stage IV patients, treatment is based on the age and health of the patient, the extent of the cancer, and the presence of any complicating abnormalities. Stages I to IIA are treated surgically; Stages IIB through III are treated with radiation. Radiotherapy is usually a combination of **brachyther-**

TABLE 28–2 International Classification of Cancer of the Cervix

The staging of cancer of the cervix is a clinical appraisal, preferably confirmed with the patient under anesthesia; it cannot be changed later if findings at operation or subsequent treatment reveal further advancement of the disease.

Stage 0	Carcinoma in situ, intraepithelial carcinoma
Stage I	The carcinoma is strictly confined to the cervix (extension to the corpus should be disregarded)
Stage Ia	Preclinical carcinomas of the cervix; that is, those diagnosed only by microscopy
Stage Ia1	Minimal microscopically evident stromal invasion
Stage Ia2	Lesions detected microscopically that can be measured. The upper limit of the measurement should not show a depth of invasion of more than 5 mm taken from the base of the epithelium, either surface or glandular, from which it originates, and a second dimension, the horizontal spread, must to exceed 7 mm. Larger lesions should be staged as Ib
Stage Ib	Lesions of greater dimensions than stage Ia2, whether seen clinically or not. Preformed space involvement should not alter the staging but should be specifically recorded so as to determine whether it should affect treatment decisions in the future
Stage II	Involvement of the vagina but not the lower third, or infiltration of the parametria but not out to the sidewall
Stage IIa	Involvement of the vagina but no evidence of parametrial involvement
Stage IIb	Infiltration of the parametria but not out to the sidewall
Stage III	Involvement of the lower third of the vagina or extension to the pelvic sidewall. All cases with a hydronephrosis or nonfunctioning kidney should be included, unless they are known to be attributable to other cause.
Stage IIIa	Involvement of the lower third of the vagina but not out to the pelvic sidewall if the parametria are involved
Stage IIIb	Extension onto the pelvic sidewall and/or hydronephrosis or nonfunctional kidney
Stage IV	Extension outside the reproductive tract
Stage IVa	Involvement of the mucosa of the bladder or rectum
Stage IVb	Distant metastasis or disease outside the true pelvis

Source: International Federation of Gynecology and Obstetrics.

apy and external pelvic radiation. **Pelvic exenteration** may be chosen for a select group of patients with cervical cancer. This procedure includes removal of all pelvic viscera, including the rectosigmoid colon and bladder.

Recurrent disease is usually treated with combination chemotherapy. The drugs used include ifosfamide and mesna, cisplatin, bleomycin, fluorauracil, doxorubicin, mitomycin, vinblastine, hydoxyurea, topotecan, and paclitaxel. Combination regimens are more effective than single agents.

Side Effects and Complications

Postoperative bladder dysfunction, lymphocyst formation, pulmonary embolism, pelvic infection, and hemorrhage are the acute postsurgical complications. Radiation side effects include skin reactions, acute radiation cystitis, proctosigmoiditis, and enteritis, all of which are transient and resolve steadily after treatment ends. Nurses can educate patients to help manage the cramping, diarrhea, or bleeding that may occur by altering their diet and using antispasmodic medications. An interruption of a week in the radiation treatment regimen may be needed.

Nursing Considerations

Nurses must take an adequate sexual history and counsel and educate both the patient and the sexual partner. The patient must be urged to continue regular follow-up care. Nurses should allow for the expression of feelings, since many patients will be overwhelmed with the diagnosis and treatment plan and the potential loss or threat to their sexual functioning. (See Chapter 18.)

Long-Term Sequelae

Vaginal cervical fibrosis, vaginal stenosis, **dyspareunia,** fistula formation, bowel obstruction, and proctitis are possible long-term side effects of cervical cancer. Depending on the complication, nursing care may be especially challenging. Fistula formation, for example, requires prevention of skin breakdown, odor control, nutritional support, and psychosocial care as the focus of the nursing care. Dilatation of the vagina, necessitated by stenosis from radiation, will require a regimen of using a dilator on a regular basis after instruction from the nurse. Women should receive anticipatory guidance regarding the management of these complications and support to deal with the psychosocial sequelae.

OVARIAN CANCER

Incidence and Risk Factors

Ovarian cancer is the deadliest of the gynecologic cancers. It was estimated that, in 1996, 26,600 women would be diagnosed with the disease and 14,500 women would die. Ovarian cancer is the fourth leading cause of cancer death in women in the United States. Incidence of this disease increases with age, and mean age at diagnosis is 59. Long-term survival is achieveable in early-stage disease, but unfortunately 75% to 80% of the time this disease is diagnosed at an advanced stage.

Ovarian cancer is not one disease, but is composed of several cell types. Epithelial, stromal, and germinal cells give rise to subsets of ovarian cancer. Epithelial tumors constitute 80% to 90% of all **malignant** neoplasms. The histologic categories of ovarian cancer include serous, mucinous, endometrioid, clear cell, Brenner, and undifferentiated carcinomas.

Risk factors fall into two categories, genetic and hormonal factors. Genetic risk includes a family history of ovarian cancer, especially for women with two first-degree relatives who were diagnosed with it. Nulliparity, early menarche, late menopause, and infertility are the associated reproductive or endocrine factors. It is thought that oral contraceptives may reduce the risk of ovarian cancer. Environmental and dietary factors are suggested as possible risk factors, but no definite correlation has been found at this time.

Prevention and Early Detection

Detection of ovarian cancer early in the disease process is hampered by a lack of knowledge regarding its pathogenesis and the absence of early-stage symptoms. Several detection modalities exist for ovarian cancer, including the pelvic examination, transvaginal or transabdominal **ultrasound,** color flow doppler, and a blood test for the antigen CA-125. Unfortunately, many ovarian tumors are not detectable early. Annual pelvic examinations for women over the age of 40 will detect some, but not all, ovarian tumors. High-risk women (i.e., women with one or more relatives with ovarian cancer) are a separate group that needs to be screened more aggressively.

Evaluation and Staging

Ovarian cancer is most often silent until late in its development. There are no common signs and symptoms. Early symptoms are vague abdominal discomfort, dyspepsia, flatulence, bloating, and digestive disturbances. It is the vagueness of these symptoms that causes the difficulty in early diagnosis, since many healthy women experience vague digestive disturbances. If these symptoms persist without explanation or apparent cause, more thorough testing should be directed at ruling out ovarian cancer. Ovarian cancer spreads by serosal seeding, direct extension, and lymphangitic or hematogenous pathways. The symptoms that appear late in the disease progression include abdominal distention and pain, ascites, and a pelvic mass. Ovarian cancer is staged surgically with an exploratory staging laparotomy. The surgery includes meticulous and thorough inspection and evaluation of the abdomen for possible sites of disease dissemination. The surgical goal is to remove as much tumor as possible and to leave no residual tumor nodule greater than 1 cm. Successful surgical reduction of disease increases the effectiveness of subsequent combination chemotherapy. The staging system for ovarian cancer is outlined in Table 28–3.

Treatment

Postoperative treatment consists of combination chemotherapy. As a result of recent clinical trials the current recommendation of the Gynecology Oncology Group is a combination of paclitaxel and platinum therapy (either carboplatin or cisplatin) for a minimum of six cycles after surgery. This is the approach for all stages of ovarian cancer except very early stage disease, which needs no further treatment after surgery. In recent years, after primary chemotherapy patients underwent a second surgical exploratory laporotomy to determine whether the

TABLE 28–3   International Federation of Gynecology and Obstetrics (FIGO)
Staging for Ovarian Carcinoma

Stage I	Growth limited to the ovaries.
Stage IA	Growth limited to one ovary; no ascites present containing malignant cells. No tumor on the external surface; capsule intact.
Stage IB	Growth limited to both ovaries; no ascites present containing malignant cells. No tumor on the external surfaces; capsules intact.
Stage IC	Tumor classified as either stage IA or IB but with tumor on the surface of one or both ovaries; or with ruptured capsule(s); or with ascites containing malignant cells present or with positive peritoneal washings.
Stage II	Growth involving one or both ovaries, with pelvic extension.
Stage IIA	Extension and/or metastases to the uterus and/or tubes.
Stage IIB	Extension to other pelvic tissues.
Stage IIC*	Tumor either stage IIA or IIB but with tumor on the surface of one or both ovaries; or with capsule(s) ruptured; or with ascites containing malignant cells present or with positive peritoneal washings.
Stage III	Tumor involving one or both ovaries with peritoneal implants outside the pelvis and/or positive retroperitoneal or inguinal nodes. Superficial liver metastasis equals stage III. Tumor is limited to the true pelvis but with histologically proven malignant extension to small bowel or omentum.
Stage IIIA	Tumor grossly limited to the true pelvis with negative nodes but with histologically confirmed microscopic seeding of abdominal peritoneal surfaces.
Stage IIIB	Tumor of one or both ovaries with histologically confirmed implants of abdominal peritoneal surfaces, none exceeding 2 cm in diameter; nodes are negative.
Stage IIIC	Abdominal implants greater than 2 cm in diameter and/or positive retroperitoneal or inguinal nodes.
Stage IV	Growth involving one or both ovaries, with distant metastases. If pleural effusion is present, there must be positive cytologic findings to allot a case to stage IV. Parenchymal liver metastasis equals stage IV.

*Notes about the staging: To evaluate the impact on prognosis of the different criteria for allotting cases to stage IC or IIC, it would be of value to know whether the rupture of the capsule was spontaneous or caused by the surgeon and if the source of malignant cells detected was peritoneal washings or ascites.

Source: International Federation of Gynecology and Obstetrics.

disease was eradicated. At present, second-look operative exploration is recommended only for certain candidates participating in clinical trials, because this procedure has not impacted overall **survival rates.**

Radiotherapy is used palliatively in ovarian cancer patients for treatment of a large mass pressing on the rectosigmoid or urinary tract and to control pain or bleeding from uterine or vaginal **metastasis.**

Many chemotherapeutic agents have been used for recurrent ovarian cancer. Often retreatment is given using the primary therapy if the patient has been disease free for 6 months or more. The most active agents used for treatment of recurrent disease (salvage therapy) are hexamethylmelamine, etoposide, ifosfamide, tamoxifen, fluorouracil, and doxorubicin. Unfortunately, no agent is curative at this stage, and response rates are between 15% and 25%. Intraperitoneal therapy, chemotherapy directly into the abdomen, has been evaluated in both early-stage and advanced-disease patients; the role of this therapy is still under investigation.

Side Effects and Complications

Postoperatively, most patients recover quickly without complications and begin chemotherapy while still recuperating in the hospital. Chemotherapy side effects depend on the regimen chosen, but may include hair loss, nausea and vomiting, neurotoxicities, **myelosuppression,** and/or arthralgias or myalgias. (See Chapter 9.) If the disease progresses without successful treatment, patients often have bowel obstructions, ascites, and **anorexia.**

Nursing Considerations

Nurses must educate healthy women to continue yearly visits to their physicians beyond the reproductive years. A yearly pelvic examination is important; it may lead to an early diagnosis of ovarian cancer. Once diagnosis is made and treatment begun, nurses are partners with patients in their care and must educate them about the potential side effects of treatment and complications that should be reported immediately. The focus of nursing care will be to promote optimal quality of life for these patients with advanced disease. Significant time should be allowed for assessment of coping skills and emotional needs as a part of the care plan for each patient.

Long-Term Sequelae

Since this disease is often diagnosed late and, as a result, is not curable, long-term sequelae may not be a major focus of assessment. As a result of chemotherapy, patients may experience peripheral neuropathies that are debilitating and painful and continue to be bothersome long after therapy has ended. Abdominal adhesions from surgery may occur, causing abdominal pain and obstruction.

VULVAR CANCER

Vulvar cancer represents about 1% of all gynecologic tumors. A variety of benign and malignant growths can occur on the vulva. Types of vulvar cancer include dystrophies, intraepithelial neoplasia, bowenoid papulosis, vulvar condyloma, and squamous cell carcinoma. Vulvar dystrophies appear as **leukoplakia,** or thick white plaques, and are treated topically. Vulvar intraepithelial neoplasias (VIN) are preinvasive grades of this disease, and the treatment is individualized but usually conservative and can include laser evaporation, cryosurgery, or local excision. Bowenoid papulosis is benign and is treated with surgical excision. Vulvar condyloma are genital warts, thought to be transmitted by the human papilloma virus.

Squamous cell carcinomas account for 90% to 95% of vulvar tumors and are more commonly seen in older women. The lesions can appear on the labia majora, clitoris, or the periurethral areas and will begin to ulcerate with growth. A vulvar biopsy confirms the diagnosis. This cancer spreads by lymphagitic dissemination, and the disease is staged surgically (see Table 28–4). A cystoscopy, sigmoidoscopy, and chest x-ray are ordered as part of the initial evaluation, and the treatment of choice is surgery. The extent of the surgery is based on the tumor size, location, and lymph node involvement. Radiation is not used alone in this disease, but it may be given pre- or postoperatively depending on the extent of the disease. Pelvic radiation is recommended if the lymph node biopsies are positive.

Complications of radical vulvar surgery can include wound separation, infection, and necrosis. Managing the pain or discomfort associated with treatment is a major focus of the nursing intervention with the vulvar cancer patient. In addition, psychosocial support is essential because of the disturbance in body image and sexual function. Peripheral lymphedema and low sexual satisfaction may be long-term sequelae of treatment for vulvar cancer. Nurses must educate patients regarding the signs and symptoms of vulvar cancer, encouraging older women to continue visiting their physicians yearly after menopause.

VAGINAL CANCER

Vaginal tumors represent only 2% of all gynecologic tumors. Squamous cell carcinomas occur most frequently, 85% of the time. Other types include adenocarcinoma, verrucous carcinoma, small-cell carcinoma. **Diethystilbestrol (DES)** exposure is associated with clear-cell adenocarcinoma, **sarcoma,** and melanoma. Vaginal intraepithelial neoplasia (VAIN) is the preinvasive form of vaginal cancer. VAIN produces no symptoms and is diagnosed by an abnormal Pap smear and further investigated by a colposcopy-directed biopsy. Treatments for the preinvasive disease include laser evaporation, cryosurgery, electrocautery, and/or intravaginal chemotherapy cream.

Two-thirds of all vaginal cancers affect women over the age of 50; it is most commonly seen in the sixth and seventh decades of life. The etiology is unknown,

TABLE 28–4 Clinical Stages of Invasive Carcinoma of the Vulva

Stage	*Tumor Classification*			*Description*
	Invasive Carcinoma of the Vulva (FIGO Classification)			
0				Carcinoma in situ
I	T1	N0	M0	All lesions confined to the vulva with a maximum diameter of 2 cm or less and no suspicious groin lymph nodes
	T1	N1	M0	
II	T2	N0	M0	All lesions confined to the vulva with a diameter greater than 2 cm and no suspicious groin lymph nodes
	T2	N1	M0	
III	T3	N0	M0	Lesions extending to the urethra, vagina, anus, or perineum, but without grossly positive groin lymph nodes
	T3	N1	M0	
	T3	N2	M0	
	T1	N2	M0	Lesions of any size confined to the vulva and having suspicious lymph nodes
	T2	N2	M0	
IV	T1	N3	M0	Lesions with grossly positive groin lymph nodes regardless of extent of primary
	T2	N3	M0	
	T3	N3	M0	
	T4	N3	M0	
	T4	N0	M0	Lesions involving mucosa of the rectum, bladder, urethra, or involving bone
	T4	N1	M0	
	T4	N2	M0	
	M1A			All cases with pelvic or distant metastases
	M1B			

Source: International Federation of Gynecology and Obstetrics.

TABLE 28–5   Clincial Staging of Invasive Cancer of the Vagina (FIGO System)

Stage 0	Carcinoma in situ, intraepithelial carcinoma
Stage I	The carcinoma is limited to the vaginal wall
Stage II	The carcinoma has involved the subvaginal tissue but has not extended on to the pelvic wall
Stage III	The carcinoma has extended on to the pelvic wall
Stage IV	The carcinoma has extended beyond the true pelvis or has involved the mucosa of the bladder or rectum. A bullous edema as such does not permit allotment of a case to stage IV.

Source: International Federation of Gynecology and Obstetrics. (Data from *Gynecology Oncology Group pathology manual* [unpublished]).

but genital viruses and chronic irritation are suggested causes. Signs and symptoms include vaginal bleeding, vaginal discharge, and pelvic pain. The most common site for this disease is the upper one-third of the posterior vaginal wall. If an abnormal vaginal Pap smear is taken, it should be investigated with colposcopy and biopsy. FIGO staging for vaginal cancer is given in Table 28–5; it is a clinical staging system. Treatment depends on the stage of disease, the location of the tumor, the patient's age, and the desire to preserve a functional vagina. Vaginal cancer spreads to the lymph nodes closest to the primary tumor. If the vaginal cancer is in the upper portion of the vagina it spreads to the deep pelvic lymph nodes; if it is in the lower portion it spreads to the groin or femoral lymph nodes. The treatment approach is radiation, external or brachytherapy. Surgery can be part of primary therapy or done prior to radiation and can include a radical hysterectomy, vaginectomy, and pelvic lymph node sampling. Pelvic exenteration, removal of the uterus, bladder, and/or rectum, is required for advanced disease.

The nursing challenges are focused on physical care in the acute stage and psychosocial care in the chronic phase of recuperation. Altered body image and altered sexual functioning need to be addressed by the nurse.

CANCER OF THE FALLOPIAN TUBE

This is a rare disease, representing 0.31% to 1.8% of all gynecologic tumors. Incidence peaks in the fifth decade, with a mean age at diagnosis of 52. Diagnosis is made during an exploratory laporotomy for an adnexal or pelvic mass. It is critical to differentiate this disease from cancer of the ovary or uterus. The most frequent type of fallopian tube cancer is a papillary adenocarcinoma. Less commonly seen are squamous cell carcinoma, **choriocarcinoma,** or sarcoma. There is no official staging system for this disease.

Treatment consists of cytoreductive surgery including a TAH and BSO, cytology of the pelvis and peritoneal organs, and biopsy of selected lymph nodes. Radiation therapy and chemotherapy may be used in the management of this dis-

TABLE 28–6   FIGO Staging System for Gestational Trophoblastic Disease

Stage I	Disease confined to the uterus
Stage II	Disease confined to the pelvis
Stage III	Disease confined to the pelvis and lungs
Stage IV	Involvement of other metastatic sites

Source: International Federation of Gynecology and Obstetrics.

ease. Nursing care is focused on the treatment plan chosen and includes psychosocial support throughout the intervention.

GESTATIONAL TROPHOBLASTIC DISEASE (GTD)

Gestational trophoblastic disease (GTD) refers to all neoplastic disorders arising from the chorionic portion of the placenta. These include partial or complete hydatiform mole, placental site tumor, invasive mole, and gestational choriocarcinoma. Partial or complete **hydatiform mole** is a benign form of GTD and is described as a pregnancy lacking an intact fetus. Advanced maternal age or a previous molar pregnancy are the most significant risk factors. Bleeding in the first trimester is a common sign, along with a discrepancy in the size and date of the pregnancy. **Human chorionic gonadotropin (hCG)** is elevated in all patients with GTD. The treatment is suction currettage. Complete hydatiform mole can lead to malignant GTD in 10% to 30% of cases, and therefore all patients need to be continually monitored after diagnosis with weekly hCG titers. As long as the titer is decreasing, no intervention is necessary.

If the hCG titer plateaus or begins to increase, a work-up for malignant GTD must be initiated. A complete work-up must be performed, including ultrasound and enhanced **computerized tomography** of the pelvis, abdomen, lungs, and brain. Staging is based on the FIGO staging system (Table 28–6) or on a simplified staging system. The simplified staging system separates patients with nonmetastatic disease from those with metastatic disease. The treatment for nonmetastatic disease and what is called low-risk metastatic disease is a single-agent chemotherapy consisting of methotrexate or actinomycin-D given at scheduled intervals. Both agents have comparable remission rates, 90% to 100%. The hCG titers are followed until three consecutive negative titers have been obtained. For patients with high-risk metastatic disease, a combined modality approach may be needed, including multiagent chemotherapy and possibly surgery. Often the agents combined are methotrexate, actinomycin, chlorambucil, etoposide, cyclophosphamide, and/or folinic acid. With aggressive therapy, high-risk patients should have a 75% cure rate.

Nursing intervention includes education concerning the unusual disease process and treatment. Often psychosocial support is an important component of nursing care, because grief over the loss of pregnancy and fear of disease and treatment are concurrent issues for these patients, and they often are young.

CONCLUSION

Gynecologic cancers can occur in women of all ages and are curable in the early stages. Women must be educated to get an annual physical with a pelvic examination and Pap smear after the age of 40. A yearly gynecologic examination is also indicated for women at the onset of sexual activity. Early detection is imperative for an impact on survival. Once a diagnosis is made, careful follow-up is important for all women with gynecologic cancer. Nurses remain the best caregivers to provide education about these diseases and to provide support for effective coping with the treatment and its side effects. It can be both challenging and rewarding to provide nursing care to women with gynecologic cancer.

BIBLIOGRAPHY

Martin, L. K., & Braly, P. S. (1991). Gynecologic cancers. In S. Baird, R. McCorkle, & M. Grant (Eds.), Cancer Nursing (pp.502–535). Philadelphia: W. B. Saunders.

Qazi, F., & McGuire, W. P. (1995). The treatment of epithelial ovarian cancer. CA—A Cancer Journal for Clinicians, 45(2), 88–101.

Ozols, R. F. (1992). Ovarian cancer, Part II: Treatment. Current Problems in Cancer, 15(2) (entire issue).

Walczak, J. R. (Ed.). (1990). Gynecologic cancers. Seminars in Oncology Nursing, 6(3) (entire issue).

29

Central Nervous System Cancers

Betty Owens

Although primary cancers of the central nervous system (CNS) comprise a small percentage (1.5%) of all cancers, they are devastating because of their effect on the individual's mind and personality. The prognosis is poor, and quality of life can be greatly affected by neurological deficits caused by the **tumor** and/or subsequent treatments.

INCIDENCE

In 1996, 17,900 primary brain tumors were expected to be diagnosed, with the **incidence** slightly higher in males than in females. In the same year, 13,300 deaths were expected from CNS cancer. Peak incidence in adults occurs between the ages of 45 and 70. Recent studies suggest that the incidence of brain tumors in elderly adults is truly increasing and is not just the result of improved imaging techniques; however, this is controversial and needs additional study. Brain tumors are the second most common malignancy in children. Peak incidence in children is between the ages of 4 and 9 years. Tumor location, as well as **histology,** differs between adults and children. The majority of tumors in children are located in the cerebellum, brain stem, optic nerve, parasellar region, and pineal gland. Adult tumors are located in the cerebrum, meninges, and nerve roots. Primary CNS tumors rarely metastasize outside of the CNS.

The majority of primary CNS tumors occur in the brain; less than 15% originate in the spine. Of patients with systemic cancers, 20% to 40% will develop brain metastases. The most common primary cancers in these cases are lung, breast, and melanoma. In all patients diagnosed with brain metastases, 50% have a single **metastasis,** 20% have two metastases, and 10% have more than five

TABLE 29-1   All Brain and CNS Tumors: Frequencies and Percent Distribution
by Histology; Surveillance, Epidemiology, and End Results (SEER)
1973–1987

Histology	Frequency	Percent
Glioma (mixed and other)	728	4.7
Ependymoma	458	3.0
Astrocytoma, not otherwise specified	5,459	35.3
Protoplasmic and gemistocytic astrocytoma	276	1.8
Fibrillary and astrocytoma	267	1.7
Pilocytic astrocytoma	223	1.4
Glioblastoma	6,197	40.1
Oligodendroglioma	530	3.4
Medulloblastoma	553	3.6
Other	771	5.0
Total	15,462	100.0

Source: Copyright © Polednak, A. P., Flannery, J. T. (1995). Brain, other central nervous system,
and eye cancer. CANCER *Supplement, 75,* 332. Reprinted by permission of Wiley-Liss, A Division
of John Wiley and Sons, Inc.

metastatic tumors. Some systemic cancers metastasize to the bony structure of
the spine.

CLASSIFICATION

Many, but not all, primary brain tumors are gliomas (see Table 29–1). **Glioma** is
a general term for tumors that arise from glial cells, which provide supporting
structure for the neurons. The types of glial cells are astrocyte, oligodendrocyte,
and ependymocyte, and subsequent tumors are called astrocytoma, oligodendroglioma, and ependymoma. Gliomas infiltrate normal brain tissue and,
although they are usually located in a single area of the brain, may be multifocal.

Common Adult Brain Tumors

Astrocytoma   **Astrocytoma** is the most common brain tumor in adults. Two
grading scales are commonly used, the Kernohan and the World Health
Organization (WHO) (see Table 29–2). These tumors are frequently described as
low- or high-grade tumors. A low-grade astrocytoma can, and often does, degen-
erate into a high-grade tumor. Mixed grades can be found within a tumor, but
final pathology and subsequent treatment are determined by the tumor's most
aggressive component. Astrocytomas, except pilocytic or cerebellar astrocytoma,
are infiltrative, invading surrounding normal tissue, and cannot be surgically
removed.

Prognosis for pilocytic or cerebellar astrocytoma in children is extremely
good, and many are cured with surgery alone. However, high-grade astrocytomas

TABLE 29-2 Grading Scales for Astrocytoma

	Kernohan	World Health Organization (WHO)
Low grade	Astrocytoma I	
	Astrocytoma II	Astrocytoma
High grade	Astrocytoma III	Anaplastic astrocytoma
	Astrocytoma IV	Glioblastoma multiforme

have a very poor prognosis even with surgery, radiotherapy, and **chemotherapy.** Survival for anaplastic astrocytoma is about 18 to 24 months and for **glioblastoma** 9 to 12 months. Survival for Grade II astrocytoma varies but averages 6 to 7 or more years. Over all, younger patients with a good performance status at diagnosis have a better prognosis than older patients who have many neurological deficits.

Oligodendroglioma Pure oligodendroglioma grows more slowly than astrocytoma. The WHO scale grades these tumors as **oligodendroglioma** (low grade) and anaplastic oligodendroglioma (high grade). Oligodendroglioma rarely exists as a pure entity; it is usually a mixed histology. An oligodendroglioma/astrocytoma is expected to behave as its most aggressive astrocytic component. The prognosis for oligodendroglioma is usually slightly better than that for astrocytoma.

Meningioma A meningioma is a slow-growing tumor that arises from the dural covering of the brain, usually not infiltrating normal brain tissue but pushing it aside. A meningioma is **benign** by histology, but it can be **malignant** by location—that is, located in an area where the tumor cannot be removed and where it can cause neurological deficit and eventual death. This can be true of other benign tumors as well. Rarely, a histologically malignant meningioma can occur.

Common Pediatric Brain Tumors

Cerebellar Astrocytoma The benign and often cystic cerebellar astrocytoma (also called *pilocytic astrocytoma*), is potentially curable by surgery alone. No further therapy is needed, and recurrence is low (see Table 29-3). Astrocytomas located in the cerebrum or within or near the brain stem are usually much more aggressive and follow the grading scale described for adult astrocytoma.

Medulloblastoma Medulloblastoma arises in the cerebellum and frequently disseminates through the cerebrospinal fluid (CSF) pathway. Rare in adults, medulloblastoma may present at any age but occurs most frequently in children 3 to 8 years of age. Extent of tumor at **diagnosis** and extent of resection are factors in survival. Imaging of the entire spine is imperative for an appropriate treatment decision. Survival has greatly improved in recent years with combined modality treatment using surgery, radiotherapy, and chemotherapy (see Table 29-3). If this tumor is located above the tentorium, it is called a *primitive neuroectodermal tumor (PNET)*.

TABLE 29-3   Manchester Children's Tumor Registry: Survival for Childhood Cancer

Histology	1954–1963		1964–1973		1974–1983	
	n	Percent 5-Year Survival	n	Percent 5-Year Survival	n	Percent 5-Year Survival
Ependymoma	30	20	30	23	30	29
Juvenile astrocytoma	50	66	66	74	50	83
Medulloblastoma	44	25	50	40	56	41

Source: Adapted from Birch, J. M., et al. (1995). Improvements in survival from childhood cancer: Results of a population based survey over 30 years. *Epidemiology, 296,* 1373. Reprinted with permission from the British Medical Association.

Ependymoma   Ependymoma occurs most commonly in children, and although it can be found anywhere in the CNS, it usually develops in the fourth ventricle, obstructing the flow of cerebral spinal fluid (CSF) and causing hydrocephalus. A ventriculoperitoneal (VP) shunt may be needed on an emergency basis before resection is attempted. An ependymoma may seed down the spine, and thus the entire spine should be imaged. Although usually relatively slow growing, an ependymoma can become aggressive, and because of its critical location, long-term survival is poor (see Table 29–3).

Spine Tumors

Spine tumors develop more frequently in adults than in children. Primary tumors of the spine are classified according to their location in relation to the dura (membrane that covers the spinal cord) and the spinal cord itself, and by histopathology. The following are the locations and histologies of common spine tumors:

1. Intradural extramedullary—**schwannoma,** meningioma.

2. Intradural intramedullary—astrocytoma, ependymoma.

3. Extradural—metastatic.

Approximately half of primary spine tumors are schwannoma or meningioma; both are benign by histology. Only 20% are gliomas, with the majority of those being ependymoma. Most primary spine tumors are slow growing, causing pain and neurological deficits but not usually death. Metastases to the spine from systemic cancers may also cause spinal instability from vertebral destruction.

RISK FACTORS

The etiology of primary brain tumors is not known. Although many causes have been investigated, only a few genetic conditions and exposure to ionizing radiation have an association. A person with Von Hippel Lindau disease develops multiple benign vascular tumors called *hemangioblastoma*. A person with neurofibromatosis develops multiple benign peripheral nerve tumors called *neurofibroma* and is predisposed to develop meningioma, acoustic neuroma, and glioma. Also, gliomas may be associated with tuberous sclerosis. Some chromosomal changes have been discovered in certain tumors. Although meningioma at one time was thought to be related to head trauma, research has not shown this to be true. Although some chemicals cause brain tumors in animals, definitive clinical studies have not been done; however, some occupations with a higher than average incidence of brain tumors have been studied. In 1992 The Central Brain Tumor Registry of the United States was established as a nonprofit corporation to try to collect data from state cancer registries on both benign and malignant brain tumors.

PREVENTION

There is no known means to prevent CNS tumors, although it would be best to avoid excessive exposure to ionizing radiation and chemicals.

EARLY DETECTION

With only 17,900 brain tumors diagnosed each year, it is not cost effective to scan the general public routinely for **screening** purposes only. Families with known genetic risk factors should be followed closely in a genetic clinic.

CLINICAL PRESENTATION

Children can be difficult to diagnose because of their inability to describe their symptoms. Similarly, diagnosis is difficult in many adults because patients are often unaware of their deficits and do not seek—and even refuse—medical evaluation.

Adults

In adults the most common presenting symptoms are headache and seizure. Initially headaches are mild, but they increase in frequency and intensity. A scan is usually not obtained with the first complaint of a headache unless other neurological signs are present. Types of seizures range from a brief staring episode (petit mal) to a generalized tonic-clonic seizure involving the whole body (grand mal). Other presenting symptoms include neurological deficits, especially in the areas of sensation/movement, vision, and speech. If the tumor is located near the motor strip, mild weakness to paralysis may occur on the opposite side of the body. A patient with a tumor located near the speech center may experience expressive and/or receptive aphasia ranging from mild word-finding problems to complete inability to speak and/or understand. Focal symptoms are related to the area of the brain where the tumor is located. Tumors have no predilection for any particular area of the brain.

Cognitive symptoms, more subtle than physical deficits, may range from mild memory problems to significant mental confusion. Impaired memory, judgment, and decision making affect personal, social, and work relationships. Relationships may be broken and employment lost before the tumor is diagnosed.

Children

In children, headache, vomiting, ataxia, poor coordination and balance, and nystagmus occur due to the infratentorial location of most tumors. The age of the child also influences presenting signs and symptoms. An infant may have a bulging fontanel from increased intracranial pressure and may be very irritable. School-age children may demonstrate a decline in school performance. Arrest, delay, or even acceleration in growth and development is possible with some tumors, especially those located in the parasellar region such as craniopharyngioma or germinoma.

Late symptoms of a brain tumor result from increased intracranial pressure and include severe headache, nausea and vomiting, and decreased level of consciousness. Death will occur if intracranial pressure is not alleviated.

DIAGNOSIS

A computerized axial tomography (CAT) or magnetic resonance imaging (MRI) scan is obtained if a brain tumor is suspected. The entire spine is imaged if disseminated disease is suspected. A cerebral angiogram is rarely performed unless the tumor is expected to be highly vascular and the surgeon needs this information to plan treatment. Lumbar puncture (LP) may be dangerous in the face of increased intracranial pressure, with the risk of precipitating brain herniation. It is performed to obtain a specimen of CSF for cytology when dissemination into the CSF is expected and risk of brain herniation is negligible. Positive emission tomography (PET) scans are available in some centers. They are useful in evaluating recurrent tumors to distinguish between necrosis as a result of treatment and live tumor. For deep and inaccessible tumors, a stereotactic biopsy can precisely locate the tumor and obtain a tissue specimen by the most direct route, disturbing as little normal brain tissue as possible and avoiding critical structures. The greatest risk of stereotactic biopsy is hemorrhage.

TREATMENT

Brain Tumors

The majority of malignant tumors show evidence on MRI of edema around the tumor. Initially, the patient's symptoms are treated with a corticosteroid (usually dexamethasone) if edema is present, an anticonvulsant if a seizure has occurred, and a VP shunt if hydrocephalus is a problem.

Surgery   After ameliorating immediate symptoms, surgery is the primary treatment for most brain tumors. The goal of surgery is to make a diagnosis and to remove as much tumor as possible without causing neurologic deficits. If the tumor is benign by histology and is surgically accessible, the surgeon will attempt a complete resection. If it is malignant and/or in a critical area, as much tumor as is safe will be removed. New neurosurgical technologies are improving patient outcomes. Brain mapping locates critical structures prior to surgery. Stereotactic guided craniotomy (by standard stereotactic frame or new computerized robotic microscopes or wands) assists the surgeon to locate the borders of the tumor. If all of a low-grade tumor has been removed and the patient can be relied on to return for follow-up scans, no further treatment may be recommended until the tumor recurs. If residual tumor remains, radiation therapy is generally recommended.

Radiotherapy   After surgery, radiotherapy is the next standard therapy for primary brain tumors. All high-grade gliomas receive radiotherapy postoperatively. Some centers still recommend whole brain radiotherapy, but usually focal therapy is administered. The maximum dose is approximately 6,000 centigray (cGy) given in daily fractions (180–200 cGy) over 5 to 6 weeks. Radiation in children is delayed as long as possible (until at least 2 to 3 years of age) because of concerns regarding the action of the radiation on normal white matter with subsequent long-term effects, especially on intelligence. Both adult and pediatric patients with tumors that disseminate down the spine receive craniospinal radiation.

Other forms of radiotherapy and delivery methods are being evaluated. These include drugs to enhance the effect of radiotherapy, radiosensitizing agents. Hyperfractionization, two treatments per day, is a technique used to administer a higher total dose without additional toxicities. **Brachytherapy,** temporary radioactive implants into the tumor bed, delivers radiation directly to the tumor. Radiosurgery is a means to precisely deliver a lethal dose of radiation to a well-defined area in the brain with minimal adverse consequences or risks to the surrounding brain tissue. The value of radiosurgery for glioma is still being evaluated, but radiosurgery for small metastases and small, well-defined benign tumors has shown benefit.

Chemotherapy   After radiotherapy, chemotherapy is the next standard therapy for primary brain tumors; it may be given concurrently with radiotherapy, after radiotherapy, or when the tumor recurs. For astrocytoma, the standard drug is carmustine (BCNU) used as a single agent. For oligodendroglioma or mixed oligodendroglioma/astrocytoma, preliminary studies suggest that PCV [procarbazine, lomustine (CCNU), vincristine] may be slightly more beneficial than BCNU. A key problem in chemotherapy for brain tumors is finding an agent that is lipid soluble and small enough to pass through the blood brain barrier and yet effective. Because of this, techniques for regional delivery are being evaluated. Other standard chemotherapy drugs, new combinations, and newly developed agents are being evaluated. Chemotherapy is a primary treatment for children because of the need to delay radiation as long as possible. Drugs used with children differ from those used with adults.

Metastatic Brain Tumors

Recommended treatment of metastatic brain tumors depends on several factors, including number, size, and location of metastases; histology; sensitivity to other therapies; condition of the patient, and expected survival. Therapies that may be recommended are surgery, radiotherapy, chemotherapy, and **stereotactic radiosurgery.** An aggressive approach to the treatment of brain metastases can improve quality of life for most patients.

Spine Tumors

Surgery alone for benign primary tumors of the spine is usually sufficient to relieve the pressure on the spinal cord and spinal nerves. Radiotherapy may be recommended for aggressive tumors. Radiotherapy alone is needed for radiosensitive metastatic spine tumors. Surgery in metastatic spine tumors is only required if a mass is causing an acute neurological deficit or if the spine needs stabilization to avoid neurologic deterioration during radiotherapy.

SIDE EFFECTS AND COMPLICATIONS

A patient receiving corticosteroids to reduce cerebral edema can experience many side effects; thus, the goal of therapy is to give the patient as small a dose as necessary to maintain maximum neurologic function. Side effects include weight gain, increased appetite, fluid retention, increased susceptibility to infection, excessive hair growth, irritability, insomnia, and gastric irritation. Fortunately, these resolve when the medication is tapered off.

A patient receiving an anticonvulsant may experience different side effects depending on the individual drug; however, most patients complain of fatigue until they adjust to the medication. The most commonly prescribed anticonvulsant is phenytoin.

Potential complications of surgery for a brain tumor include infection, bleeding, neurologic deficit, and death. The greatest surgical risk related to maintaining the patient's preoperative neurologic status is proximity of the tumor to areas of the brain that control critical functions.

Radiotherapy is well tolerated, with minimal toxicity. Side effects include temporary (depending on surface dose) hair loss, fatigue, mild bone marrow depression, headache, nausea, and vomiting. During radiotherapy cerebral edema may temporarily increase, and the patient's neurological problems may worsen, requiring an increase in steroid dose. The long-term effects of radiation on intelligence and cognition are a major concern. This is especially true in very young children, and therefore radiation is not recommended for children under 2 years of age. In treating very aggressive gliomas, often the risk of the growing tumor outweighs the long-term potential toxicity of radiotherapy.

Chemotherapy—BCNU and PCV—is usually well tolerated in adults. Toxicities are those of the individual drugs used (see Chapter 9). Concurrent chemotherapy with radiotherapy seems to increase the toxicities.

LONG-TERM SEQUELAE

Of greatest concern in the adult population is the worsening of neurologic deficits, both physical and cognitive. Patients who experience short-term memory problems (a common complaint in adults) and their families express much frustration with this deficit. This is one of the more difficult symptoms to resolve.

Children can have many long-term sequelae from treatment, such as delayed or arrested growth and development, cognitive impairments, socialization and relationship problems, and endocrine problems including infertility and growth retardation.

A patient whose high-grade tumor is recurring will usually experience the same or worsening of the original presenting symptoms. If the tumor does not respond to treatment, the symptoms will continue to worsen. Death is usually not sudden. The patient will sleep more hours each day, become lethargic, and eventually lapse into a coma. Death may result from increased intracranial pressure or an opportunistic infection related to the patient's depressed immune status, immobility, and lack of adequate fluid intake and nutrition. Fortunately, the patient is often unaware of his or her deficits, but observing the patient's deterioration is difficult for the family.

NURSING CONSIDERATIONS

In addition to dealing with a life-threatening illness, newly diagnosed adult brain tumor patients and their families are struggling with new physical and cognitive impairments. Nurses should provide information regarding the tumor type, potential problems, symptom management, safety issues, and treatment expectations. Booklets are available from national brain tumor organizations. Seizure management information can be obtained from the Epilepsy Foundation. Children should be followed very closely, and appropriate referrals should be made, especially for school and growth and development issues. Long-term sequelae affect a pediatric patient into adulthood, including social relationships, independence, and employment. Family counseling and support are often needed.

Rehabilitation plays an important role for both adult and pediatric patients. Families should be an integral part of each treatment plan, and they need to be provided with a resource person to call whenever new problems arise over the months and years after diagnosis and treatment. Brain tumor support groups offer information and **support** (see Appendix).

CONCLUSION

Unfortunately, the incidence of brain tumors may be increasing in the elderly adult population. Little progress has been made in treating the most aggressive tumor, glioblastoma multiforme, but new directions in research (gene therapy, tumor vaccines, immunotherapy) provide hope for the future. The goal of new therapies is to lengthen survival without sacrificing quality of life. Both patients and their families need information and support over the continuum from diagnosis until death.

BIBLIOGRAPHY

Albright, A. L. (1993). Pediatric brain tumors. CA—A Cancer Journal for Clinicians, 43, 272–288.

Amato, C. A. (1991). Malignant glioma: Coping with a devastating illness. Journal of Neuroscience Nursing, 23, 20–23.

Birch, J. M., Marsden, H. B., Jones, P. H. M., Pearson, D., & Blair, V. (1995). Improvements in survival from childhood cancer: Results of a population based survey over 30 years. Epidemiology, 296, 1372–1376.

Black, P. M. (1991). Brain tumors. The New England Journal of Medicine, 324, 1471–1476.

Brem, S., Rozental, J. M., & Moskal, J. R. (1995). What is the etiology of human brain tumors? Cancer, 76, 709–713.

Bronstein, K. S. (1995). Epidemiology and classification of brain tumors. Neuro-Oncology, 7, 79–89.

DeAngelis, L. M. (1994). Management of brain metastases. Cancer Investigation, 12, 156–165.

Laperriere, N. J., & Bernstein, M. (1994). Radiotherapy for brain tumors. CA—A Cancer Journal for Clinicians, 44, 96–108.

Laws, E. R., & Thapar, K. (1993). Brain tumors. CA—A Cancer Journal for Clinicians, 43, 263–271.

Miller, R. W., Young, J. L. Jr., & Novakovic, B. (1995). Childhood cancer. CANCER Supplement, 75, 395–405.

Polednak, A. P., & Flannery, J. T. (1995). Brain, other central nervous system, and eye cancer. CANCER Supplement, 75, 330–337.

Shiminski-Maher, T., & Shields, M. (1995). Pediatric brain tumors: Diagnosis and management. Journal of Pediatric Oncology Nursing, 12, 188–198.

30

Skin Cancers

Anne Marie Maguire

INCIDENCE

Skin cancers account for about one-third of all diagnosed cancers; they are more prevalent than any other type of cancer in Americans. About 77% of all skin cancers are basal cell carcinomas, and another 20% are squamous cell carcinomas. The remaining 3% are melanomas and rare skin cancers. The ratio of basal to squamous cell cancers is 5:1 in males and 10:1 in females.

In 1996, the American Cancer Society (ACS) estimated that over 800,000 new cases of nonmelanoma skin cancers (NMSC) and 38,300 cases of melanoma would be diagnosed. Of the melanomas, approximately 21,800 cases would occur in males and 16,500 cases in females. Incidence is 10 times higher in Caucasians than in African Americans. Rare invasive nonmelanoma skin cancers (e.g., cutaneous T-cell lymphomas and Kaposi's sarcomas) were estimated to account for another 16,000 new cases.

Mortality rates for NMSC in the past 25 years have decreased approximately 20% to 30% because of early detection and treatment. NMSCs are curable, but it was still estimated that about 2,100 persons would die from them in 1996. Most of these deaths would be caused by squamous cell carcinoma, which has a metastatic rate of 1% to 2%. Basal cell carcinoma metastases or deaths are rare. Another 7,300 persons were expected to die from melanoma in 1996. The melanoma mortality rate for males is almost double that for females. The estimated cumulative lifetime risk for developing melanoma will be 1 in 75 by the year 2000.

Classical Kaposi's sarcoma was first described in elderly Mediterranean, Middle Eastern, or Jewish men in 1872. Today, most cases are diagnosed in HIV-positive patients. About one-third of all homosexual men with HIV infection develop Kaposi's sarcoma. Table 30–1 lists the incidence and characteristics of the major skin cancers.

RISK FACTORS

The leading cause of NMSC, especially squamous cell carcinoma, is cumulative excessive exposure to **ultraviolet radiation (UVR)** from the sun. It is estimated that regular use of sunscreen (SPF 15) during childhood and adolescence would decrease the lifetime incidence of NMSC by 78%. Excessive UVR, particularly ultraviolet B (UVB), can occur in those with outdoor occupations, such as farmers, sailors, or fishermen, or in those who enjoy weekend recreational activities such as skiing, swimming, or mountain climbing. **Risk** increases when the majority of the sun's rays are reflected on the earth's surface. Maximal exposure occurs between 11 A.M. and 3 P.M. (daylight saving time), with almost 100% of UVR being reflected at noon. Those living in latitudes close to the equator are also at increased risk. Ultraviolet A (UVA) produced at tanning booths and by sun lamps causes the same types of skin changes, putting users at increased risk for developing skin cancers.

Other factors associated with UVR exposure that increase the risk of NMSC and melanoma include fair skin, blue or green eyes, blonde or red hair, sun-induced freckles, previous NMSC, inability to tan, actinic keratoses, albinism, and **xeroderma pigmentosa** (a genetic disorder in which DNA is damaged by UVR and is unable to repair itself). Actinic keratoses are red, scaly lesions that are smaller than 1 cm in diameter and can be found on the skin of fair-skinned older adults. Immune suppression secondary to organ transplant, **chemotherapy,** or HIV infection is also a factor. Finally, the thinning ozone layer is expected to greatly increase the number of NMSCs in the future.

Some factors are not associated with UVR exposure. They include ionizing radiation; chronic exposure to tar, soot, shale, petroleum lubricating oil, paraffin, or creosote oil; and arsenic ingestion from well water and insecticides. Chronic ulcers, human papilloma virus, psoralen plus UVA (PUVA) therapy for psoriasis, radiation dermatitis, and scars from heat or chemical burns are examples of skin damage that can also lead to NMSC development.

Although the sun-related risks described earlier can contribute to the development of melanoma, the following risk factors are more significant. Melanoma occurs more often in those with new moles or existing moles that are undergoing changes in appearance; those with dysplastic nevi, congenital nevi, or lentigo maligna; those with a personal or family (first-degree relative) history of melanoma; immunosuppressed persons; and Caucasians.

Dysplastic nevi are pigmented lesions 5 to 12 mm in diameter; they are larger than common nevi (freckles, moles, and beauty marks). Their borders are irregular, ill-defined, and have a macular and papular component. Colors range from tan to dark brown on a pink background. They are especially common on the trunk, but also appear on covered areas of the body such as the scalp, breast, and buttocks. There may be more that 100 nevi on the body; they usually begin

TABLE 30–1 Incidence, Clinical Characteristics, and Common Sites
of Principal Cutaneous Cancers

Incidence	Clinical Characteristics	Common Sites
Basal Cell Carcinoma		
Most common form of skin cancer; occurs primarily in patients exposed to prolonged or intense sunlight, especially whites with light eyes, light hair, and fair complexions.	Nodulo-ulcerative basal cell cancer: Elevated lesions with umbilicated, ulcerated centers; raised waxy or "pearly" borders; moderately firm. Superficial basal cell cancer: Barely elevated plaques, usually with crusted and erythematous centers and raised, threadlike pearly borders; often multiple.	Nose, eyelids, cheeks, and trunk. Uncommon on palms and soles. Metastases are extremely rare.
Squamous Cell Carcinoma Less common than basal cell carcinoma; occurs primarily on areas exposed to actinic radiation and on vermilion border of lips.	Appearance varies from an elevated nodular mass to a punched-out ulcerated lesion to a fungating mass. Unless basal cell carcinomas, squamous cell carcinomas are opaque.	75% occur on head, 15% on hands, and 10% elsewhere. Can metastasize to regional lymph nodes; in more advanced lesions, visceral (especially pulmonary) metastases can occur.
Malignant Melanoma Far less common than basal cell carcinoma or squamous cell carcinoma.	Usually irregularly pigmented (black, gray, white, blue, brown, red); usually more than 6 mm in diameter and asymmetric. May be flat or elevated, eroded or ulcerated; outline usually irregular, often with notch; frequently mildly symptomatic (e.g., pruritic). Characteristic clinical features can be easily remembered by thinking of ABCD: A = Asymmetry B = Border irregularity C = Color variegation D = Diameter generally greater than 6 mm.	Any cutaneous area, although the trunk in men and the legs in women are common; less common in areas unexposed to sun. Metastasizes, often first to regional lymph nodes.

Source: From O. F. Roses., S. L. Gumport, M. N. Harris, & A. W. Kopf. (1989). *The diagnosis and management of common skin cancers* (p. 5). Atlanta, GA: American Cancer Society. Reprinted with permission of publisher.

appearing in adolescence and continue through adulthood. Their presence increases the lifetime risk of melanoma to 5% to 10% versus 0.7% in the general population.

Congenital melanocytic nevi (birthmarks) are present at birth, although they may not be immediately apparent. Large and medium nevi usually have grossly irregular surfaces, varying shades of brown colors, and perhaps hair. Small lesions have smooth surfaces and more uniform color, and they lack hair. The 1% of newborns who have these lesions have approximately a 6% chance of developing melanoma.

PREVENTION AND EARLY DETECTION

The incidence, morbidity, and mortality from skin cancers can be reduced by eliminating exposure to known **risk factors** or by diagnosing lesions at an early stage, when they are small and thin and when cure is possible.

The Skin Cancer Foundation offers patient education guidelines to protect skin from exposure (Figure 30–1). In general, regular application of sunscreens (SPF 15) year round and wearing protective clothing from age 6 months through old age can help prevent most skin cancers. Those who are allergic to PABA-based formulas should use a non-PABA formula. Children can be taught to stay out of the sun when their shadow is shorter than they are. The elderly should be instructed to take a daily vitamin D supplement (200 IU), because sunscreens can block vitamin D synthesis during sun exposure. Some drugs and cosmetics (e.g., quinolones, tetracycline, chlorpromazine, amiodarone, and oral contraceptives) increase sensitivity to sun exposure. Patients taking these medications should consult a physician, nurse, or pharmacist before going in the sun.

Routine self-examination of the skin is a strongly recommended means of detecting skin cancer, particularly melanoma, in the early stage. Three pamphlets, *The Diagnosis and Management of Common Skin Cancers, Malignant Melanoma in the 1990s: The Continued Importance of Early Detection and the Role of Physician Examination and Self-Examination of the Skin,* and *Why You Should Know About Melanoma* are professional and public education materials published by the American Cancer Society that nurses can use as teaching guides. The pamphlets contain colored photographs of NMSC, melanoma, and dysplastic nevi and illustrate skin self-examination techniques (Figure 30–2). Nurses should encourage individuals, particularly those at high risk, to perform skin self-examination once a month and also have an annual skin examination by a physician or nurse practitioner.

When examining the skin, it is important to differentiate abnormal moles from common, **benign,** pigmented lesions. The ABCD rule given in Table 30–1 is the easiest method for recalling the danger signs associated with melanomas. It should be emphasized that a melanoma may not have all of these characteristics. Patients should consult a health care professional if they discover any abnormal findings during their skin assessment.

Limit time in the sun, regardless of the hour or season.
- Avoid the midday hours between 10:00 A.M. and 3:00 P.M., when the sun's rays are the strongest.
- Keep track of the time spent in full sunlight; do not stay in an unshaded spot for long stretches of time.

Use a sunscreen of SPF 15 or higher whenever spending time outdoors.
- This applies to all outdoor activities: athletics, shopping, picnicking , walking or jogging, gardening, even waiting for a bus.
- Choose a sunscreen with ingredients that block both UVB and UVA rays.
- Apply liberally and evenly to all exposed skin. The average adult in a bathing suit should use approximately one ounce of sunscreen per application. Using too little will reduce the product's SPF, and its protection.
- Be sure to cover often-missed spots: lips, ears, around eyes, neck, scalp if hair is thinning, hands, and feet.
- Reapply at least every 2 hours, more often if some of the product may have been removed while swimming, sweating, or towel-drying.
- Choose a product that suits the skin and the activity. Sunscreens are available in lotion, gel, spray, cream, and stick forms. Some are labeled as waterproof, sweat proof, or especially for sports; as fragrance-free, hypoallergenic, or especially for sensitive skin or children.

Cover up.
- Wear long-sleeved shirts and long pants. The more tightly woven the fabric and the darker the color, the more protection given. If light can be seen through a fabric, UV rays can get through too. Water makes fabrics more translucent, so do not rely on a wet T-shirt for sun protection.
- A broad-brimmed hat goes a long way toward preventing skin cancer in often-exposed areas like the neck, ears, scalp, and face. Opt for a three-inch brim that extends all around the hat. Baseball caps and visors shade the face but leave the neck and ears exposed.
- UV-blocking sunglasses with wraparound or large frames protect eyelids and the sensitive skin around eyes, common sites for skin cancer and sun-induced aging. Sunglasses also help reduce the risk of cataracts later in life.

Seek the shade.
- Be aware, however, that sunlight bouncing off reflective surfaces can reach even beneath an umbrella or a tree.

Never seek a tan.
- There is no such thing as a healthy tan. A tan is a skin's response to the sun's damaging rays.

Stay away from tanning parlors and artificial tanning devices.
- The UV radiation emitted by indoor tanning light is many times more intense than natural sunlight. Dangers include burns, premature aging of the skin, and the increased risk of skin cancer.

Protect children and teach them sun safety at an early age.
- Healthy habits are best learned by the young. Because skin damage occurs with each unprotected exposure and accumulates over the course of a lifetime, sun safety for children should be a priority.

FIGURE 30–1   Guidelines for the Prevention of Skin Cancer

Source: Adapted from the Skin Cancer Foundation. (1992).

Step 1.
Make sure the room is well lighted, and that you have nearby a full-length mirror, a hand-held mirror, a hand-held dryer, and two chairs or stools. Undress completely.

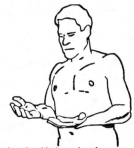

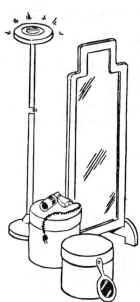

Step 2.
Hold your hands with the palms face up, as shown. Look at your palms, fingers, spaces between the fingers, and forearms. Then turn your hands over and examine the backs of your hands, fingers, spaces between the fingers, fingernails, and forearms.

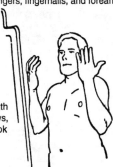

Step 3.
Now position yourself in front of the full-length mirror. Hold up your arms, bent at the elbows, with your palms facing you. In the mirror, look at the backs of your forearms and elbows.

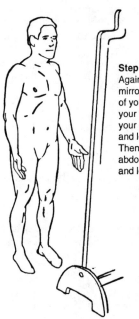

Step 4.
Again using the full-length mirror, observe the entire front of your body. In turn, look at your face, neck, and arms. Turn your palms to face the mirror and look at your upper arms. Then look at your chest and abdomen, pubic area, thighs, and lower legs.

Step 5.
Still standing in front of the mirror, lift your arms over your head with the palms facing each other. Turn so that your right side is facing the mirror and look at the entire side of your body: your hands and arms, underarms, sides of your trunk, thighs and lower legs. Then turn, and repeat the process for your left side.

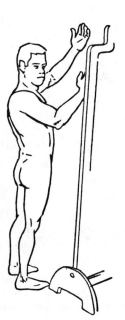

FIGURE 30–2   Skin Self-Examination Techniques

Source From R. J. Friedman, D. S. Rigel, & A. W. Kopf. (1990). *Early detection of malignant melanoma: The role of physician examination and self-examination of the skin* (pp. 20–23). Atlanta, GA: American Cancer Society. Reprinted with permission of the publisher.

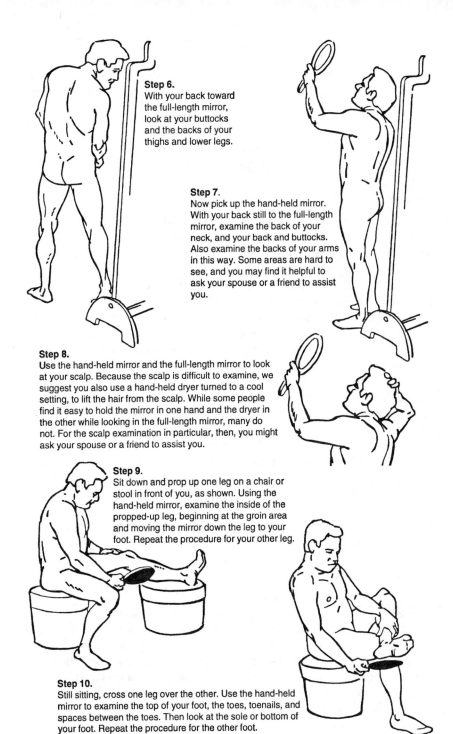

Step 6.
With your back toward the full-length mirror, look at your buttocks and the backs of your thighs and lower legs.

Step 7.
Now pick up the hand-held mirror. With your back still to the full-length mirror, examine the back of your neck, and your back and buttocks. Also examine the backs of your arms in this way. Some areas are hard to see, and you may find it helpful to ask your spouse or a friend to assist you.

Step 8.
Use the hand-held mirror and the full-length mirror to look at your scalp. Because the scalp is difficult to examine, we suggest you also use a hand-held dryer turned to a cool setting, to lift the hair from the scalp. While some people find it easy to hold the mirror in one hand and the dryer in the other while looking in the full-length mirror, many do not. For the scalp examination in particular, then, you might ask your spouse or a friend to assist you.

Step 9.
Sit down and prop up one leg on a chair or stool in front of you, as shown. Using the hand-held mirror, examine the inside of the propped-up leg, beginning at the groin area and moving the mirror down the leg to your foot. Repeat the procedure for your other leg.

Step 10.
Still sitting, cross one leg over the other. Use the hand-held mirror to examine the top of your foot, the toes, toenails, and spaces between the toes. Then look at the sole or bottom of your foot. Repeat the procedure for the other foot.

FIGURE 30–2 Continued

Other signs and symptoms of melanoma include a change in the size, color, or surface of a nevus; development of an irregular border; and oozing, bleeding, itchiness, tenderness, or pain.

BASAL CELL CARCINOMA AND SQUAMOUS CELL CARCINOMA

Pathology

Basal cell carcinoma occurs primarily on sun-exposed areas of the body—the head, neck, and arms. It frequently appears as a raised, nodular lesion with a smooth, clear border and telangiectasia. Ulceration, bleeding, and pruritus may be present. Lesions appear during the middle years or old age. Recurrence can appear within the treatment scar, at the edge of a skin graft, or within the suture line. This type of skin cancer rarely metastasizes.

Squamous cell carcinoma commonly arises on sun-damaged skin or from preexisting skin lesions (e.g., actinic/solar keratoses or burns). Approximately 1% of untreated actinic keratoses develop into squamous cell carcinomas. A squamous cell carcinoma appears as a scaly, keratotic, slightly elevated nodule. Oval or circular in shape, the lesion may ulcerate and, if not treated, may become a fungating mass. **Metastases** can occur in proximal lymph nodes or visceral organs such as the lungs. **Tumors** on the lips, ears, vulva, or penis, or those that deeply invade the dermal layers, are more likely to metastasize.

Diagnosis of both cancers is made by histologic examination. An incisional, shave, or punch biopsy may be obtained to confirm the diagnosis. Basal and squamous cell carcinomas are classified as Grade 1 through 4 depending on the histologic **differentiation.** Grade 1 has the highest differentiation and lowest metastatic potential, Grade 2 is moderately well **differentiated,** Grade 3 is poorly differentiated, and Grade 4 has the least number of differentiated cells and the most number of atypical cells.

Treatment

Both cancers have a favorable prognosis. About 90% to 95% of basal cell and 75% to 80% of squamous cell carcinomas can be cured. Surgery and radiation therapy produce comparable results. The most significant treatment risks include disfigurement and functional impairment of the head and neck.

Several types of surgeries are used for treatment, including curettage and electrosurgery (electrodesiccation, electrocoagulation or electrocautery), cryosurgery (liquid nitrogen) alone or with curettage and electrosurgery, excision, Mohs surgery, and laser surgery. In **Mohs surgery,** the tumor is removed and each layer is microscopically examined to ensure a complete resection of cancerous tissue while preserving normal tissue. This technique is frequently used for aggressive or recurrent tumors where cosmetic appearance is important (e.g., eyelid, nose, helix of the ear, or lips). Depending on the size and location of the tumor, flaps or full- or split-thickness skin grafts may be necessary following excisional or

Mohs surgery. Lymph node involvement is treated with dissection and, when needed, radiation therapy.

Wound care routines include cleansing with diluted hydrogen peroxide or soap and water, followed by application of antibiotic ointment and a Telfa™ dressing. Complications such as scarring, delayed wound healing, or occasional bleeding, if desiccated tissue separates from the wound, can occur.

Radiation therapy can be effective in treating primary or recurrent tumors or as palliation of inoperable tumors in some patients. Patients may be considered for radiation if they are elderly, medically debilitated, or poor surgical risks, or if they have large lesions that might create a cosmetic defect if removed surgically. Patients receive 4,000 to 6,000 cGy in fractionated doses depending on tumor size. If there is a recurrence, subsequent surgery is difficult to perform because of gradual skin changes following radiation.

The use of topical chemotherapy (5-fluorouracil) is limited to actinic keratoses and superficial basal cell carcinomas on the face, trunk, or extremities because the drug does not penetrate to tumor cells below the epidermis. Researchers are currently studying the effects of injecting agents such as alpha interferon and 5-fluorouracil directly into the lesions. This research may identify new ways to treat patients who are not surgical candidates.

Follow-up should be individualized and scheduled regularly to assess for recurrence or metastases from the treated tumor or for the development of additional tumors. Approximately 95% of all recurrences and metastases of squamous cell carcinomas occur within 5 years of initial treatment. High-risk patients need lifelong follow-up.

MALIGNANT MELANOMA

Pathology

Malignant melanoma originates in proliferative, single melanocytes in the lower epidermis. Lesions can arise on any epithelial surface (e.g., gall bladder, esophagus, meninges, vagina, or upper respiratory tract), but they usually occur on the skin. Growth can proceed radially or vertically. These cancers are found predominantly on the trunk, head, and neck of males and on the lower and upper extremities of females. When African Americans develop melanomas, they are commonly located on less-pigmented skin areas, such as the palms of the hands and the soles of the feet, and on subungual areas.

Excisional or incisional biopsy is performed to obtain tissue for pathologic examination. In 1988, the American Joint Committee on Cancer revised the **staging** system for melanoma. They combined the Clark system and the Breslow system, which examined level of invasion (epidermis to subcutaneous tissue) and tumor thickness, respectively (see Table 30–2). Together the two systems are a highly significant prognostic indicator. The 5-year **survival rate** is 93% for localized disease and 57% for regional disease; distant metastatic disease survival is only 15%. About 82% of melanomas are localized at the time of diagnosis. Melanoma metastasizes to lymph nodes, skin, lung, brain, liver, and bone.

TABLE 30–2   Revised Staging System for Malignant Melanoma:
American Joint Committee on Cancer*

Stage	Criteria	TNM
IA	Localized melanoma < 0.75 mm or Level II	T1N0M0
IB	Localized melanoma 0.76–1.5 mm or Level III	T2N0M0
IIA	Localized melanoma 1.5–4 mm or Level IV	T3N0M0
IIB	Localized melanoma > 4 mm or Level V	T4N0M0
III	Nodal metastases involving only one regional lymph node basin or fewer than 5 in-transit metastases in the absence of nodal disease	any T, N1M0
IV	Advanced regional metastases or distant metastases	any T, any N, M1 or 2

*When thickness and level of invasion do not coincide within a T classification, thickness takes precedence.

Source: From M. N. Harris, R. L. Shapiro, & D. F. Roses. (1995). Malignant melanoma. Cancer, 75, 716. Copyright © 1995. Reprinted with permission of Wiley-Liss, a division of John Wiley and Sons, Inc.

Researchers have examined the relationship between melanoma development and menstruation, pregnancy and exogenous hormones. Studies have noted that women diagnosed during pregnancy have shorter disease-free survival time and greater likelihood of lymph node metastases. Long-term survival rates, however, are the same for each group. The single most important prognostic indicator is tumor thickness. Additional studies have been unable to link melanoma development to menstrual or exogenous hormone factors.

Treatment

The primary therapy for localized melanomas is wide excisional surgery. Margins of normal tissue are usually excised at this time to prevent recurrence at the surgical borders. Biopsy and definitive surgery may be performed as a one- or two-stage procedure. Lymph node dissection is performed when thicker lesions (1–4 mm) are excised to determine regional lymph node involvement. Larger excisions may require skin grafting. Melanomas of the fingers and toes, regardless of thickness, are treated by amputation of the involved digit.

Adjuvant chemotherapy and **immunotherapy** continue to be studied to improve survival or to palliate Stage IV disease. Dacarbazine (DTIC) alone has about a 20% response rate and is used to treat metastatic skin lesions, subcutaneous tissue, and lymph nodes. Combination regimens include DTIC with cisplatin, carmustine or vinblastine and tamoxifen. The main side effects are nausea and vomiting and can be treated with antiemetics (see Chapter 9).

Limb perfusion may be used for patients with multiple recurrences or local nodal metastases. In this procedure, the major artery and vein of the affected extremity are isolated with a tourniquet and then temporarily oxygenated and perfused by a corporeal bypass machine. Extremely high doses of chemotherapy (6–10 times the usual systemic dose) are infused into the tumor. The tourniquet prevents systemic distribution of the drug. After 1 hour, the chemotherapy is stopped and the tourniquet is removed. The most common drug used for limb perfusion is melphalan.

Biologic response modifiers such as alpha **interferon** and **interleukin-2** alone and with **lymphokine-activated killer (LAK) cells** have been studied with varying results. Currently, infiltrating tumors with **tumor-infiltrating lymphocyte (TIL) cells** that contain the gene for cytokines, i.e., the **tumor necrosis factor (TNF)**, is being investigated. A melanoma vaccine to prevent the disease has been successfully developed in an animal model. It has been shown to slow the progression of metastatic lesions in some patients, but it is still in the experimental phase and its efficacy is not known at this time.

Since most melanomas are not radiosensitive, the use of radiation therapy is reserved for palliating symptoms of pain and obstruction in the brain, bone, and lymph nodes.

Lifelong follow-up is needed for all patients with early diagnosed disease. They are at risk for developing additional lesions. Those diagnosed with advanced disease need follow-up for treatment-related side effects and may need referral to hospice care.

KAPOSI'S SARCOMA

Pathology

The classical form of **Kaposi's sarcoma (KS)** appears as dark blue to reddish-purple spots or nodules on the arms (25%) or legs (75%). Patients exhibit edema and may have involved lymph nodes or viscera. In those who are HIV-positive, epidemic KS is the most common malignancy and is characterized by smaller pink to purple lesions on the trunk, head, and neck. Most patients have multiple lesions and edema secondary to lymph node blockage. Visceral lesions can occur on the gastrointestional (GI) tract, lungs, liver, pancreas, gingiva, pharynx, tongue, soft palate, adrenal glands, spleen, testes, and larynx. GI lesions result in diarrhea. Pulmonary lesions cause **dyspnea,** orthopnea, and cough, which may be incorrectly attributed to pneumocystis carinii pneumonia. Many patients have additional symptoms that may be related to immunodeficiency and infection, such as fever, weight loss, malaise, and **anorexia.** Both forms are rarely curable, but they are not life threatening.

Treatment

Treatment for both forms of KS is palliative and aimed at improving quality of life. Therapy may be limited because of side effects that may not be well tolerated by elderly or immunocompromised patients. Patients with classical KS have a 10 to 15-year life expectancy, while those with the epidemic form have shorter life spans and usually die of opportunistic infections.

Radiation is used to treat facial lesions or those that cause local problems such as plantar lesions that limit mobility or pharyngeal lesions that result in dysphagia.

Treatment regimes in HIV-positive patients with systemic disease include chemotherapy and alpha interferon, antiretrovirals (e.g., zidovadine), prophylaxis for opportunistic infection, and hematological support (e.g., GM-CSF). Chemotherapy agents such as vinblastine, vincristine, etoposide, bleomycin, or doxorubicin are used alone or in combination. Patients need careful monitoring for symptoms of immunosuppression. Research in the use of navelbine, paclitaxel, beta and gamma interferon, angiogenic inhibitors, and retinoids is continuing and may help future patients.

NURSING CONSIDERATIONS

All nurses, regardless of their area of practice, can aid in the prevention and early detection of NMSC. Pediatric and school nurses can educate children, adolescents, and their parents about the dangers of overexposure to the sun in early life and the need for protective clothing, sunblocks, and sunglasses. Those working with adult and geriatric populations can teach monthly skin self-examination and emphasize avoidance of tanning booths and use of protective barriers. When skin self-examination is practiced, NMSC and melanomas are detected early and cure rates are high.

Nursing care of patients undergoing radiation or chemotherapy for all types of skin cancer consists of interventions to minimize treatment-related side effects. Some patients require cosmetic surgery to correct defects and improve their appearance. All patients need encouragement to continue periodic follow-up, because they are at increased risk for recurrence or the development of additional skin cancers. Terminally ill patients with advanced melanoma or Kaposi's sarcoma will also need referral to a hospice program.

CONCLUSION

As rates of skin cancer continue to climb, researchers are looking for newer interventions to offer patients. The use of biological response modifiers, intralesional chemotherapy, and the development of a melanoma vaccine for humans are some of the potential interventions that may become available in the next century.

BIBLIOGRAPHY

Fleming, I. D., Amonette, R., Monaghan, T., & Fleming, M. D. (1995). The principles of management of basal and squamous cell carcinoma of the skin. *Cancer, 75,* 699–704.

Friedman, R. J., Rigel, D. S., Silverman, M. K., Kopf, A. W., & Vossaert, K. A. (1991). *Malignant melanoma in the 1990s: The continued importance of early detection and the role of the physician examination and self-examination of the skin.* Atlanta, GA: American Cancer Society, 1–26.

Harris, M. N., Shapiro, R. L., & Roses, D. F. (1995). Malignant melanoma. *Cancer, 75,* 715–725.

Johnson, T. M., Rowe, D. E., Nelson, B., & Swanson, N. A. (1992). Squamous cell carcinoma of the skin (excluding lip and oral mucosa). *Journal of the American Academy of Dermatology, 26,* 467–484.

Lilenbaum, R. C., & Ratner, L. (1994). Systemic treatment of Kaposi's sarcoma: Current status and future directions. *AIDS, 8,* 141–151.

Loescher, L. J., Buller, M. K., Buller, D. B., Emerson, J., & Taylor, A. M. (1995). Public education projects in skin cancer. *Cancer, 75,* 651–656.

Marks, R. (1995). An overview of skin cancers. *Cancer, 75,* 607–612.

Rhodes, A. R. (1995). Public education and cancer of the skin. *Cancer, 75,* 613–636.

31

Cancers of the Bone

Michele V. Bennett

In the 1960s, when surgery alone was used for the treatment of primary bone cancer, only 15% to 20% of patients experienced long-term survival. The current outlook is much more optimistic. New surgical limb-sparing techniques, in conjunction with new **chemotherapy** regimens and radiation (for certain **tumors**), have decreased the need for amputation in many cases, and overall **survival rates** have improved dramatically. When the treatment regimen includes pre- or postoperative chemotherapy, survival can increase to up to 80%.

INCIDENCE

Primary malignant bone tumors are uncommon, comprising approximately 0.2% of all new cancer cases in the United States. In 1996, it was estimated that 2,500 new primary bone malignancies would be diagnosed. The **incidence** of primary bone cancer is highest in children and adolescents. Cancer **metastases** to bone from other primary tumors are more common than primary bone malignancies in all age groups.

RISK FACTORS

Although the precise cause of bone cancer is not known, several factors are known to contribute to its development. Periods of rapid skeletal growth seem to be associated with at least some bone cancers, since the incidence of bone cancer is highest during the adolescent growth spurt. Individuals with conditions that stimulate increased bone metabolism, such as Paget's disease and hyperparathyroidism, are also at increased **risk** for bone cancer, as are patients with certain congenital abnormalities such as Ollier's disease or multiple enchondromatosis. The role of the P53 gene in bone cancer is presently being studied.

CLINICAL MANIFESTATIONS

Symptoms of bone cancer vary according to the type and location of the tumor. Pain is the prevailing symptom. Typically, the pain is unrelated to position or activity and is more intense at night. Some patients may also exhibit a palpable mass. Other signs and symptoms include a fracture that does not heal, a pathological fracture, weight loss, fever, and generalized malaise. The lungs are the most common site for metastases to occur because the cells spread through a hematogenous route. Symptoms of pulmonary involvement range from cough to **dyspnea** to pleural effusion.

Laboratory tests may reveal some common abnormalities. Patients may present with an elevated alkaline phosphatase (osteogenic sarcoma), an elevated lactate dehydrogenase (LDH) (Ewing's sarcoma), abnormal blood count, **anemia,** or an elevated erythrocyte sedimentation rate.

DIAGNOSIS AND EVALUATION

X-ray is the best and least expensive diagnostic tool that exists today. Almost all primary bone tumors can be found on an x-ray. Commonly, a lesion is found on x-ray, and if it is suspicious for a malignancy, the patient usually undergoes either **magnetic resonance imaging (MRI)** or a **computerized axial tomography (CT)** scan, and possibly angiography. A bone scan is done to evaluate for metastases or skip lesions, which are lesions in the same bone but are not at the primary site of the lesion. The patient then undergoes a surgical biopsy, which can be performed through a CT-guided needle biopsy or open surgical biopsy. Once the cellular **histology** is known, a treatment plan is determined for the specific tumor. This plan may include pre- and postoperative chemotherapy, surgery, radiation, or all three types of treatment. The type of surgery, limb sparing or amputation, depends on the results of the work-up as well as the patient's response to chemotherapy, if necessary.

Patients with a newly diagnosed bone cancer, especially adults, should be evaluated for an undiagnosed primary tumor, since metastatic lesions to the bone are more common than primary cancers. Cancers of the lung, breast, prostate, kidney, and thyroid are the most common sites of origin that metastasize to bone.

TYPES OF BONE CANCER

Bone tumors are named according to the cell type from which they originate.

Osteosarcoma

The most common primary bone-forming tumor, **osteosarcoma,** primarily affects children and young adults. Osteosarcoma arises from **osteoblast cells,** cells that multiply rapidly during periods of skeletal growth. Osteosarcoma is diagnosed in 20% of patients with a primary bone tumor and affects males more commonly than females (1.5:1). A majority of these tumors are located around the knee joint, in either the distal femur or the proximal tibia. The proximal humerus is also a common site for this tumor.

Many patients with osteosarcoma can be treated successfully with new surgical techniques that salvage the affected limb. With this approach, the segment of bone containing the tumor, as well as margins of unaffected tissue, including bone, muscles, tendons, ligaments, and even nerves on all sides of the tumor, are surgically removed. Bone can be reconstructed using autologous bone (fibula), cadaveric allografts, or endoprostheses.

Not all patients are candidates for limb salvage. The major contraindications are major neurovascular involvement or the presence of pathologic fractures or infection before surgery. Also, young children whose linear growth is incomplete frequently will have better functional results with amputation and prostheses than with resection. Tumors can be controlled locally with surgery, but they frequently metastasize to the lungs if no other therapy is utilized.

Some patients who undergo an amputation may experience postoperative phantom pain, the perception of sensation in the amputated portion of the limb. While some degree of this sensation is common after amputation, severe or prolonged phantom pain occurs only in a very small percentage of amputees. Once the incision is healed, wearing a prosthesis or wrapping an elastic bandage around the stump and pulling on the ends may help alleviate phantom sensation by providing a tactile reminder of where the limb ends. Medication such as amitryptilline is presently being used with success to help control phantom pain. Calcitonin, a drug used in the treatment of osteoporosis, is also effective in control of phantom pain.

Combination chemotherapy has proven effective against osteosarcomas and is now a routine part of treatment. The use of chemotherapy before surgery has become widespread and permits intraoperative assessment of tumor response to the chemotherapy regimen. Modifications of the regimen can then be made postoperatively if tumor response has been inadequate. Patients undergoing treatment for a **malignant** bone tumor should be informed that it may take up to a year to complete a specific protocol if it includes chemotherapy.

High-dose methotrexate infusions, doxorubicin, cyclophosphamide, and cisplatin are among the most commonly used chemotherapeutic agents. However, new therapies, including ifosfamide and other agents, are being tested throughout the United States to help improve the survival rate for this condition. Patients receiving infusions of high-dose methotrexate must be well hydrated and be given oral or intravenous sodium bicarbonate to keep the urine alkaline (pH > 7) to promote excretion of the methotrexate. Side effects of methotrexate can be severe, and they include bone marrow depression, **mucositis,** nausea and vomiting, **alopecia,** and renal impairment. **Citrovorum factor** (leucovorin calcium) must be administered at specified intervals after the high-dose methotrexate infusion to "rescue" normal cells from the toxic effects of methotrexate. Further information on chemotherapy and chemotherapeutic agents is found in Chapter 9.

Chondrosarcoma

Chondrosarcoma is the second most common bone malignancy, occurring in 17% to 22% of all patients diagnosed with a primary bone tumor. It occurs more frequently in males than in females (1.8:1) and is seen most frequently in adults between 30 and 60 years of age. This tumor arises from cartilage and is usually located in the pelvis, femur, proximal humerus, or ribs. Since this tumor responds poorly to radiation and chemotherapy, surgery remains the treatment of choice. Radical resection of the tumor, including amputation, is the treatment of choice except for patients with low-grade chondrosarcoma who are candidates for local excision and bone reconstruction. Five-year survival rates range from 55% to 75%, depending on whether any soft tissue or lymph nodes are involved. High-dose radiotherapy may be given to patients with unresectable or metastatic disease; it is used in combination with surgery for patients with disease in the facial bones or skull. Chemotherapy also is utilized for patients with metastases.

Ewing's Sarcoma

Ewing's sarcoma is a marrow-originating tumor consisting of small round cells. It is seen in 10% to 14% of patients diagnosed with a malignant bone tumor, primarily children and adolescents. It affects males twice as frequently as females. This tumor arises most commonly in the diaphysis of long bones and in flat bones. Five-year survival rates range from 50% to 75%. Late relapse, more than 10 years after treatment, is not uncommon for patients with Ewing's sarcoma.

These patients may present with an anemia or a tumor fever. In addition, the LDH is a **tumor marker** for these patients.

In the past, standard therapy for this radiosensitive tumor consisted of megavoltage radiation followed by chemotherapy. Recently, patient outcomes have been improved by a treatment regimen that includes surgical excision of the tumor combined with pre- and postoperative chemotherapy. Radiation is still used in the management of surgically inaccessible tumors or tumors whose removal would result in significant disability.

The chemotherapeutic agents most commonly used to treat Ewing's sarcoma are adriamycin®, cytoxan®, vincristine, VP16, and ifosfamide. Doxorubicin and dactinomycin administered following irradiation can potentiate local skin toxicity. Commonly called *radiation recall*, the reaction consists of erythema, vesicle formation, or wet desquamation in the area that was irradiated.

Fibrosarcoma

Fibrosarcoma is a rare type of bone tumor consisting of interlacing bundles of collagen cells. This tumor is five times less common than osteosarcoma and most commonly affects persons from 20 through 60 years of age. It affects males slightly more frequently than females. Fibrosarcoma most commonly affects the femur and tibia, is radioresistant, and is generally treated with surgical resection or amputation. The 5-year survival rate is 25%.

METASTATIC BONE CANCER

Metastatic lesions to bone are more common than primary bone tumors. Breast, lung, prostate, kidney, and thyroid are the most common tumors that metastasize to bone. It is important to understand that although a patient may have a tumor in the bone, it does not mean the patient has primary bone cancer. The cells that make up the tumor originate from the primary site of the cancer. Metastasis to bone indicates disseminated disease. A suspected lesion is evaluated by x-ray, MRI or CT, and bone scan. Patients may complain of pain in a joint or bone, indicating impending or microfractures, or they may present with a pathological fracture. If the site of metastatic bone disease is a weight-bearing area or if the patient has fractured the bone, stabilization surgery needs to be performed before any further treatment can take place. When a lytic bone lesion is documented by diagnostic tests, often 50% of the bone has already been destroyed.

The goals of surgical intervention for bone metastases are to control local and progressive disease, maintain joint or extremity function, and prevent fracture of the bone. Such treatment enables the patient to continue **adjuvant therapy** without interruption.

For spinal lesions, external splinting may be used, alone or along with surgery. Patients with metastases to the spine are at high risk for spinal cord compression (see Chapter 17).

Radiotherapy may be used before surgery or for palliation of pain. It is also used following surgery to kill the bone tumor. Chemotherapy may be used to reduce the tumor mass; however, if used in conjunction with surgery, its administration will usually be delayed until wound healing is complete, since it can disrupt wound healing.

New drugs and isotopes are being utilized to help relieve symptoms associated with metastatic bone disease. Bisphosphanates such as pamidronate are used to help treat **hypercalcemia** associated with metastatic bone disease. Calcitonin, a hormone, helps to treat bone pain. It is now available as a nasal spray. Strontium 89 is a radioisotope that relieves pain as well. Although this drug can give symptom relief for up to 4 months, it is not without serious side effects.

NURSING CONSIDERATIONS

Cancers of the bone occur in patients of widely different age groups. Because developmental stage and lifestyle alterations have a major impact on a patient's adjustment to the diagnosis and treatment of bone cancer, it is important that the nurse consider these variables when planning interventions and assessing responses.

A major consideration for patients with metastatic bone cancer is quality of life. This includes issues such as pain, mobility, ability to participate in activities of daily living, emotional trauma, and identification of **support** systems.

Patients should be knowledgeable about their disease and its course. Nurses teach patients about the various tests and procedures such as x-rays, CT/MRI, bone scan, biopsy, chemotherapy, and radiation. Nurses also help patients to identify support systems that will help them to manage and cope with their disease. Patients should also be informed about mobility restrictions, pain, skin integrity problems, infection risks, and the importance of emotional support and nutrition.

Many patients experience some degree of pain, which is usually treated with opioids. Patients who have undergone amputation may experience phantom limb pain. This pain can be treated with analgesic medication and tactile stimuli, such as rubbing the "stump" or the distal end of the amputated limb.

Impaired mobility is experienced by patients who have undergone either amputation or limb salvage procedures. The goal of nursing care is to maximize the patient's functional ability. Patients should be taught preoperatively how to ambulate with assistive devices such as a walker, cane, or crutches, and to perform activities of daily living with the use of assistive devices. Referral to physical or occupational therapists helps the patient learn and practice the use of assistive devices.

Nurses should understand that surgery for bone tumors differs from surgery for **benign** conditions. Protecting the surgical site for a lengthy period of time while the patient completes radiation or chemotherapy is essential. Crutches are required for ambulation until the prosthetic bone is stabilized, the surrounding tissue has healed, and muscle strength is restored. Proper body mechanics, the use of assistive devices, and comfort measures in the form of pain medication are necessary prior to physical and occupational therapy sessions.

Patients suffering from bone cancer are prone to develop impaired skin integrity and infections. These patients are frequently immunosuppressed and may require additional therapy in the form of antibiotics. Maintaining a clean environment and proper handwashing technique before and after patient contact is imperative. Although identical precautions should be maintained for nontumor patients, they generally have an intact immune system.

Almost all patients have a fear of the unknown. Identifying support systems early after diagnosis is essential to help the patient and family cope with the meaning of a new cancer diagnosis, the loss or disfigurement of a body part, or the treatment protocol, which itself can be devastating.

Proper nutrition is important to maintain adequate caloric, fluid, and electrolyte balance. Amputees burn more calories than nonamputee patients. The side effects of chemotherapy are many, including mucositis, nausea, vomiting, diarrhea, constipation, and changes in taste. Patients need to be taught the importance of a balanced, healthy diet. They should be taught to eat fresh fruits and vegetables, and any other foods or fluids to increase caloric intake. Nurses should monitor weight, fluid intake and output, and eating habits. If nutritional or hydration status declines, nurses should recommend nutritional support. Meticulous oral care, use of topical anesthetics for mucositis, and dietary alterations may help alleviate nutritional problems.

CONCLUSION

The treatment of primary bone cancers and metastases to bone continues to evolve. It is important for the nurse to understand the many diverse needs of this patient population, enabling the patient and family to make knowledgeable decisions and participate in the treatment for this disease.

BIBLIOGRAPHY

Abeloff, M. D., Armitage, J. O., Lichter, A. S., & Niederhuber, J. E. (Eds). (1995). *Clinical oncology.* New York: Churchill Livingston.

Harris, J., Hellman, S., Henderson, I., & Kinne, D. (1991). *Breast diseases* Philadelphia: J. B. Lippincott.

Huvos, A. G. (1991). *Bone tumors: Diagnosis, treatment, and prognosis* (2nd ed). Philadelphia: W. B. Saunders.

Lane, J., & Healey, J. (1993). *Diagnosis and management of pathologic fractures.* New York: Raven.

Piasecki, P. (1993). Bone and soft tissue sarcoma. In S. Groenwald, M. H. Frogge, M. Goodman, & C. H. Yarbro (Eds.), *Cancer nursing* (3rd ed., pp. 877–902). Sudbury, MA: Jones and Bartlett.

Racolin, A. (1992). Metastases to bone: Incidence, issues, and implications for nursing. *Current Issues in Cancer Nursing Practice Updates, 1*(5), 1–12.

Rounseville, C. (1992). Phantom limb pain: The ghost that haunts the amputee. *Orthopaedic Nursing, 11,* 67–71.

Strang, P., & Qvarner, H. (1990). Cancer related pain and its influence on quality of life. *Anticancer Research, 10,* 109–112.

Williamson, V. C. (1992). Amputation of the lower extremity: An overview. *Orthopaedic Nursing, 11,* 55–65.

32

Leukemia

Colette N. Chaney
Patricia Jassak

The leukemias are a complex collection of hematologic **malignant** disorders of the blood and blood-forming organs (the spleen, lymphatic system, and bone marrow). **Leukemia** is characterized by a proliferation of abnormal blood cells that infiltrate the bone marrow, peripheral blood, and other organs.

CLASSIFICATION

Leukemia is classified into two types: acute and chronic, depending on the onset of symptoms and the differentiation (maturity) of the cells involved. Acute and chronic leukemia are similar, since both diseases result from dysfunctional bone marrow. However, they are strikingly different in disease presentation, treatment, and prognosis. In acute leukemia, there is a rapid onset of symptoms resulting from an overproduction of cells arrested in the blast (early nonfunctional) stage of maturation. These immature blast cells are incapable of performing the normal function of mature hematopoietic cells. In chronic leukemia, the maturation process is arrested at a later stage, but these cells also are ineffective and highly proliferative.

The two types of leukemia are further **differentiated** by the predominant cell line affected, which is either lymphocytic or myelocytic. Leukemic cells that belong to the myeloid (granulocytic) cell line, such as promyelocytes, myelocytes, and granulocytes, are classified as a nonlymphocytic or myelocytic leukemia. Leukemia cells produced in the lymphoid cell line cause lymphocytic leukemia.

Lymphocytic leukemia is further classified by the presence of antigens on the cell surface of the lymphocyte. Nonlymphocytic leukemia is subclassified according to the hematopoietic cell type that predominates. Figure 32–1 identifies the

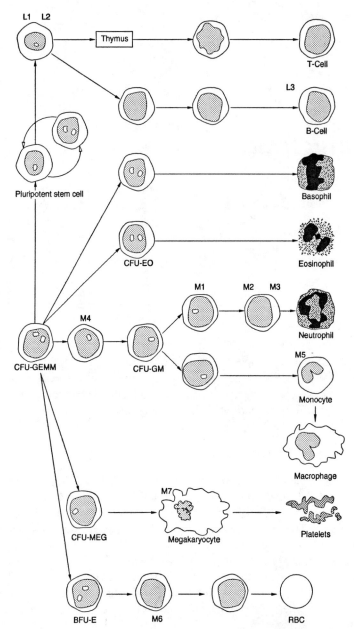

FIGURE 32–1 Hematopoietic Cascade with FAB Classification of Aute
Nonlymphocytic Leukemia and Acute Lymphocytic Leukemia
at Proposed Levels of Arrested Cell Maturation.

BFU = burst-forming unit, CFU = colony-forming unit, GM = granulocyte-macrophage, E = erythrocyte, EO = eosinophil, EPO = erythropoietin, GEMM = granulocyte-erythrocyte-macrophage-
megakaryocyte, L1 = childhood, L2 = adult, L3 = Burkitt's type, M1 = undifferentiated myelocytic,
M2 = myelocytic, M3 = promyelocytic, M4 = myelomonocytic, M5 = monocytic, M6 = erythro-
leukemia, M7 = megakaryocytic, MEG = megakaryocyte.

Source: Wujcik, D. (1993). Leukemia. In S. L. Greenwald, M. H. Frogge, M. Goodman, & C. H.
Yarbro (Eds.), *Cancer nursing: Principles and practice* (3rd ed., p. 1152). Sudbury, MA: Jones and
Bartlett. Reprinted with permission.

levels of arrested cell **differentiation** for acute lymphocytic and myelocytic leukemia.

INCIDENCE

Leukemia accounts for approximately 2.1% of all cancer cases in the United States. It was estimated that 27,600 new cases of leukemia would be diagnosed in 1996. Approximately 40% of leukemia cases are lymphocytic leukemia (acute and chronic), while myelocytic leukemias (acute and chronic) account for 46%. The remaining 14% of leukemia cases are unspecified.

Chronic lymphocytic leukemia (CLL) accounts for approximately 25% of all leukemias and occurs predominately in the older population. **Chronic myelocytic leukemia (CML)** affects patients at any age, with a peak **incidence** between the ages of 40 and 60. CML accounts for 10% to 15% of the annual incidence of leukemia.

In the United States 11,000 new cases of acute leukemia are diagnosed annually. Of acute leukemias, 25% occur in children and 75% occur in adults. Further delineation based on predominant cell type and population affected reveals that 80% of **acute lymphocytic leukemia (ALL)** cases occur in children, with a peak incidence at 3 to 4 years of age. ALL is rare in adults after 40 years of age.

Acute myelocytic (nonlymphocytic) leukemia (AML or ANLL) occurs most often in adults (90%), with the incidence gradually increasing with age; 30% of patients with AML are more than 60 years old.

RISK FACTORS

The etiology of leukemia is not fully understood, but several predisposing factors have been identified. Exposure to ionizing radiation remains the most conclusively identified leukemogenic factor in humans. Recently, attention has focused on exposure to electromagnetic fields as a contributor to cancer. However, to date, no form of electromagnetic energy at frequency levels below those of ionizing radiation and ultraviolet radiation has been shown to cause cancer.

Prior drug therapies that have demonstrated an increased **risk** in the subsequent development of leukemia include the antibiotic chloramphenicol, phenyl butazone, and alkylating agents. In addition, certain chemicals have the ability to mutate or ablate the bone marrow **stem cells** and produce acute leukemia. Benzene (found in unleaded gasoline, rubber cement, and cleaning solvents) has been implicated in the development of acute leukemia. Exposures to hair dye and paint and other occupational exposures to chemicals remain under investigation.

Several hereditary syndromes are associated with chromosomal abnormalities that demonstrate an increased risk for the development of acute leukemia. They include, but are not limited to, Bloom's syndrome, Down syndrome, Kleinfelter's syndrome, and Fanconi's anemia. Familial risk factors also exist. A fivefold risk increase for the development of acute leukemia exists if a family member has been previously diagnosed with AML. Hematologic diseases such as myelodys-plastic syndrome (MDS) and CML are known to transform over the course of the disease into acute leukemias. Viruses, especially a group of RNA viruses that can cause leukemia in animals, possibly play a role in the etiology of human leukemia. This remains unproven. Increasing age is a **risk factor** for the development of chronic leukemias as well as AML.

EARLY DETECTION

Manifestations of acute leukemia are the result of an abnormal proliferation of cells that are arrested in an early stage of the maturation process. This increased proliferation causes crowding and inhibits the functional ability of normal hematopoietic cells.

The most common symptoms of the acute leukemias include nonspecific fatigue and weakness, bruising, fever, persistent infection, and weight loss. Abdominal fullness related to hepatosplenomegaly, headaches, nausea, vomiting, and blurred vision from central nervous system involvement are also initial symptoms reported.

Chronic leukemias are often discovered by chance on a routine complete blood count (CBC) evaluation. Chronic fatigue and reduced exercise capacity are usually the first symptoms. Other clinical manifestations develop as the leukemic cells infiltrate the bone marrow, lymph nodes, spleen, and liver. These symptoms present as fever and night sweats, bone pain, easy bruising and petechiae, abdominal fullness, and early satiety with weight loss from splenomegaly or hepatomegaly.

DIAGNOSIS

A thorough diagnostic workup for leukemia is imperative so that the specific classification and the predominant cell type involved can be identified. CBC results and peripheral blood smears may suggest a **diagnosis** of leukemia, but confirmation is based on a full examination of the bone marrow. This is accomplished by a bone marrow procedure in which specimens are obtained for morphology, pathology, immunology, and cytogenetic evaluations. (Generally the bone marrow procedure is an aspirate. A small core of the bone is removed, bone marrow fluid is taken, and a biopsy is performed.)

Morphologic evaluations include an assessment of cellularity, cell type, and stage of differentiation. Special stains such as Sudan black or myeloperoxidase (MPO) permit the designation of **French-American-British (FAB) morphology** classification categories. Immunophenotyping complements morphology and is especially useful in discriminating AML from ALL. It is also helpful in correctly diagnosing subgroups of each classification by determining the lineage and stage of differentiation of the leukemic cells.

Cytogenetic analysis in leukemia can be used to predict prognosis and enables the health care team to choose treatment related to the prognosis. For example, in AML a translocation of chromosomes 8 and 21 or an inversion of chromosome 16 is predictive of a high complete remission rate, a long complete remission duration, or both (See Chapter 2). A chromosome anomaly can also confirm a diagnosis, such as in the identification of a translocation between chromosomes 15 and 17 in AML, FAB type M3, or of the translocation occurring between chromosomes 9 and 22, also known as the **Philadelphia chromosome** (Ph') in CML. Chromosome evaluation also can be useful in monitoring for disease progression. In CML, the appearance of secondary chromosome anomalies occurs approximately 3 to 6 months before **blast crisis** (transformation of chronic leukemia cells to acute leukemia due to increased proliferation and differentiation stage). Pathology evaluations determine the cellularity of the bone marrow and the percentages and presence of cell types.

Lumbar puncture is performed to assess the presence of leukemic cells in the central nervous system (CNS). This diagnostic tool is especially important in patients with ALL and AML, FAB types M4 or M5, which are known to present with a higher incidence of CNS involvement.

EVALUATION AND STAGING

Leukemias are staged using the classification systems shown in Table 32–1. The FAB classification system for acute leukemias is universally accepted and is based on analysis of cellular morphology and histochemical staining of blast cells. Unfavorable prognostic factors are identified in Figure 32–2.

TREATMENT

The goal of treatment for acute leukemia is the eradication of the leukemic stem cell. The course of therapy is divided into two stages: induction and postremission, or consolidation. With current **induction chemotherapy,** 60% to 80% of adults with acute nonlymphocytic leukemia and 70% to 80% of adults with acute lymphocytic leukemia achieve complete remission.

In AML, standard remission induction therapy is a combination of the antimetabolite cytosine arabinoside given for 7 days plus an anthracycline (daunorubicin, doxorubicin, idarubicin) or mitoxantrone. All trans-retinoic acid, a derivative of vitamin A, is a recently approved therapeutic option for patients with AML, FAB type M3 (promyelocytic). ALL remission induction therapy includes vincristine, prednisone, and an anthracycline, alone or in combination with L-asparaginase.

In postremission **(consolidation) therapy,** the goal of treatment is to prevent recurrence. Examples of AML treatment options include consolidation with higher doses of the drugs used in remission induction, intensification with different drugs in the hope that they will be effective in leukemic cells that may have become resistant, and bone marrow transplant. Several options also are available for the postremission treatment of ALL. These include such drugs as cytarabine, thioguanine, methotrexate, cyclophosphamide, and 6-mercaptopurine.

TABLE 32–1   Staging of Leukemias

Rai's Staging Classification of CLL

Stage 0	Absolute lymphocytosis > 15 × 109/1
Stage I	As stage 0 + enlarged lymph nodes (adenopathy)
Stage II	As stage 0 + anaemia (Hgb < 10g/L) ± organomegaly
Stage III	As stage 0 + anaemia (Hgb < 10g/L) ± adenopathy
Stage IV	As stage 0 + thrombocytopenia (platelets < 100 × 109/1) ± adenopathy ± organomegaly

Staging of CML

Chronic phase	≤ 15% blasts and promyelocytes in the peripheral blood and/or bone marrow
Accelerated	≥ 15% blast cells in the peripheral blood ≤ 30% blasts and promyelocytes in the peripheral blood and/or bone marrow
Blast crisis	≥ 30% blasts and promyelocytes in the peripheral blood and/or bone marrow

French-American-British (FAB) Classification of Acute Myeloid Leukemia

---

M1	Undifferentiated myelocytic
M2	Myelocytic
M3	Promyelocytic
M4	Myelomonocytic
M5	Monocytic
M6	Erythroleukemia
M7	Megakaryocytic

French-American-British (FAB) Classification of Acute Lymphocytic Leukemia

---

L1	Childhood (Pre B- and T-cell)
L2	Adult (Pre B- and T-cell)
L3	Burkitt's type (B-cell)

Maintenance chemotherapy is the prolonged use of low-dose treatment, primarily with ALL. In ALL, the drugs commonly used are methotrexate and 6-mercaptopurine, often in combination with brief courses of vincristine and prednisone. Maintenance therapy prevents relapse in children with ALL but has not been proven effective in adults with either AML or ALL.

Bone marrow transplant (BMT) is indicated as a treatment option for patients with AML who have achieved an initial remission induction (see Chapter 11).

CLL

1. Stage 3 or 4
2. Infection
3. Progressive enlargement of spleen
4. Leukemic infiltration of the bone marrow

CML

1. Ph^1 negative
2. Pancytopenia
3. Increasing leukocytosis
4. Progressive basophilia
5. Secondary chromosome abnormalities (Double Ph^1, inversion 17 + 8, + 19)

ALL

1. Male
2. Age > 10 years
3. FAB L3
4. B-cell immunophenotype
5. Leukocyte count > 50,000
6. CNS involvement
7. Cytogenetic abnormalities (t(9:22), t(4:11), t(8:22), t(8:14))

AML

1. Age > 60 years
1. FAB M0, M5, M6, M7
3. Biphenotypic
4. Infection at diagnoses
5. Poor performance status
6. Low serum albumin levels
7. High LDH
8. Antecedent hematologic disorder (MDS or CML)
9. Previous chemotherapy or radiation
10. CD34 expression
11. Chromosomal abnormalities (t(9:22), t(6:9), inversion 3, trisomy 8, deletions or monosomies of chromosomes 5 and 7)

FIGURE 32–2 Unfavorable Prognostic Factors

Patient age and availability of a **human-leukocyte antigen (HLA)** donor for **allogeneic BMT** limit eligibility. Other types of BMT, matched unrelated donor (MUD), purged **autologous BMT** (the source of bone marrow is the patient), or **peripheral blood stem cell transplantation** also may be used. However, these types of transplants carry more risk of complications (MUD) or increased risk of relapse than an HLA allogeneic BMT. In ALL, BMT is indicated after the patient experiences a first relapse of the disease. The difference in timing for the inclusion of a BMT is related to the responsiveness of the disease in achieving a durable remission.

Unfortunately, most patients with AML experience a relapse of their disease within a short time frame. *Relapse* refers to the reappearance of clinical or hematological evidence of leukemic cells in the bone marrow or extramedullary sites, such as the CNS, testes, or skin. Patients may undergo second or multiple relapsed induction therapy. Response of second and subsequent remissions is influenced by the duration of the previous remission and prior therapy. Leukemic cells change their cellular structure over time; therefore, chemotherapy becomes less effective.

There is a great deal of interest in the therapeutic potential of **hematopoietic growth factors** in supportive care and the treatment of acute leukemia (see Chapter 10). They have been used to reduce the period of **myelosuppression** following intensive chemotherapy. Additionally, researchers are currently exploring whether or not leukemic cells stimulated by hematopoietic growth factors are more susceptible to antitumor drugs.

CML is a chronic disease for which the only known cure is the ablation of the Ph[1] chromosome by BMT following high-dose chemotherapy. Since only 25% of patients have matched-HLA BMT donors, suppression of disease progression is the most common form of treatment. This is attempted by the use of chemotherapeutic agents such as hydroxyurea or busulfan. In patients with early disease, alpha **interferon** alone has produced a complete hematologic response in 30% to 70% of cases. With advanced disease, effectiveness has been noted when interferon is given after cytotoxic therapy has decreased the tumor load. Blast crisis CML requires intensive chemotherapy, similar to that used in acute leukemia, and has a poor prognosis.

For patients with CLL, treatment is initiated once they become symptomatic. The alkylating agent chlorambucil is given orally to control disease progression. Prednisone or cyclosporin is used if the patient has bone marrow infiltration or autoimmune hemolytic anemia. Fludarabine and cladribine, recently available nucleoside analogs, have produced positive responses in patients refractory to chlorambucil.

SIDE EFFECTS

Complications of leukemia are related to the increased cell proliferation (tumor burden) and treatment therapy. **Leukostasis** is a syndrome of vascular sludging from aggregation by excessive numbers of circulating leukemic blast cells. It is most prevalent at initial diagnosis when the white blood cell (WBC) count is 100,000 cells/mm^3 or greater. Vascular occlusion, rupture, or hemorrhage may occur anywhere in the body as a result of this condition. Leukostasis is prevented with administration of hydroxyurea to lower the WBC count or with the initiation of **leukophoresis** in patients who present with WBC counts greater than 150,000 cells/mm^3. Antileukemic therapy is initiated once the danger of leukostasis is eliminated.

Infection, bleeding, and anemia result from tumor burden, as immature cells crowd out normal hematopoietic cells or as a result of treatment. Antileukemic therapy produces bone marrow aplasia and therefore places the patient at risk for complications resulting from a nonfunctional bone marrow. Infection is the major complication for leukemic patients, since there is a prolonged period (3–6 weeks) of neutropenia. **Neutropenia** is a decreased WBC (neutrophil) count and exists when the absolute neutrophil count (WBC × (% neutrophils + % bands) is less than 1,000 cells/mm^3. Most infections are due to organisms endogenous to the host or present in the environment. Patients with leukemia are especially susceptible to fungal and viral infections due to their prolonged immunocompromised state. Patients should be consistently monitored for increased temperatures and other changes in routine vital signs. Once fever is present in a neutropenic state, antimicrobial therapy should be initiated immediately.

Bleeding episodes occur when there is a decrease in the number of circulating platelets. Minor bleeding may be characterized by oozing from the gums or nose or the development of petechiae or ecchymosis. Major bleeding can occur if platelet levels fall below 20,000/mm³. Platelet (PLT) transfusions may be necessary if the platelet count falls between 10,000 and 20,000/mm³ or if the patient has active bleeding. **Anemia,** resulting from a lack of circulating hemoglobin, may cause fatigue, shortness of breath, pallor, and tachycardia. The administration of packed red blood cells (PRBCs) is given for symptom relief or if the patient's hemoglobin drops below 8 gm/dl.

Blood products that are leukocyte poor and irradiated are used to decrease the antibody production against antigens on the leukocytes. These blood products minimize transfusion reactions and may prevent PLT refractoriness. Often patients who receive a large number of platelet transfusions become refractory or unresponsive to subsequent platelet transfusions due to a build-up of exposure to multiple antigens. HLA typing should be done on patients who are potential candidates for bone marrow transplant prior to the initiation of chemotherapy. This typing can also be used to provide HLA-matched platelets to patients who become refractory to random or single-donor platelet products.

When tumor cells are destroyed, large amounts of intracellular by-products are released into the extracellular circulation. This process is referred to as **tumor lysis syndrome.** Subsequent hyperkalemia, hypocalcemia, hyperphosphatemia, and hyperuricemia can result. Renal complications occur if uric acid crystallizes in the renal tubules and collecting ducts. Allopurinol and intravenous fluids are usually administered to assist the body in clearing these intracellular by-products.

Some leukemic cells (promyelocytes—M3) release procoagulants that are associated with a disorder of uncontrolled clotting called **disseminated intravascular coagulation (DIC).** Coagulation factors are frequently monitored in patients who are at risk for the development of DIC.

Neurotoxicity can be a result of disease involvement in the CNS or as a side effect of high-dose cytosine arabinoside. Neurotoxicity related to drug toxicity generally consists of cerebellar dysfunction and can be mild or severe. Once neurotoxicity is suspected, further doses of cytosine arabinoside are withheld. The incidence of neurotoxicity increases with patient age and higher doses of cytosine arabinoside. If detected early, this toxicity may be reversible. Patients with low platelet counts also are at risk for CNS hemorrhage. Confusion or changes in orientation may alert the nurse to suspect intracranial hemorrhage. Confirmation is obtained via a CT scan of the brain.

Treatment with anthracyclines (daunorubicin, doxorubicin, or idarubicin) or mitoxantrone carries the risk of cardiotoxicity because in cumulative doses these drugs may directly damage the heart muscle. Patients will undergo a baseline MUGA scan. Subsequent MUGA scans may be repeated if clinically indicated. Signs and symptoms are similar to those seen with congestive heart failure.

LONG-TERM SEQUELAE

Five-year relative **survival rates** are commonly used to monitor progress in the treatment of cancer. It was estimated that in 1996 that 21,000 people would die as a result of leukemia. Patients with AML have a median survival duration of 1 year and a long-term (5-year) survival rate of 20%, whereas adults with ALL who complete therapy have up to a 40% long-term survival rate.

Survival in CLL depends largely on the patient's disease stage. Rai stage 0 patients have a mean survival of 12 years or more, while Rai stage IV patients have a mean survival of only 2 years. People with CLL usually die because of infection due to bone marrow failure and immune deficiency.

CML is divided into three phases. The natural course of the disease is an initial chronic phase, which transforms into an accelerated phase within 30 to 65 months, depending on the type of therapy given. The disease then progresses to the blastic phase (acute proliferation of immature cells), which has a median survival rate of 3 months.

NURSING CONSIDERATIONS

The care of individuals with leukemia requires a multidisciplinary team approach in which nurses play a pivotal role. Knowledge of the disease process, treatment regimens, and side effects enables the nurse to identify and institute prompt medical interventions for patients experiencing life-threatening complications.

Patient education regarding diagnosis, treatment, and symptom management is a vital aspect of the nurse's role. Psychosocial **support** for the patient and family is continuous as the patient progresses through the disease continuum (see Chapter 19).

Over the past 3 decades, survival of patients with leukemia has increased. Major influencing factors contributing to the increased survival trend include multimodality treatment and milestones in supportive therapies such as blood banking, nutritional support, and antimicrobial therapy.

Increased survival trends have also impacted late effects of therapy. Late effects of therapy are primarily related to treatment and include neuropsychiatric problems, cardiac dysfunction, delayed growth and development in children, infertility, development of second malignancies, and psychosocial adaptation.

Nurses are also in key positions to make valuable contributions in the implementation of medical and companion nursing research studies. Research will identify the best treatment regimens to ensure durable responses to treatment and to effectively identify and control the immediate and long-term complications.

CONCLUSION

A multidisciplinary approach is mandatory for the care of the individual with a diagnosis of leukemia. Acute or chronic and myclocytic or lymphocytic leukemias require diverse treatment plans and supportive care regimens. Prognoses among the different classifications of leukemia remain quite variable. The nurse is responsible for coordinating all aspects of direct patient care, including chemotherapy and supportive care, medication administration, assessment and evaluation of symptom management, patient and family education, and psychosocial support.

Clinical research continues to identify favorable and high-risk prognostic factors among subsets of individuals with leukemia. Nurses effectively participate in the research process through adherence to protocol requirements and consistent and clear documentation of the individual's response to therapy. The treatment of leukemia continues to evolve as more effective treatment regimens are identified and supportive care interventions become available. The ultimate goal is to increase response and survival duration while maintaining an improved quality of life for the individual with leukemia.

BIBLIOGRAPHY

Bain, B. J. (1995). Routine and specialized techniques in the diagnosis of hematological neoplasms. *Journal of Clinical Pathology, 48*, 501–508.

Copelan, E. A., & McGuire, E. A. (1995). The biology and treatment of acute lymphoblastic leukemia in adults. *Blood, 85*, 1151–1168.

Dewald, G. W., & Wright, P. I. (1995). Chromosome abnormalities in the myeloproliferative disorders. *Seminars in Oncology, 22*, 341–354.

Estey, E. H. (1995). Treatment of acute myelogenous leukemia and myelodysplastic syndromes. *Seminars in Hematology, 32*, 132–151.

Lawrence, J. (1994). Critical care issues in the patient with hematologic malignancy. *Seminars in Oncology Nursing, 10*, 198–207.

Purandard, L. (1995). Caring for patients with chronic leukaemia. *Nursing Times, 91*, 27–28.

Wujcik, D. (Ed.). (1995). Pharmacia. *Nursing care issues in adult acute leukemia.* New York: PRR.

Wujcik, D. (1993). Leukemia. In S. L. Groenwald, M. H. Frogge, M. Goodman, & C. H. Yarbro (Eds.), *Cancer nursing: Principles and practice* (3rd ed.). Sudbury, MA: Jones and Bartlett.

33

Lymphomas

Margie Graff Anderson

Primary **tumors** originating in the lymphatic system were first identified in 1832. Now these tumors are known as Hodgkin's disease and non-Hodgkin's lymphoma. Since the early 1970s incidence rates for non-Hodgkin's lymphoma have increased while the incidence of Hodgkin's disease has declined. **Lymphomas** have been seen with increasing frequency in individuals testing positive for human immunodeficiency virus (HIV). Since the clinical course and response to treatment of patients with HIV are different from those of patients not infected with HIV, they are discussed separately in this chapter.

HODGKIN'S DISEASE

Incidence

An estimated 7,500 new cases of Hodgkin's disease are diagnosed annually, occurring in a bimodal age-incidence distribution with the **incidence** peaking in the mid 20s, then declining until the mid 40s, and then increasing with age. The decline in the overall incidence of Hodgkin's disease is seen primarily in the older population. Hodgkin's disease is rare before age 5, and in children under age 10 it is much more common in males than in females. In adults it is slightly more common in males. An estimated 1,450 individuals die of Hodgkin's disease annually. Since the advent of combination **chemotherapy,** adult Hodgkin's disease has become one of the most curable malignancies.

Etiology

Data on familial aggregation suggest that there may be genetic factors associated with the disease development. Although the exact etiology of Hodgkin's disease is not known, it has been suggested that viruses play a role in its development. A slightly greater incidence of Hodgkin's disease has been observed in individuals who previously had infectious mononucleosis. In addition, defects in immune responses that occur in Hodgkin's disease are similar to those seen in patients with other diseases caused by human **retroviruses.** Studies suggest that the origin may be of the **B-lymphocyte, T-lymphocyte,** or **macrophage** cell line. The presence of large multinucleated Reed-Sternberg cells in the tumor is characteristic of the disease. The origin of the Reed-Sternberg cell and the identity of its normal counterpart remains unclear. Hodgkin's is thought to originate from a single focus, usually a lymph node. Patients with Hodgkin's disease exhibit defects in immune system function throughout the course of the disease, although to a lesser degree after remission is obtained.

Clinical Presentation

Patients are often asymptomatic and may present with painless lymphadenopathy. Lymphadenopathy is most commonly found in the supraclavicular, cervical, and mediastinal lymph node regions. The spread of disease is contiguous and predictable, first involving adjacent lymph nodes before spreading to other organs. The spleen, liver, and retroperitoneal lymph nodes may also be involved, although patients may not exhibit clinical signs of involvement at **diagnosis.** Associated symptoms of unexplained weight loss of more than 10% of body weight in the 6 months prior to diagnosis; frequent, drenching night sweats; and fever with temperatures above 38 degrees C may also be present. Pruritis, an additional systemic symptom, significant if it is recurrent, is otherwise unexplained, and parallels disease activity. These symptoms, defined as "B" symptoms for **staging** purposes, occur with greater frequency in older patients and have a negative impact on prognosis.

Diagnosis and Staging

Diagnostic criteria for Hodgkin's disease include a thorough history and physical examination plus hematology and chemistry profiles. Diagnosis is confirmed by lymph node and bone marrow biopsy. A chest x-ray to evaluate complaints of persistent cough or **dyspnea** may identify mediastinal involvement, which is present in up to 50% of patients. The extent of disease is determined by **computerized tomography (CT)** scans of the thoracic, abdominal, and pelvic areas, Gallium scans of mediastinal or hilar lymph nodes, and lower extremity **lymphangiograms.** If the extent of disease cannot be determined by other diagnostic tests and confirmation of abdominal disease would alter the choice of therapy, a staging laparotomy may be performed. Treatment recommendations vary depending on the extent or stage of disease. The widely used Ann Arbor Staging Classification, shown in Table 33–1, is used to determine treatment and prognosis and to enable the clinician to compare patients enrolled in various treatment protocols.

TABLE 33–1   Ann Arbor Staging Classification

Stage 1	Involvement of a single lymph node region or of a single extralymphatic organ or site.
Stage II	Involvement of two or more lymph node regions on the same side of the diaphragm or of an extralymphatic organ or site on the same side of the diaphragm.
Stage III	Involvement of lymph node regions or structures on both sides of the diaphragm.
Stage IV	Diffuse involvement of extralymphatic organs or tissue with or without associated lymph node enlargement. Reasons for classifying the patient as Stage IV should be identified.
For All Stages	A—No symptoms B—Presence of symptoms (fever, sweats, weight loss of > 10% of body weight).

Treatment

Therapy for Hodgkin's disease has improved over the last 30 years, resulting in a long-term **survival rate** of nearly 70% today. The role of surgery in Hodgkin's disease is limited to diagnostic biopsy, staging procedures, or to splenectomy in selected cases. Accurate staging is critical to the development of the most effective treatment plan.

Radiation Therapy   Radiation therapy alone is curative in most patients with Stage I or Stage II disease. The addition of chemotherapy to the treatment plan may be indicated in patients with poor prognostic factors such as "B" symptoms or in those with Stage III or Stage IV disease. The radiation therapy fields, designed to treat all involved lymph nodes with the same radiation dose, are illustrated in Figure 33–1. Radiotherapy may also be given to chains of clinically uninvolved nodes to limit the spread of disease along its predictable routes. When used in combination with chemotherapy, the total dose of radiation may be decreased. Therapy is usually administered over a period of 4 to 6 weeks.

Complications of radiotherapy for Hodgkin's disease are related to the dose given and the volume of tissue irradiated. Careful treatment technique and shielding reduce the risk of cardiac complications, but radiation pneumonitis is seen in up to 20% of patients. Other complications include nausea, weight loss, esophagitis, skin reactions, **myelosuppression,** and fatigue. Hypothyroidism requiring hormone replacement is not uncommon. The risks of long-term complications need to be assessed, and follow-up for early detection of potential sequelae is essential.

Chemotherapy   Intensive chemotherapy is used in most patients with Stage III and Stage IV disease and in some patients with earlier-stage disease. Combinations of at least four chemotherapeutic drugs are needed to achieve a

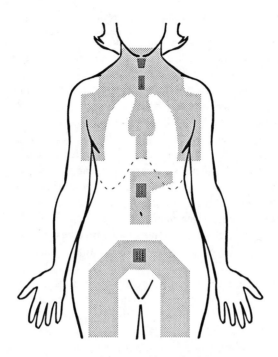

FIGURE 33-1   Radiation Fields for Hodgkin's Lymphoma

I = mantle, I + II = subtotal nodal irradiation, I + II + III = total nodal irradiation

cure. The most commonly used combinations are MOPP (nitrogen mustard, vincristine, procarbazine, and prednisone) and ABVD (doxorubicin, bleomycin, vincristine and dacarbazine). These regimens have induced complete remission in over 80% of patients treated. Cycles of MOPP are often alternated with ABVD or other combination chemotherapy regimens in an attempt to overcome drug resistance that may develop to a single combination or to reduce the risk of late effects of therapy such as secondary **leukemia.**

The most frequently observed acute side effects of chemotherapy include nausea and vomiting, myelosuppression, **alopecia,** and mood changes associated with steroid therapy. Neurotoxicity related to treatment with vincristine is also seen. Chemotherapy increases the risk for secondary malignancies, particularly acute leukemia. The risk appears to be greatest in patients over the age of 40. The risk of acute leukemia 10 years after therapy with MOPP is about 3%. For those treated with ABVD the risk for the same period is about 1%.

Bone Marrow Transplant   The use of high-dose chemotherapy and **autologous bone marrow** and/or **peripheral stem cell** rescue may be considered as an optional treatment for refractory and relapsed Stage III and Stage IV Hodgkin's disease. This treatment approach is currently considered an investigational therapy.

Side Effects, Long-Term Sequelae, and Nursing Considerations

Treatment approaches for Hodgkin's disease are frequently complex. Nurses may need to help patients and families to understand the therapy and its impact. Nurses also play a crucial role in the management of chemotherapy and radiation side effects, and in explaining the importance of long-term surveillance. Issues related to long-term effects of radiation and chemotherapy are particularly relevant to the large proportion of patients who are young adults. Two major concerns are the effects on reproductive ability and the risk of a second malignancy.

The occurrence of infertility is age dependent in females. Of female patients over age 35, 40% to 50% experience ovarian dysfunction following MOPP therapy. Although younger women may not initially experience this difficulty, they may be at risk for premature menopause as a result of ovarian failure. If the abdomen is irradiated during treatment, the ovaries can be shielded or surgically displaced to maintain fertility. Since fertility cannot be assured following treatment, patients should be encouraged to discuss their concerns before therapy begins.

Males who receive MOPP have a greater than 80% chance of irreversible sterility. These patients may wish to consider storing sperm through a banking program prior to treatment. Because patients may still be able to conceive during therapy, all sexually active patients undergoing treatment should be advised to use contraceptives during and for 6 months following treatment.

The increased incidence of a secondary malignancy should be discussed. Patients need to be informed of the risk and assisted in balancing the long-term risks of therapy with the benefits of treating a life-threatening disease. Long-term follow-up after treatment is essential.

NON-HODGKIN'S LYMPHOMA

Non-Hodgkin's lymphoma (NHL) is seven times more common than Hodgkin's disease. Of the estimated 52,700 new cases of NHL diagnosed annually, as many as 23,300 will die of the disease. Overall survival at 5 years with optimum treatment for all patients with NHL is approximately 50% to 60%. Over the past 25 years, the incidence of NHL has increased by over 65%. Non-Hodgkin's lymphoma can occur in any age group, but an increase in incidence is seen beginning in the fourth decade. Males are more often affected than females. Individuals with congenital or acquired immunodeficiencies, including individuals with AIDS, those undergoing organ transplantation, and those with autoimmune diseases, are at increased risk for developing NHL.

Etiology

Non-Hodgkin's lymphoma is a malignancy of the B- and T-lymphocytes. Clones of the malignant cells may infiltrate the lymph nodes, bone marrow, peripheral blood, or other organs. As with Hodgkin's disease, a viral etiology has been implicated. Most NHLs fall into two broad categories related to their clinical behavior: the nodular, indolent type and the diffuse, aggressive lymphomas. The pat-

TABLE 33–2 Rappaport Staging Classification

Low Grade	Diffuse, lymphocytic, well differentiated
	Nodular, lymphocytic, poorly differentiated
	Nodular, mixed, lymphocytic and histiocytic
Intermediate Grade	Nodular, histiocytic
	Diffuse, lymphocytic
	Diffuse, mixed, lymphocytic and histiocytic
High Grade	Diffuse, histiocytic
	Diffuse, lymphoblastic
	Diffuse, undifferentiated

tern of spread is less predictable with NHL than with Hodgkin's disease, and disease is frequently disseminated at the time of diagnosis.

Clinical Manifestations

Patients with NHL present with localized or generalized lymphadenopathy, which they may identify as having waxed and waned over a period of several months. Early involvement of the oropharyngeal lymphoid tissue or infiltration of the bone marrow is common. With gastrointestinal involvement, an abdominal mass may be detected or the patient may describe vague symptoms of back pain or abdominal discomfort. Patients may also exhibit systemic "B" symptoms, including night sweats, fever, and/or weight loss. Approximately one-third of patients will have splenomegaly or hepatomegaly. Central nervous system involvement in immunocompetent individuals is uncommon at diagnosis.

Diagnosis and Staging

In addition to careful examination of all lymph node regions, a CBC, bone marrow, and lymph node biopsy are utilized to diagnose NHL. Serum chemistry may reflect elevated uric acid and calcium levels. The Ann Arbor Staging Classification employed in Hodgkin's disease is used, but it is of less value with NHL because it does not account for the **histology,** or type of tumor. Several classification systems have been proposed for NHL; the most commonly employed Rappaport classification is shown in Table 33–2. For treatment purposes, lymphomas may also be classified as low, intermediate, or high-grade. The histology of the tumor is more important to prognosis than the extent of disease.

Treatment

Surgery The primary role of surgery is to establish diagnosis and to assist with staging. Rarely, surgery is utilized to resect areas of the gastrointestinal tract to prevent bowel obstruction, or for splenectomy in patients exhibiting hypersplenism.

Radiation and Chemotherapy   Unlike the contiguous node extension seen in Hodgkin's disease, NHL is disseminated via the vascular system. Consequently, radiation therapy is generally used in conjunction with chemotherapy as opposed to being the primary treatment. Radiation therapy may be used alone in Stage I **diffuse histiocytic lymphoma,** although it is more common to combine radiation with chemotherapy. The patient's age and clinical condition may affect the choice of treatment. Therapy for low-grade lymphomas is controversial, because they are not curable with current regimens. These indolent lymphomas do have a long natural history with a median survival approaching 10 years in untreated patients. Patients with intermediate and high-grade, aggressive lymphomas are routinely treated with combination chemotherapy with or without radiation therapy. Combination chemotherapy with a variety of regimens such as MOPP or CHOP (cyclophosphamide, doxorubicin, vincristine, and prednisone) have led to high rates of remission, although the remission usually lasts for less than 5 years. Following relapse, the remissions achieved are generally shorter. Unfortunately, only about 50% of patients with aggressive lymphomas are cured. **Colony-stimulating factors** may be utilized to enable the delivery of more intensive chemotherapy, but studies have not confirmed an overall decrease in drug toxicity (other than **neutropenia)** or increased survival rates. Bone marrow transplant following high-dose chemotherapy has resulted in long-term remissions for patients with relapsing lymphomas.

Side Effects, Long-Term Sequelae, and Nursing Considerations

The nurse can help the patient and family understand various treatment approaches and manage side effects of radiation and chemotherapy. Many patients remain neutropenic for prolonged periods of time during treatment and must be provided with the education necessary to protect them when they are vulnerable to infection. In addition, a bulky tumor may cause obstruction and pressure, resulting in complications such as spinal cord compression, **superior vena cava syndrome,** ascites, or gastrointestinal or ureteral obstruction. These oncology complications are discussed in Chapter 17. Permanent sterility associated with radiation and cumulative doses of cyclophosphamide is a risk. A significantly elevated risk of a second primary malignancy exists for up to 2 decades following diagnosis and treatment. As with Hodgkin's disease, the nurse should help the patient balance the risk of therapy with the benefit of treatment.

AIDS-RELATED LYMPHOMA

Incidence

Central nervous system (CNS) lymphoma was included along with certain opportunistic infections in the earliest definitions of AIDS. In the revised 1985 definition of AIDS, other specific types of non-Hodgkin's lymphoma (NHL) were included. The incidence of lymphoma has nearly paralleled the course of the AIDS epidemic. While in the majority of cases the diagnosis of AIDS precedes the development of NHL, in as many as 30% the diagnosis of AIDS is made at the time of the diagnosis of NHL. Unlike **Kaposi's sarcoma,** which affects primarily homosexual men and seems to be declining in incidence, NHL affects all risk groups and is increasing in incidence. Estimates of the approximately 36,000 cases of NHL diagnosed in the United States in 1992 suggest that up to 25% were in patients who were HIV positive. As improved therapies extend the survival of patients with HIV, increased incidence of NHL in this population is likely to be seen.

Etiology

The relationship between AIDS and NHL, although not completely understood, is not surprising considering the relationship of NHL with other states of immune deficiency, congenital or acquired. The malignancies that develop in organ transplant patients receiving medications associated with an increased risk of various cancers tend to regress spontaneously when immunosuppression is eliminated, underscoring the importance of immune function in inhibiting the development of cancer. If immunosuppression alone were responsible for the predilection to the development of malignancy, one would expect to see a variety of neoplasms in this patient population. In fact, 95% of all HIV-associated malignancies are either Kaposi's sarcoma or NHL. In the patient who is HIV positive, numerous factors have been suggested to address the increased incidence of NHL, including **B-cell** proliferation uncontrolled by **T-cells,** or the presence of oncogenic viruses. AIDS-related primary CNS lymphoma is reported to have nearly a 100% association with the Epstein-Barr virus. Patients with CNS lymphoma generally have advanced AIDS, are severely debilitated, and are usually considered to be in the terminal phase of their disease.

Clinical Manifestations

Clinical presentation with AIDS-related lymphoma is different from that seen in patients who are not HIV positive. The patient most often presents with advanced-stage disease, which is frequently extranodal. The central nervous system is the most common extranodal site, followed by the bone marrow and bowel. The possibility of brain lesions attributable to fungal infection or tuberculosis may obscure the diagnosis of primary brain lymphoma. The diagnosis of NHL outside the central nervous system is complicated by a history of fevers, night sweats, and significant weight loss in nearly all patients who are HIV positive. Lymphoma should be considered in any HIV-positive patient with progressive lymphadenopathy.

Diagnosis and Staging

Diagnosis of AIDS-related lymphoma is based on lymph node and bone marrow biopsy. CT scans of the chest and abdomen, gastrointestinal endoscopic exams, and cultures to rule out complicating opportunistic infections are important in determining lymphoma stage. When CNS lymphoma is suspected, a CT or MRI of the head may be appropriate. Unfortunately, imaging cannot distinguish between CNS lymphoma and toxoplasmosis, a far more common finding in HIV-associated illness, which may occur simultaneously. Patients whose clinical findings deteriorate in the presence of toxoplasmosis therapy are candidates for brain biopsy to identify NHL. Meningeal involvement is present in up to 20% of patients. Therefore, a lumbar puncture with administration of intrathecal methotrexate may be appropriate to reduce the risk of CNS relapse. The Ann Arbor Staging Classification is used, although the majority of patients present with advanced disease with high-grade lymphoblastic histology. Prognosis is related to a number of important factors not included in the staging system, including (a) severity of the immune deficiency (CD4 + lymphocyte cell counts < 200/mm^3); (b) history or presence of opportunistic infections; (c) bone marrow involvement; (d) performance status (Karnofsky < 70%); and (e) presence of extranodal disease.

Treatment

Treatment of NHL poses a challenge imposed by the presence of AIDS, currently an incurable illness. The underlying immunodeficiency of AIDS limits the potential for dose-intensive regimens of chemotherapy. The lymphomas themselves are aggressive, frequently involve the bone marrow and central nervous system, and are usually in an advanced stage at the time of diagnosis. Optimal therapy has yet to be determined.

Surgery　Due to the diffuse nature of CNS lymphoma, surgical decompression with or without removal of the tumor is of no benefit to the patient. Surgical intervention is typically limited to diagnostic biopsy or treatment of complications such as obstructions.

Radiation and Chemotherapy　The role of radiation therapy is limited to patients with primary CNS lymphoma. In addition to having advanced disease, these patients are usually extremely debilitated and demonstrate focal neurologic symptoms such as seizures and paralysis. Many patients show partial improvement in neurologic symptoms following therapy. Disease recurs in the brain in over 90% of patients following high doses of radiation. Median survival for this group of patients is generally less than 6 months. Survival is somewhat better in the absence of concurrent opportunistic infections and in patients with better performance status.

Administration of chemotherapy compromises the immune system, increasing the likelihood of opportunistic infection. Response rates following administration of multiple chemotherapeutic agents tend to be lower than for the non-HIV-positive population, and periods of remission are shorter. Because the curative potential is so low and the treatment-related morbidity and mortality so high in the presence of aggressive treatment, low-dose chemotherapy is most often employed. One study employing a dose-attenuated version of M-BACOD (methotrexate, bleomycin, adriamycin®, cyclophosphamide, vincristine, and dexamethasone) followed by pneumocystis prophylaxis following four to six cycles of chemotherapy reported a median survival of 6 to 15 months. The addition of the **hematopoietic growth factor** GM-CSF to a CHOP (cyclosphosphamide, doxorubicin, vincristine, and prednisone) regimen indicated that patients receiving GM-CSF tolerated the chemotherapy better, as evidenced by shorter periods of neutropenia and shorter periods of hospitalization. No increase in survival time was achieved in spite of complete response rates of nearly 70%. Median survival ranged from 8 to 11 months. A number of strategies have been suggested to maximize the benefit of therapy in this patient population, including (a) intrathecal **central nervous system prophylaxis;** (b) systemic chemotherapy, even in patients with localized disease; (c) low-dose chemotherapy with or without growth factors; and (d) opportunistic infection prophylaxis with antibiotics and antifungal agents.

Side Effects and Nursing Considerations

Treating the side effects of radiation and chemotherapy common to *any* patient with lymphoma is a challenge. Care of AIDS-related lymphoma is further complicated by the fact that patients are often severely debilitated and have advanced-stage disease. The immunosuppressive nature of HIV infection and the incidence of coexisting opportunistic infection limit the treatment options available. The patient is often dealing with depression and loss, the financial burden imposed by the illness, isolation, and at times rejection by friends and family. In addition to dealing with patient and family concerns regarding various treatment options and management of side effects of therapy, the nursing care must also include the often overwhelming emotional consequences of AIDS.

CONCLUSION

The lymphomas are a unique group of malignancies that present many challenges to nurses caring for patients with these cancers. Complications of the disease and/or treatment are often complex, requiring knowledgeable and highly skilled nursing care. Often these diseases can be controlled for many years, and cure rates are climbing, giving patients, families, and nurses hope for the future.

BIBLIOGRAPHY

Aboulafia, D. (1994). Human immunodeficiency virus-associated neoplasms. In G. V. Foley (Ed.), *Cancer Practice* (pp. 297–306). Philadelphia: J. B. Lippincott.

Erickson, J. (1994). Update on Hodgkin's disease. *The Nurse Practitioner, 19*(11), 63–68.

Gomez, E. (1995). A teaching booklet for patients receiving mantle field irradiation. *Oncology Nursing Forum, 22,* 121–126.

Lundquist, D., & Stewart, F. M. (1994). An update on non-Hodgkin's lymphomas. *The Nurse Practitioner, 19,* 41–54.

PDQ (Physician Data Query). [Database on-line] Bethesda, MD: National Cancer Institute; 1995, November. *Adult Hodgkin's disease.* Available from National Cancer

Institute; National Library of Medicine, Bethesda, MD; OVID Technologies, Inc., New York, NY; Lexis-Nexis, Miamisburg, OH.

PDQ (Physician Data Query). [Database on-line] Bethesda, MD: National Cancer Institute; 1995, November. *Adult non-Hodgkin's lymphoma*. Available from National Cancer Institute; National Library of Medicine, Bethesda, MD; OVID Technologies, Inc., New York, NY; Lexis-Nexis, Miamisburg, OH.

PDQ (Physician Data Query). [Database on-line] Bethesda, MD: National Cancer Institute; 1993, November. *AIDS-related lymphoma*. Available from National Cancer Institute; National Library of Medicine, Bethesda, MD; OVID Technologies, Inc., New York, NY; Lexis-Nexis, Miamisburg, OH.

PDQ (Physician Data Query). [Database on-line] Bethesda, MD: National Cancer Institute; 1995, March. *Primary CNS lymphoma*. Available from National Cancer Institute; National Library of Medicine, Bethesda, MD; OVID Technologies, Inc., New York, NY; Lexis-Nexis, Miamisburg, OH.

Rosenthal, D. S., & Eyre, H. J. (1995). Hodgkin's disease and non-Hodgkin's lymphomas. In G. Murphy, W. Lawrence Jr., & R. Lenhard Jr. (Eds.), *American Cancer Society textbook of clinical oncology* (pp. 451–469). Atlanta, GA: American Cancer Society.

Weinshel, E., & Peterson, B. (1993). Hodgkin's disease. CA—A *Cancer Journal for Clinicians, 43*(6), 327–346.

34

Multiple Myeloma

Bonny Libbey Johnson

Multiple myeloma is a **malignant** disease involving excessive proliferation of plasma cells, the antibody-producing cells derived from B-lymphocytes. It is an incurable disease that derives its name from an autopsy description in 1873 of multiple tumors of "large round cells" located in the bone marrow. The clinical signs and symptoms of multiple myeloma are related to the accumulation of these malignant plasma cells and the protein secreted by them. Thus, the disease has the potential to affect almost every system in the body.

While advances have been made in the supportive care of patients with this disease, the prognosis for survival has not changed in the past 30 years. The median survival for patients with multiple myeloma remains 30 to 36 months from the time of diagnosis. New technology may facilitate earlier diagnosis; however, the impact of this on survival is not yet known.

EPIDEMIOLOGY

The estimated **incidence** of multiple myeloma for 1996 was 14,400 cases (7,700 men and 6,700 women), accounting for about 1% of all cancers in the United States. The rate of death per year is approximately 10,000. The rate of myeloma among the African-American population is much higher than for whites; African-American men have the highest incidence at 9.6 cases per 100,000, compared to 2.8 per 100,000 white men. Over the past 2 decades, there has been a rising incidence of myeloma, which probably reflects more sensitive **screening** tests rather than a true increase in the disease. Myeloma remains a disease of the elderly, with a peak age at diagnosis between 50 and 70 and a median age of 68 for men and 70 for women.

TABLE 34–1   Immunoglobulin Production and Function

Class	Normal Serum Level	Function
IgG (gamma)	12 mg/dl	Confers passive immunity by crossing placenta; produced after initial IgM production; binds to complement and mononuclear cells.
IgA (alpha)	1.8 mg/dl	Primary immunoglobulin in saliva, tears, and gastrointestinal and respiratory tract secretions; protects mucous membranes as first line of defense.
IgM (mu)	1.0 mg/dl	Produced as first response to antigenic stimulation; first immunoglobulin produced by infants.
IgD (delta)	0.03 mg/dl	Acts as cell-surface receptor; binds with antigen and triggers further immune response.
IgE (epsilon)	.0003 mg/dl	Stimulates mast cells; responds to allergenic exposure and parasitic infection.

ETIOLOGY

There are no known etiologic factors for multiple myeloma in most cases, although selected factors are implicated in the development of the disease. The higher incidence among men and African Americans suggests a role for genetics, and there are several reports of myeloma among siblings. Exposure to petroleum products and asbestos or a history of chronic infections or repeated allergenic stimulation may increase **risk** for the disease. As with other hematologic malignancies, a history of radiation exposure is associated with the diagnosis of myeloma, with cases occurring up to 20 years later. The fact that multiple myeloma is a disease of the elderly suggests that the known effect of aging on the immune system plays a role in its development.

PATHOPHYSIOLOGY

Normal Plasma Cells

Myeloid and lymphoid cells are derived from a **pluripotent stem cell** in the bone marrow. Lymphoid cells, or **lymphocytes,** differentiate into either T-lymphocytes or B-lymphocytes. The primary function of **T-lymphocytes** is to regulate the immune system and confer cell-mediated immunity. **B-lymphocytes** mature into plasma cells, which are uniquely capable of producing and secreting immunoglobulins, or antibodies, necessary for humoral immunity. The functions of the various classes of immunoglobulins are listed in Table 34–1.

Malignant Plasma Cells

The unrestricted proliferation of malignant **plasma cells,** or myeloma cells, arises in the bone marrow after a single cell has undergone malignant transformation. These cells infiltrate bone, most commonly the thoracic and lumbar vertebrae and also the ribs, skull, pelvis, and proximal bones. All myeloma cells excessively secrete a homogeneous class of immunoglobulin, determined by the original malignant cell, resulting in a **monoclonal gammopathy.** The abnormal immunoglobulin produced by the malignant plasma cell clone is unable to function as normal antibody and participate in humoral immunity. Immunoglobulins are easily detectable in the serum by protein electrophoresis and immunoelectrophoresis techniques. Thus, the occurrence of an abnormal accumulation of one immunoglobulin will be reflected as a "spike," referred to as an *M-spike, M-protein,* or *M-component* (M = myeloma, malignant, or monoclonal protein). Secretion of excessive free proteins is measured in urine as **Bence-Jones proteinuria.**

The immune system is regulated with significant interplay between T-lymphocytes and B-lymphocytes. **Cytokines,** which are produced by T-lymphocytes or monocytes, specifically interleukin-6 (IL-6), may stimulate the growth of myeloma cells. In addition, both plasma cells and myeloma cells secrete the cytokines interleukin-1 (IL-1) and **tumor necrosis factor (TNF),** which in turn stimulate secretion of IL-6. All of these cytokines are capable of acting as **osteoclast-activating factors (OAFs),** which contribute to the bone destruction seen in multiple myeloma.

CLINICAL FEATURES

The presenting symptoms of multiple myeloma result from (a) direct effect of the malignant cell population within the marrow, causing bone marrow depression; (b) increased osteoclastic activity, causing bone destruction; and (c) the accumulation of immunoglobulins throughout the body. The course of the disease is variable and can be categorized as "smoldering," "indolent," or overt multiple myeloma, depending on the degree of bone disease, immunoglobulin secretion, and bone marrow plasmacytosis. Approximately 20% of patients are diagnosed without symptoms. **Monoclonal gammopathy of unknown significance,** or MGUS, is a diagnosis given to patients who have a serum monoclonal protein detected on electrophoresis with no bone lesions, no excess of bone marrow plasma cells, and a low M spike. Some, but not all MGUS patients eventually develop the full clinical picture of myeloma.

The severity of presenting signs and symptoms depends on the number of **tumor** cells present, or *tumor burden.* The most common presentation of multiple myeloma is bone pain together with anemia. Bone pain results from either destructive bone lesions or bone tenderness due to extensive bone marrow involvement. Skeletal lesions may result in pathologic fractures (especially of the vertebra), spinal cord compression, and hypercalcemia. The common symptoms

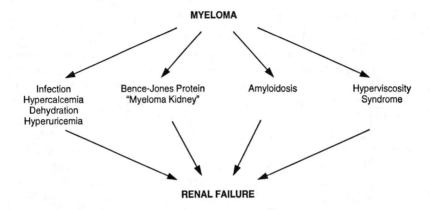

FIGURE 34-1   Factors Predisposing to Renal Failure in Multiple Myeloma

of hypercalcemia (nausea, constipation, mental status changes, dehydration) can be vague and misleading, especially in the elderly population.

Bone marrow depression with anemia and/or leukopenia and **thrombocytopenia** signifies replacement of normal marrow by tumor cells. Examination of the bone marrow by biopsy may reveal plasma cells in excess of normal (normal $\leq$ 10%). This, together with deficient normal plasma cell function and the bone marrow suppressive effects of cytotoxic therapy, places the patient at enormous risk for infection, especially by encapsulated organisms such as *Streptococcus pneumoniae*, *Hemophilus influenza*, *Staphylococcus aureus*, and gram-negative rods. The risk for infection increases throughout the course of disease as the patient is treated with cytotoxic and steroid therapy.

Renal dysfunction is present in one-third of patients at diagnosis, and up to 50% of patients will experience renal failure during the course of the disease. Its pathogenesis is related to many factors (Figure 34-1), including direct tumor effects as well as the secondary effects of treatment and disease. The most common causes of renal failure are hypercalcemia and Bence-Jones proteinuria. *Myeloma kidney* denotes infiltration of the kidney by proteins, which form precipitates that damage the tubules. Other exacerbating conditions include hyperuricemia, due to tumor cell lysis and excretion, and infection with concomitant antibiotic therapy.

Hyperviscosity syndrome is a rare complication of myeloma, occurring in 5% of patients. It is more common in patients with IgM myeloma, but occurs also in IgG and IgA myeloma (Table 34-1). The high concentration of serum proteins, or *serum viscosity*, causes sludging in the circulation and in specific organs such as the kidney, brain, and eye. Clinical effects include blurred vision, irritability, headache, drowsiness, and confusion.

Amyloid protein deposits, or *amyloidosis*, occur in the organs of 15% of patients with myeloma, resulting from free light chains deposited in sheets. While amyloid deposition can adversely affect many organs (liver, spleen, heart, peripheral nerves), renal dysfunction due to impaired protein resorption by the kidney is the most common complication for patients with myeloma.

TABLE 34–2 Myeloma Staging System

Stage	Criteria

I	All of the following:
	Hgb value > 10 g/dl
	Serum calcium value normal (< 12 mg/dl)
	On roentgenogram, normal bone structure or solitary bone plasmacytoma only
	Low M-component production rates
	    IgG value < 5 g/dl
	    IgA value < 3 g/dl
	    Urine light chain M-component on electrophoresis < 4 g/24 hr

II	Overall data not as minimally abnormal as shown for Stage I and no single value as abnormal as defined for Stage III

III	One or more of the following:
	Hgb value < 8.5 g/dl
	Serum calcium value > 12 mg/dl
	Advanced lytic bone lesions (scale 3)
	High M-component production rates
	    IgG value > 7 g/dl
	    IgA value > 5 g/dl
	    Urine light chain M-component on electrophoresis > 12 g/24 hr

Subclassification
    A = relatively normal renal function (serum creatinine value < 2.0 mg/dl)
    B = abnormal renal function (serum creatinine value > 2.0 mg/dl)

Examples
    Stage IA = low cell mass with normal renal function
    Stage IIIB = high cell mass with abnormal renal function

Source: Alexanian, R., Balcerzak, S., Bonnet, J. D., et al. (1975). Prognostic factors in multiple myeloma. *Cancer, 36,* 1192–1201. Adapted by permission of Wiley-Liss, A Division of John Wiley and Sons, Inc. Copyright © 1975 Wiley-Liss.

A minority of patients (7%) with myeloma present with a solitary lesion, or **plasmacytoma.** This may occur in the bone or in soft tissue, and it signifies a much smaller tumor burden. Symptoms are related directly to the area involved, with local pain and swelling. These patients generally have a more favorable prognosis and survive longer.

DIAGNOSIS

The **diagnosis** of multiple myeloma is made by examination of the blood and bone marrow, urine, and radiographic assessment of bone involvement. These measures, together with history and physical examination help determine the amount of disease and extent of involvement. The **staging** system for myeloma quantifies the tumor cell mass (Table 34–2) and allows prediction of survival, as

TABLE 34–3   Diagnostic Evaluation of Multiple Myeloma

Diagnostic Tests	Purpose
Bone marrow aspirate/biopsy	Degree of marrow plasmacytosis and normal hematopoiesis
Blood work	
CBC	Degree of cytopenia
Serum chemistry	Ca^{++}, uric acid, renal function
Serum B_2 microglobulin	Protein shed by myeloma cells
Serum protein electrophoresis (SPEP)	Quantifies M-protein spike
Immunoelectrophoresis (IEP)	Specifies M-protein
Skeletal x-rays	Extent and character of bone lesions ("punched-out" lesions)
24-hour urine	Presence/absence of Bence-Jones
Urine protein	protein, renal function
Urinalysis	

well as comparison of patient groups for clinical treatment trials. The diagnostic work-up is summarized in Table 34–3.

TREATMENT

Antitumor Treatment

Systemic treatment for myeloma is usually withheld until patients develop symptoms of the disease. Currently, the standard treatment regimen consists of oral melphalan and prednisone given for 4 days every 4 weeks. This oral regimen can easily be administered on an outpatient basis; however, patients must be closely monitored for bone marrow suppression, renal failure, infection, and steroid toxicity. Skeletal lesions may be treated with local radiation therapy. While most patients respond to this initial regimen with a fall in the M-protein level and improvement of symptoms, the goal remains palliation, and the median duration of response is 2 to 3 years.

If the patient does not respond to initial treatment or relapses, the most effective regimen to date is VAD (vincristine, doxorubicin, dexamethasone). The vincristine and doxorubicin (adriamycin®) are administered intravenously for 4 days every 28 days, and the dexamethasone is given orally over 4 days on a weekly basis. Dose modifications are indicated for severe bone marrow suppression, steroid toxicity, paresthesia or severe constipation, hepatotoxicity, or other severe untoward reactions. Table 34–4 summarizes the common side effects of agents used in the treatment of myeloma; however, the nurse caring for patients receiving treatment should consult a more detailed drug reference.

Radiation therapy is curative treatment only in the case of a solitary plasmacytoma. In addition, radiation therapy is given as palliative treatment to control

TABLE 34–4   Side Effects of Treatment for Multiple Myeloma

Treatment	Side Effects
Melphalan	Bone marrow suppression
	Renal insufficiency
	Myelodysplastic syndrome; secondary leukemia
Prednisone	Dyspepsia
	Hyperglycemia; fluid and sodium retention
	Steroid psychosis
	Myopathy
Interferon	Anorexia, fatigue, flu-like syndrome
	Thrombocytopenia
	Hepatic toxicity
	Mental status changes
VAD	
Vincristine	Neuropathy (peripheral and autonomic)
	Alopecia
	Constipation
Doxorubicin	Bone marrow suppression
	Nausea/vomiting; stomatitis; hepatic toxicity
	Alopecia
	Cardiomyopathy
Dexamethasone	Dyspepsia
	Hyperglycemia; fluid and sodium retention
	Myopathy
	Steroid psychosis
Radiotherapy (site-specific)	Nausea/vomiting; diarrhea
	Bone marrow suppression
	Pneumonitis
	Fatigue

pain and prevent pathologic fractures in osteolytic bone lesions and to improve mobility and decrease pain in the case of spinal cord compression caused by vertebral tumors.

Biologic response modification provides a new direction for treatment, due to the inadequacy of current treatment regimens and recent understanding of the role of cytokines in stimulating myeloma cell growth. **Interferon** has been used as maintenance therapy following response to **induction chemotherapy,** with some improvement in duration of response and survival. Methods to interrupt the production of IL-6, such as the use of **monoclonal antibodies,** are under investigation.

Bone marrow transplant following high doses of chemotherapy, with or without total body irradiation (TBI), is currently under investigation as a means of eradicating myeloma cells. The potential for this strategy may be limited due to severe toxicity in the elderly myeloma patient population. **Graft-versus-host** disease and the limited availability of matched donors make **allogeneic transplantation** difficult. In addition, because myeloma is a disease of the bone marrow, adequate purging of the marrow prior to **autologous transplant** is technically difficult. The use of **hematopoietic growth factors** and **peripheral blood stem cells** to rescue patients after transplant-conditioning regimens may improve the feasibility of this approach.

Nursing Considerations

In the absence of curative treatment for multiple myeloma, supportive care to prevent or ameliorate complications and optimize the patient's quality of life assumes paramount importance.

Management of pain due to bone involvement and pathologic fracture involves preventive as well as therapeutic approaches. Effective analgesia must be provided utilizing both narcotic and nonnarcotic agents. Nonsteroidal anti-inflammatory drugs should be avoided because of potential renal effects. Sudden episodes of acute pain may signal pathologic fractures, especially compression fractures of the vertebrae. Surgical stabilization procedures or proper positioning and support of limbs and back with braces or slings may be employed to relieve pressure and stress. A goal of pain management should be maintenance of mobility, because this will also decrease bone resorption and hypercalcemia.

A sudden change in the pattern of back pain or the onset of radicular pain, with or without paresthesia, may signify impending spinal cord compression. Immediate attention must be paid to early signs of cord compression, because early detection allows prompt treatment with radiation therapy and helps prevent permanent neurological damage.

Hypercalcemia occurs as a result both of bone destruction by myeloma cells and of secretion of **lymphokines** that activate osteoclastic activity, resulting in bone demineralization. Early detection is essential in order to avoid hypercalcemic crisis: severe nausea and vomiting, dehydration, confusion, and renal failure. The most effective means of controlling hypercalcemia is to reduce the number of myeloma tumor cells with effective antitumor regimens. However, as the disease progresses, management will include efforts to maintain mobility and adequate hydration (up to 2 to 3 liters per day), together with pharmacologic agents such as mithramycin, calcitonin, steroids, or bisphosphonates.

Bone marrow suppression results in anemia, thrombocytopenia, and leukopenia. **Anemia,** especially in the elderly, causes significant fatigue and weakness. Blood transfusions may provide significant temporary improvement, and erythropoietin, a red blood cell growth factor, has recently been shown to raise the hemoglobin level. Patients and families may be instructed about energy conservation, adequate nutrition, and rest periods. Platelet transfusions may be indicated for signs of bleeding and platelet counts below normal.

Infection remains the most common cause of death in patients with myeloma. The most common sites of infection are the respiratory tract, urinary tract, skin, sinuses, and blood. Supportive care includes patient and family education about recognizing and reporting early signs of infection and the importance of such measures as coughing and deep breathing, adequate fluid intake, maintenance of mobility, avoidance of crowds or actively ill family members, and avoidance of vaccines produced with live organisms. Antibiotics must be used judiciously in view of potential renal compromise. The use of intravenous immunoglobulins is controversial.

The management of renal failure requires effective antitumor treatment to decrease the Bence-Jones proteinuria, as well as attention to each of the exacerbating factors described in Figure 34–1. Plasmapheresis, to lower the circulating immunoglobulin level, or dialysis may be used to avoid irreversible damage until the myeloma is brought under control. *Hyperuricemia*, or high serum levels of uric acid, results in precipitates that damage the renal tubules. This may be a result of tumor cell lysis due to cytotoxic chemotherapy, excess protein breakdown, and inadequate renal clearance. The administration of allopurinol, which prevents the formation of uric acid, and hydration with urine alkalinization may be indicated when treatment is initiated. In addition, nurses should be alert to the possible renal toxicity of all medications, especially antibiotics.

CONCLUSION

Multiple myeloma is a disease that, while incurable, extends over a prolonged period of time with varying degrees of symptoms that can have a significant impact on a patient's quality of life. Specific anticancer therapy will benefit most patients initially. Scientific investigation continues to define the underlying pathophysiologic cause and behavior of the disease, and, hopefully, will result in more effective antitumor treatment. Until then, supportive care, both medical and nursing, will provide the greatest benefit to the patient and family.

BIBLIOGRAPHY

Alexanian, R., & Dimopoulos, M. (1994). The treatment of multiple myeloma. *The New England Journal of Medicine, 330*, 484–489.

Gautier, M., & Cohen, H. J. (1994). Multiple myeloma in the elderly. *Journal of the American Geriatric Society, 42*, 653–664.

Gross, J., & Johnson, B. L. (1994). *Handbook of oncology nursing* (2nd ed.). Sudbury, MA: Jones and Bartlett.

Lawrence, J. (1994). Critical care issues in the patient with hematologic malignancy. *Seminars in Oncology Nursing, 10*, 198–207.

Lokhorst, H. M., & Dekker, A. W. (1993). Tumor review: Advances in the treatment of multiple myeloma. *Cancer Treatment Reviews, 19*, 113–128.

Salmon, S. E., & Cassady, J. R. (1993). Plasma cell neoplasms. In V. T. DeVita, S. Hellman, & S. A. Rosenberg (Eds.), *Cancer: Principles and practice of oncology* (4th ed., pp. 1984–2025). Philadelphia: J. B. Lippincott.

Sheridan, C. (1994). Multiple myeloma. In S. Groenwald, M. H. Frogge, M. Goodman, & C. H. Yarbro (Eds.), *Cancer nursing: Principles and practice* (3rd ed., pp. 1229–1237). Sudbury, MA: Jones and Bartlett.

35

Other Cancers

Deborah Lowe Volker

This chapter discusses the less common cancers, including esophageal, gastric, pancreatic, hepatobiliary, and endocrine malignancies, as well as metastatic cancers in which the primary site is unknown. Although these cancers occur less frequently than others, they may present even greater challenges to patients and caregivers because many are especially difficult to treat and, in most instances, carry a poor prognosis.

ESOPHAGEAL CANCER

Incidence

Cancer of the esophagus is a disease of middle to older age, with three times as many cases occurring in men than in women. **Incidence** in the United States is about 12,000 new cases per year. There is a disproportionate incidence among African Americans, with rates three times higher than that of whites. The most common type of esophageal cancer is **squamous cell carcinoma**; however, the **adenocarcinoma** subtype is increasing at a rate of 5% to 10% each year. The reason for this increase is not clear, but it may be associated with an increasing incidence of Barrett's esophagus, a condition of epithelial changes that occur in the lower esophagus secondary to chronic exposure to refluxing gastric fluids. Incidence of esophageal cancer fluctuates worldwide, with the highest incidence observed in China and Japan. Unfortunately, the 5-year **survival rate** for esophageal cancers is poor; 11,200 deaths from this cancer were predicted in the United States in 1996.

Risk Factors and Prevention

The exact cause of esophageal cancer is unknown, but many cases are associated with chronic irritation of the esophageal tissue. Such irritants include tobacco, alcohol, gastric acid, and hot drinks. Of note, tobacco and alcohol have an additive and cumulative effect. Other predisposing factors include radiation therapy, lye ingestion, and a genetic condition, tylosis (characterized by hyperkeratosis of the palms and soles). Dietary factors, including absence of fruits and vegetables and consumption of smoked, nitrate-cured, and salt-cured foods, are implicated in esophageal cancer.

Measures to prevent esophageal cancer include avoidance or limited intake of alcohol, cessation of smoking and smokeless tobacco products, inclusion of fruits and vegetables in the daily diet, and avoidance of cured foods.

Early Detection and Diagnostic Evaluation

Early detection is best achieved by screening and following high-risk patients. The typical patient who develops esophageal cancer is a male in his 50s or 60s with a history of cigarette smoking and heavy alcohol use. Patients usually experience a 3- to 6-month history of progressive weight loss and dysphagia prior to diagnosis, and they often present with locally advanced disease. Other presenting symptoms may include pain upon swallowing, anorexia, and supraclavicular adenopathy. Patients with advanced disease may experience hoarseness due to recurrent laryngeal nerve involvement, hematemesis, melena, and cough due to tracheoesphageal fistula.

Diagnostic evaluation begins with a chest x-ray and barium esophagogram, which will reveal a narrowing of the esophagus. Endoscopy and biopsy must then follow in order to determine invasiveness of the tumor, integrity of the esophageal wall, and tumor tissue type. Once the diagnosis is confirmed, extent of disease is evaluated via computerized tomography (CT) scan of the chest and abdomen, bone scan, and bronchoscopy. Such staging is important in order to identify patients who can benefit from surgical resection of the tumor, and those with metastatic disease who will not benefit from surgery, and to assess response to treatments. Unfortunately, most esophageal cancers are not detected until the tumor is large and invasive, because the esophagus is quite distensible and thus compensates for partial blockage by the tumor.

Treatment

Treatment goal plans (cure versus palliation) are based on the clinical stage of the disease and the feasibility of surgical resection of the tumor. Surgery, radiation, and chemotherapy are all useful treatment modalities, with surgery as the primary approach whenever possible. Usually, local tumor control is best achieved by surgical resection. Because the esophagus has no mesenteric support structure, tumor resection with end-to-end anastomosis (as is done in many colorectal malignancies) is not feasible. Instead, most tumors require a partial esophagogastrectomy (removal of the affected part of the esophagus, the remaining distal end, and the upper portion of the stomach). The remaining esophagus is then reconstructed using the stomach or a segment of intestinal tissue.

Chemotherapy and radiation may be used both to palliate disease and as a part of the primary treatment program in conjunction with surgery. Cisplatin,

5-FU, and mitomycin are effective drugs; clinical trials involving other compounds are underway. Radiation therapy can be used as curative treatment for very small tumors; however, more typically, it is indicated for relief of the obstructive effects of bulky tumors.

Other palliative techniques may be used to maintain esophageal patency. These may include esophageal dilation, insertion of a funnel tube (such as the Celestin®), or direct tumor ablation using laser techniques.

Side Effects/Complications

Complications associated with surgical resection include anastomotic leaks, fistulae, and respiratory complications. Chemotherapy-related side effects are drug specific. Potential complications of radiation therapy include fistulae, strictures, hemorrhage, radiation pneumonitis, and pericarditis. Patients may experience side effects of esophageal radiation, including esophagitis and local skin reactions. Radiation side effects will vary according to the anatomical structures in the therapy field.

Nursing Considerations

Nursing care is particularly challenging because most patients present with advanced disease and treatments cause numerous complications. The goals of care include educating patients about treatment options and their side effects and assisting patients with managing complications of the disease and treatments. Difficulty managing oral secretions is particularly problematic, and it can precipitate respiratory complications due to aspiration, as well as malnutrition. Social isolation can be another problem arising from difficulty in managing oral secretions. Throughout the course of the disease, nurses play a key role in helping patients and families cope with the many challenges and fears associated with a debilitating, often terminal disease.

GASTRIC CANCER

Incidence

Although about 23,000 new cases of gastric cancer arise in the United States each year, the incidence has decreased substantially over the past several decades. Conversely, stomach cancer remains a major cause of death in Japan. Stomach cancers are more common in males than females, and a disproportionate number of cases occur in African Americans. Although the incidence of stomach cancer has declined, the death rate is still substantial, at 14,000 per year. As with many other types of cancers, stomach cancer can be cured when diagnosed and treated at an early stage.

Risk Factors and Prevention

Although the etiology of stomach cancer is unknown, several dietary factors are linked with the disease. Smoked or salted foods, foods contaminated with aflatoxin (e.g., some grains or peanuts), and low intake of fruits and vegetables are all associated with stomach cancer. The increased use of refrigeration, resulting in less need to add preservatives (e.g. salt, smoking, pickling) to food, may well account for the declining stomach cancer mortality rates over time. The bacterium associated with gastric ulcers, *Helicobacter pylori*, may also play an etiologic role; however, the exact link remains unclear. Other potential **risk factors** include pernicious anemia, peptic ulcers, adenomatous gastric polyps, achlorhydria atrophic gastritis, and low socioeconomic status.

Preventive measures for stomach cancer include following a diet rich in fruits and vegetables and low in cured foods. Individuals with the precursors described in the previous paragraph should have regular medical follow-up and receive an endoscopy should symptoms arise.

Early Detection and Diagnostic Evaluation

Typically, stomach cancer does not produce detectable symptoms until it has advanced to a late stage. The most common symptoms include loss of appetite, stomach pain, dyspepsia, dysphagia, nausea, and vomiting. Because many of these symptoms mimic benign gastric ulcers and other common stomach disorders, patients may self-treat with antacids and other over-the-counter remedies and delay seeking medical intervention for several months. As the disease progresses, weight loss, **anemia,** melena, and hematemesis may occur.

Diagnosis is usually confirmed by upper GI barium studies and tumor visualization and biopsy via endoscopic gastroscopy. Abdominal CT is also useful for evaluating liver, nodal, and other extragastric involvement.

Treatment

Surgical resection of the tumor and any involved nodes may be curative in early stages of the disease. Most often a radical subtotal gastrectomy is performed, unless the tumor is quite advanced. Either a Billroth I (gastroduodenostomy) or a Billroth II (gastrojejunostomy) procedure is selected. The Billroth II is preferred, but it is more radical in that it involves resection of 75% of the stomach and removal of the antrum, pylorus, proximal end of the duodenum, and surrounding lymph nodes and vascular support.

Unfortunately, disease often recurs after surgery; therefore, **adjuvant therapies** may be considered. When used alone, chemotherapy and radiation do not improve survival rates. However, when used in combination with surgery or each other, these treatments do improve survival. Radiation is especially useful for palliating advanced or recurrent disease. A variety of chemotherapeutic approaches may be used, including 5-FU alone or in combination with other drugs, such as leucovorin, doxorubicin, and mitomycin. Cisplatin, etoposide, and the nitrosureas have also been used with varying success.

Side Effects/Complications

Potential complications of radical gastric surgery include infection, anastomotic leak, pneumonia, reflux aspiration, and bleeding. The patient may experience problems associated with having a substantially smaller stomach. Both nutritional problems and **dumping syndrome** may occur. Side effects of abdominal irradiation may include nausea, vomiting, cramping, diarrhea, and anorexia. Chemotherapy side effects will depend upon the agents used.

Nursing Considerations

Small, frequent feedings and fluid restriction directly before and after meals may decrease the likelihood of dumping syndrome. Because most gastric tissue is removed, vitamin B deficiency will also ensue, and replacement therapy to prevent pernicious anemia is warranted. Poor nutritional intake is a substantial problem in gastric cancer and must be managed from the outset of diagnosis (see Chapter 16).

CANCER OF THE PANCREAS

Incidence

Cancer of the pancreas accounts for 2% of all new cancers, with approximately 26,000 new cases occurring each year. However, pancreatic cancer is the fourth leading cause of cancer deaths in the United States. In 1996 it was estimated that 27,800 Americans would die of pancreatic cancer. The incidence increases with age and is more prevalent in males and African Americans. Because most patients are diagnosed with locally advanced or metastatic disease, the 5-year survival rate for pancreatic cancer is 3%.

Risk Factors and Prevention

Cigarette smoking is a risk factor. Dietary factors are also implicated, with fat and meat consumption associated with higher rates of pancreatic cancer. Conversely, diets rich in fruits and vegetables are associated with lowered risk. Other conditions that may be linked with the disease include history of gastric resection for benign peptic ulcer disease, diabetes mellitus, and chronic pancreatitis.

Early Detection and Diagnostic Evaluation

Because presenting symptoms are initially vague, most pancreatic cancers are diagnosed in later stages. Symptoms include weight loss, abdominal pain, and jaundice. Other symptoms may include weakness, food intolerance, and anorexia. Of note, almost one-half of all patients are reported to have depression prior to diagnosis. Scientists postulate that this may indicate that the tumor has a neuroendocrine influence. Unless the patient is experiencing obstructive jaundice, physical examination may reveal few or no findings. Diagnostic evaluation includes abdominal CT, cholangiography, and surgical exploration. The ERCP (endoscope retrograde cholangiopancreatogram) is used to determine blockage of the pancreatic ducts; if blockage is present, a percutaneous biliary drainage tube may be inserted to facilitate drainage. Fine-needle aspiration biopsy of the tumor may be substituted for surgery, with laparoscopy to identify metastatic sites. Most pancreatic cancers are located at the head of the pancreas and are ductal adenocarcinomas. Metastatic sites include regional lymph nodes, liver, peritoneum, lung, and viscera.

Treatment

If the disease is localized, surgical resection of the tumor via total pancreatectomy or the Whipple procedure (pancreaticoduodenectomy) is warranted. The Whipple procedure involves removal of the head of the pancreas, duodenum, gastric antrum, bile duct, and gall bladder. If the tumor is advanced, other palliative surgical options are available. Biliary obstruction may be relieved via either a biliary bypass cholecystojejunostomy or a choledochojejunostomy. A gastroenterostomy may be performed to relieve gastric outlet obstruction. Biliary tract decompression can be accomplished via placement of a endoscopic stent.

Combination therapy with radiation and chemotherapy may prolong survival slightly for some patients; radiation alone is especially helpful for palliating symptoms in advanced cases.

Side Effects/Complications

Although potential surgical complications depend upon the specific operative procedure selected, typical problems include anastomotic leakage, fistula formation, abscess, and pneumonia. As with any major abdominal surgery, infection, hemorrhage, and hypovolemia may occur. Pancreatic resection also results in disruptions of both exocrine and endocrine functions. Metabolism of fat, protein, and glucose may all be disrupted. Similarly, insulin secretion and glucagon production will be altered. Thus, oral pancreatic enzyme supplements and insulin replacement therapy are necessary.

Nursing Considerations

Postoperative care includes careful monitoring and prompt intervention for surgical complications. Rigorous nutritional management is critical, given that the patient now has difficulty absorbing fat and protein. Patients experience marked alterations in dietary habits, necessitating intensive teaching regarding insulin therapy, enzyme supplements, and dietary changes. Most patients do best on small, frequent feedings of a bland, low-fat diet rich in carbohydrates and protein. Consultation with a clinical dietitian is strongly advised.

Unfortunately, most forms of pancreatic cancer progress rapidly, and most patients die within the first year after diagnosis. Palliative care via aggressive symptom management is critical. Clinical problems typically include pain, nausea, jaundice with associated pruritus (related to liver damage or ductal obstruction), ascites, hemorrhage, and hepatic failure.

LIVER CANCER

Most cancers detected in the liver are metastatic deposits, not primary tumors. Liver **metastases** are associated with many primary cancers, including lung, breast, kidney, and gastrointestinal tumors. However, primary liver cancer can occur

Incidence

Liver and biliary cancers combined represent about 19,900 new cases each year in the United States. **Mortality** is high, with 15,200 deaths estimated per year. Specifically, primary liver cancer, or *hepatocellular carcinoma*, is uncommon in the United States, yet it represents one of the most common cancers among men in the world. Approximately 1 million new cases arise worldwide each year, with most cases occurring in Asia and Africa. The 5-year survival rate for patients with primary liver cancer is less than 2%.

Risk Factors and Prevention

A number of environmental and host risk factors are associated with liver cancer. In particular, viral infection with hepatitis B and hepatitis C is strongly implicated. Other risk factors include ethanol ingestion, cirrhosis, malnutrition, aflatoxin ingestion, use of thorotrast (a biliary contrast medium), occupational exposure to vinyl chloride, and certain hereditary liver diseases. Prevention can be achieved through avoidance of risk factors, and in particular, immunization against hepatitis B virus may mitigate incidence rates once it becomes more widely available.

Early Detection and Diagnostic Evaluation

Much like other cancers of the gastrointestinal tract, the onset of liver cancer is insidious. Symptoms may include dull right upper quadrant abdominal pain, fatigue, weakness, constipation or diarrhea, epigastric fullness, anorexia, and weight loss. Abdominal mass and increased girth due to ascites may be present. Typically, serum liver function tests are abnormal, with elevations in alkaline phosphatase, asparate aminotransferase, and alanine aminotransferase. Only a minority of patients present with an elevated bilirubin. **Alpha-fetoprotein (AFP)** is typically elevated upon diagnosis and is a useful marker for monitoring response to treatment.

Diagnostic imaging studies include abdominal ultrasound, CT of the abdomen and lungs, and MRI. **Radionuclide** scanning of the liver is also helpful. Ultimately, needle biopsy under ultrasound or CT is usually done to confirm diagnosis, but it may be avoided if surgical resection is planned.

Treatment

Surgery, chemotherapy, and radiotherapy are all options for control and potential cure. Localized, early disease is best treated via surgical resection. Presence and extent of cirrhosis will mediate this decision. Liver transplantation has been attempted, but it is associated with high incidence of recurrence in the new liver. Because most patients are not candidates for curative or palliative surgery, chemotherapy may be offered. Approaches include systemic or regional perfusion (via hepatic artery or portal vein) of single or combination agents. Drugs used include FUDR, 5-FU, cisplatin, streptozotocin, etoposide, mitomycin-C, folinic acid, and mitoxantrone. Regional perfusion of drugs into the tumor vasculature is of great interest. This procedure may allow for the administration of concentrated dosages directly into the tumor bed while decreasing systemic toxicity.

Side Effects/Complications

Complications of liver resection may include hemorrhage, infection, metabolic aberrations, biliary fistula formation, abscess, pneumonia, portal hypertension, and coagulation abnormalities. Side effects of chemotherapy depend on the specific agents in use. Regional drug administration typically involves temporary (or permanent) placement of an arterial catheter directly into the tumor vasculature. Infusion of drugs via this method can precipitate both hepatic and gastric toxicity.

Nursing Considerations

Nursing care is twofold: A focus on management of treatment-induced complications and supportive care over the disease trajectory are both important. Postoperative care after liver resection includes assessment and early intervention for the complications listed earlier. Chemotherapy side effects depend on the agents in use. Because most patients die within 6 months of diagnosis, emphasis must be placed on supportive care of the patient and family. Clinical problems associated with advanced liver cancer include pain, hepatic failure, ascites, bleeding, infection, weakness, anorexia, weight loss, and pneumonia. Aggressive pain management is critical, coupled with other palliative measures to control discomfort associated with nausea, vomiting, ascites, pruritus, and other manifestations of liver failure.

BILIARY CANCER

Epidemiology

Cancer that arises in the intrahepatic or extrahepatic bile ducts is termed *cholangiocarcinoma*. This unusual subset of liver cancers accounts for about 10% of all cases. Cholangiocarcinoma is typically diagnosed in patients 50 to 70 years old; male cases predominate slightly over female cases. Cholangiocarcinoma is most prevalent in Southeast Asia and is associated with parasitic infection with liver flukes. Such biliary parasites may be etiologic agents due to their precipitation of hyperplasia of biliary epithelium. Other risk factors include chronic inflammation of the biliary tree, which can be due to polycystic liver disease, choledochal cysts, sclerosing cholangitis, hepatolithiasis, cholelithiasis, and injection of the diagnostic imaging contrast thorotrast.

Detection and Diagnosis

Most patients with cholangiocarcinoma present with extensive, advanced disease with regional lymph node involvement and distant metastases (lung or bone). Depending on the precise site of origin, presenting symptoms may include obstructive jaundice, hepatomegaly, upper abdominal mass, abdominal and back pain, and weight loss. Serologic studies may show increased levels of alkaline phosphatase, bilirubin, CEA, and CA19-9.

Treatment

Treatment options are limited. Liver transplantation has been attempted, but patients typically relapse within months. A very small subset of patients who are diagnosed prior to metastatic disease can have long-term survival after surgical resection. Another subset of patients, those who have extrahepatic, or hilar bile duct cholangiocarcinoma, can achieve a 3-year survival rate as high as 50%.

ENDOCRINE CANCERS

Collectively, the endocrine gland tumors represent about 14,500 new cases per year. Thyroid cancer is the most common type of endocrine tumor; other types include adrenal carcinoma, **pheochromocytomas,** pituitary tumors, parathyroid tumors, multiple endocrine neoplasia syndrome, carcinoid tumors, and pancreatic islet cell tumors. The endocrine tumors represent a diverse group of both **benign** and **malignant** disorders. Often, clinical manifestations of the tumors are first evident due to symptoms associated with either excess or deficient hormone production by the target organ. Given its relative prevalence as opposed to the other tumor types, thyroid cancer will be reviewed here.

THYROID CANCER

Incidence

Approximately 15,600 new cases of **thyroid cancer** arise in the United States each year. Overall, mortality is low, with about 1,200 deaths per year. The prevalence is greater in women than in men, and in whites than in African Americans. Most cases occur between the ages of 25 and 60. Thyroid cancers are classified according to tissue type. The four major subtypes are **papillary, follicular, medullary,** and **anaplastic.** The most commonly occurring subtype is papillary.

Risk Factors and Prevention

Although the precise origin of thyroid cancer is unknown, a number of risk factors have been identified. A primary risk factor is a history of therapeutic irradiation to the head and neck region for benign conditions. In the 1940s and 1950s, such treatment was used in children with tonsilar or thymic hyperplasia, acne, and tinea capitis. Many of these individuals now experience thyroid abnormalities in adulthood; approximately 7% will develop thyroid cancer. Other risk factors include preexisting goiter and family history of multiple endocrine neoplasia.

Early Detection and Diagnostic Evaluation

Most typically, thyroid cancer is evidenced by a mass detected upon physical examination. The presence of other symptoms is unlikely unless the disease is advanced. Symptoms such as hoarseness, dysphagia, shortness of breath, and hormonal irregularities indicate later-stage disease. The diagnosis is confirmed via tissue examination obtained by fine-needle biopsy.

Treatment

Surgical resection via total or subtotal thyroidectomy is the treatment of choice. Radiation therapy may also be used as an alternative or in addition to surgery. Typically, radiation is administered by oral ingestion of a radionuclide solution of ^{131}I. This is termed *ablative therapy*, in that it inactivates any remaining thyroid tissue, and it may be used in place of surgery for metastatic disease or as an adjunct to destroy any residual thyroid function. External beam irradiation may be useful for treatment of recurrent cancers previously treated with ^{131}I.

Side Effects/Complications

Potential complications of thyroidectomy include hemorrhage, impaired airway, and either temporary or permanent vocal cord paralysis. Because the parathyroid glands may be damaged by surgical manipulation, hypocalcemia can occur. Most patients tolerate ^{131}I treatment fairly well; potential complications include nausea and vomiting, fatigue, headache, inflamed salivary glands, and bone marrow suppression. Side effects of external beam thyroid irradiation include skin erythema, **mucositis**, dysphagia, and anorexia.

Nursing Considerations

The focus of nursing care depends on the treatment selected. Postoperatively, the focus of care is on maintaining airway patency and monitoring for bleeding, symptoms of hypocalcemia, and vocal cord impairment. Patients with little or no residual thyroid function after treatment will require thyroid hormone replacement therapy for the rest of their lives.

Replacement therapy must be discontinued 4 to 6 weeks prior to administration of ^{131}I in order to allow for thyroid hormone levels to drop and TSH levels to rise. TSH allows glandular uptake of ^{131}I. Care considerations for ^{131}I therapy include explaining and maintaining radiation precautions. It is important to remember that all body fluids will be radioactive for several days after ^{131}I therapy. Therefore, patients should be instructed about measures to prevent or reduce exposure of others to radioactivity. These measures include flushing the commode three times after each use; avoiding close physical contact; using separate eating utensils, linens, towels, and clothing; and sleeping in a bed alone until the radioactivity drops to a safe level. The amount of time that these precautions should be maintained varies according to the dose of ^{131}I administered. Patients receiving high doses of ^{131}I require hospitalization in isolation. Additional radiation precautions are necessary for these patients (see Chapter 8). Antiemetics may be needed to prevent nausea and vomiting, and patients need **support** and encouragement, especially while in isolation. The focus of care for patients receiving external beam treatment includes oral hygiene to prevent or relieve discomfort from mucositis, appropriate skin care measures for the irradiated field, nutritional support, and modification of activities due to fatigue.

UNKNOWN PRIMARY CANCER

Given the sophisticated diagnostic tools of cancer medicine, most cancers can be located and pinpointed to a primary site of origin. Occasionally, however, a patient will have a biopsy-proven metastatic site, but the primary tumor cannot be identified. This situation is termed *unknown primary cancer*, or *UPC*.

Incidence

The incidence of UPC ranges anywhere from 0.05% to 9% of all patients diagnosed with cancer. Typically, patients present with metastatic sites in the lung, liver, bone, or lymph nodes; yet, no primary disease site is apparent. Fortunately, the incidence of UPC seems to be decreasing due to improvements in diagnostic capabilities.

Risk Factors and Prevention

UPC is considered to represent a diverse, heterogeneous group of cancers; thus, it is difficult to identify particular risk factors. A history of cigarette smoking is the only identified risk factor that occurs with regularity. Not surprisingly, many patients with UPC are ultimately found to have lung cancer.

Diagnostic Evaluation

The patient with UPC must receive a meticulous history and physical examination. In essence, this patient requires a head-to-toe cancer screening work-up. Any suspicious findings help to guide the diagnostic process. Laboratory studies are conducted likewise. For example, a decreased hemoglobin/hematocrit could indicate an anemia secondary to blood loss from the GI tract. Further GI studies could then focus on that area as a potential primary site. **Tumor markers,** including beta-HCG, PSA, AFP, CEA, and CA-125, are also useful in guiding the clinician to other, more specific diagnostic studies. Chest x-ray is essential, but it may not differentiate between primary and metastatic lesions. Bilateral mammography is also paramount. Other, more sophisticated imaging studies are not warranted (unless symptoms dictate), with the exception of the abdominal and pelvic CT scan, which can reveal otherwise occult primary tumors in the pancreas, ovary, hepatoma, kidney, lung, adrenal gland, gallbladder, and stomach.

Treatment

If, despite this thorough work-up, a primary tumor cannot be found, a variety of approaches may be attempted. A small minority of patients do form a subset of six highly treatable UPCs. These include women with axillary adenopathy, women with peritoneal carcinomatosis, patients with poorly **differentiated** or undifferentiated carcinoma, men with extragonadal germ cell syndrome, patients with neuroendocrine **carcinoma,** and patients with high cervical adenopathy. This subset is known to respond well to specific treatment that can extend survival. Most patients, however, do not have any known optimal treatment and are typically treated with chemotherapy regimens. These include adriamycin®, 5-FU, and cisplatin-based combinations, which have initial response rates of 20% to 30%. Radiation may be used to palliate tumor-related symptoms. Response to treatment is typically brief; overall median survival is less than 12 months.

Side Effects/Complications

Complications of treatment depend on the specific approaches used.

Nursing Considerations

Care of the patient with an unknown primary site requires tremendous sensitivity. The patient grapples not only with a cancer diagnosis, but also with the distressing news that the primary site cannot be located. Such a situation often precipitates distrust and loss of confidence in the medical team. Patients require extensive support through the diagnostic phase and sensitive, yet frank explanation of treatment options and potential outcomes. Because median survival ranges from 9 to 12 months, patients and families require the full spectrum of the psychological, spiritual, and physical care needs of the terminally ill.

CONCLUSION

With the exception of thyroid cancer, the malignancies presented in this chapter are difficult to treat and create challenging patient care problems. Many patients who develop these cancers may well be eligible for clinical trials and need considerable assistance as they struggle with treatment decisions. Regardless of treatment outcome, patients and families require strong supportive care skills from all members of the interdisciplinary team.

BIBLIOGRAPHY

Abruzzese, J. L., & Raber, M. N. (1995). Unknown primary. In M. Abeloff, J. Armitage, A. Lichter, & J. Niederhuber (Eds.), Clinical oncology (pp. 1833–1845). New York: Churchill Livingstone.

Baker, K., & Feldman, J. (1993). Thyroid cancer: A review. *Oncology Nursing Forum, 20,* 95–104.

Curley, S., Levin, B., & Rich, T. (1995). Liver and bile ducts. In M. Abeloff, J. Armitage, A. Lichter, & J. Niederhuber (Eds.), *Clinical oncology* (pp. 1305–1371). New York: Churchill Livingstone.

Donehower, M. G. (1993). Endocrine cancers. In S. Groenwald, M. Frogge, M. Goodman, & C. Yarbro (Eds.), *Cancer nursing principles and practice* (3rd ed., pp. 984–1003). Sudbury, MA: Jones and Bartlett.

Frogge, M. H. (1993). Gastrointestinal cancer: Esophagus, stomach, liver, and pancreas. In S. Groenwald, M. Frogge, M. Goodman, & C. Yarbro (Eds.), *Cancer nursing: Principles and practice* (3rd ed., pp. 1004–1043). Sudbury, MA: Jones and Bartlett.

Held, J., & Peahota, A. (1992). Nursing care of patients with esophageal cancer. *Oncology Nursing Forum, 19,* 627–634.

36

Childhood Cancers

Marcia Rostad
Ki Moore

According to the American Cancer Society, 8,300 new cases of childhood cancer were estimated in 1996. One in every 475 children in the United States develops cancer before the age of 15 years. Randomized clinical trials have resulted in more effective treatment for many **tumors,** and long-term disease-free survival has continued to increase. **Survival rates** vary across specific tumors, but the overall 5-year survival rate is 68%. Advances in clinical supportive care such as **vascular access devices (VADs), enteral** and **parenteral nutrition,** new antimicrobial agents, and **colony-stimulating factors** have greatly reduced the number of treatment-related deaths. Despite the impressive strides in treatment and supportive care, cancer is still the leading cause of death from disease in children between the ages of 1 and 14 years. There were an estimated 1,700 cancer deaths in 1996, about one-third from **leukemia.**

The types of cancers that occur in children vary greatly from those seen in adults. Approximately 92% of pediatric cancers—leukemias, **lymphomas, sarcomas,** and embryonal tumors—arise from primitive embryonal tissue of mesodermal origin; central nervous system tumors arise from neuroectodermal tissue. In adults, approximately 87% of tumors are derived from tissue of epithelial origin and are called **carcinomas.** Carcinomas that are common in adults, such as lung, breast, or colorectal cancer, are rare in children. **Risk factors** for pediatric and adult tumors are also different. In adults, the latency period between exposure to environmental **carcinogens** and tumor development is long. In children, because the latency period is short, environmental risk factors are poorly understood; exposure may occur prior to conception or during the prenatal period. The development of many pediatric tumors parallels the peak time of cell growth and **differentiation** in the tissue of origin. For example, loss or inactivation of the gene that directs differentiation of nephroblasts into nephrons is associated with the

development of **Wilms' tumor.** The immaturity of children's organ systems also
has important implications for treatment and for delayed toxicity. Similarly, the
stage of psychosocial and cognitive development will greatly influence the child's
emotional response to the illness. Childhood cancers affecting the central nervous system are discussed in Chapter 29, bone tumors in Chapter 31, and lymphomas in Chapter 33.

ACUTE LEUKEMIA

Incidence

Acute lymphoblastic leukemia (ALL), the most common childhood malignancy, accounts for almost one third of all pediatric cancers. The **incidence** of ALL
is 1 per 23,000 children; approximately 2,000 new cases are diagnosed annually
in the United States. **Acute myelocytic leukemia (AML)** accounts for 15% to
25% of all leukemias occurring in childhood. AML occurs equally among boys
and girls and across all ethnic groups, whereas the incidence of ALL is higher in
white than in nonwhite children and higher in males than in females. The exact
cause of childhood leukemia is unknown. However, radiation, chromosomal
abnormalities, viruses, and congenital immunodeficiencies have all been associated with an increased incidence of leukemia. Early **detection** of the leukemia is
valuable in controlling associated complications.

Pathology

The pathophysiology of childhood leukemia involves unregulated proliferation
and incomplete maturation ("blasts") of either **lymphocytes** (ALL) or myeloid
cells (AML). Replacement of normal hematopoietic cells in the bone marrow by
the immature blasts accounts for the signs and symptoms usually present at diagnosis: **thrombocytopenia** with numerous bruises and petechiae; recurrent infections and fever; **anemia** with irritability and fatigue; and bone pain. The white
blood cell (WBC) count may be low (< 10,000) or high (> 100,000). Invasion
of the liver, spleen, testes, and lymph nodes by circulating blasts is manifested as
organomegaly and lymphadenopathy. The disease can also involve the central
nervous system (CNS): approximately 10% of children with ALL and 10% to
25% of children with AML have blasts in the cerebral spinal fluid at **diagnosis.**
Immature cells migrate out of the bone marrow and into the peripheral blood.
Despite the evidence of leukemic cells in the blood, a bone marrow aspiration is
usually required to confirm the diagnosis.

Large, multi-institutional clinical studies have identified factors that suggest
outcome and determine the intensity of ALL therapy. Cell morphology, initial
WBC count, and age at diagnosis are the most important prognostic factors.
Predictors of good survival include small lymphoblasts with a scant amount of

cytoplasm and regular nuclear shapes with occasional clefting, an initial WBC less than 10,000, and age of diagnosis between 2 and 10 years. Little is known about the risk factors for childhood leukemia. However, there is modest evidence that maternal alcohol consumption during pregnancy increases the risk of infant leukemia, especially AML, and paternal preconception exposure to radiation has been associated with an increased risk of leukemia in the infant. History of maternal fetal loss has been associated with an increased risk of leukemia, especially in children who are diagnosed before the age of 2 years.

It has been difficult to determine prognostic factors in AML because this malignancy is a heterogeneous group of leukemias. That is, it is made up of various immature cells from different myeloid precursors. There is a progressive increase in the risk of a poor outcome proportional to the WBC at diagnosis. The prognosis is also worse when children are under 2 years of age at diagnosis. The presence or absence of abnormal chromosomes has not been shown to affect outcome as it does in ALL.

Treatment

ALL treatment involves several phases. The goal of remission induction is to rapidly decrease the leukemia tumor burden with combination **chemotherapy. Central nervous system prophylaxis** with whole brain radiation and/or **intrathecal chemotherapy** is essential to preventing leukemia involvement of the brain and meninges. An intensification or consolidation phase to eradicate any residual tumor cells follows. Finally, up to 2 years of **maintenance chemotherapy** are required to sustain a complete remission. Common treatment regimens are outlined in Table 36–1.

Remission induction can be achieved in AML with the use of cytosine arabinoside (Ara-C) and one of the anthracyclines. CNS prophylaxis using intrathecal Ara-C and/or methotrexate with or without cranial radiation is also necessary. Continuation therapy follows, but its duration, intensity, and timing are controversial. Continuation therapy may involve several cycles of therapy over a relatively short span of time or similiar therapy extended over many months. Some treatment regimens suggest a bone marrow transplant at this point in therapy for AML rather than waiting for a relapse of the disease.

With current leukemia therapy, 95% of children with ALL and 75% of children with AML will achieve a complete remission. While 70% of children with ALL will remain in remission for 5 years or longer, only 25% with AML are long-term survivors. The bone marrow is the most common site of initial relapse, but relapses in the central nervous system or testes can also occur alone or along with marrow relapse. Relapses are treated with a repeat of **induction chemotherapy** followed by a modified regimen of **intensification therapy.** Second remissions historically are shorter than the first, especially if the relapse occurred relatively early into therapy. In these situations, a bone marrow transplant may offer the best chance for survival.

TABLE 36–1   Commonly Used Chemotherapeutic Agents for Childhood
Acute Lymphoblastic Leukemia

Treatment Phase	Chemotherapy
Remission induction	vincristine prednisone L-asparaginase*
Central nervous system prophylaxis	intrathecal methotrexate triple intrathecal therapy with methotrexate, arabinoside cytosine, and hydrocortisone intermediate or high-dose methotrexate in conjunction with intrathecal therapy cranial or craniospinal radiation**
Consolidation/ intensification	L-asparaginase vincristine prednisone methotrexate arabinoside cytosine* cyclophosphamide* VM-26*
Maintenance	6-mercaptopurine methotrexate vincristine prednisone

* Used to improve duration of remission, especially for patients with poor prognostic features.
** Used in conjunction with intrathecal chemotherapy for patients with CNS disease or in some patients with poor prognostic features.

WILMS' TUMOR

Incidence

Wilms' tumor is the most common primary malignant renal tumor of childhood. The incidence rate is 8.1 cases per million in white children less than 15 years of age and is slightly higher in females than males. There are approximately 460 new cases each year, accounting for 5% to 6% of all childhood cancers in the United States.

Pathology

The Wilms' tumor suppressor gene has been isolated on the short arm of chromosome 11, band 13. Loss or inactivation of the gene on both copies of chromosome 11 is required for tumor development, and it has been observed in at least one-third of children with Wilms' tumor. The majority of tumors are sporadic; however, in familial cases, the loss or inactivation of one copy of the gene

TABLE 36-2 National Wilms' Tumor Study Grouping Criteria

Group	Features
I	Tumor limited to kidney and completely excised. Surface of renal capsule is intact. Tumor was not ruptured before or during removal. No residual tumor apparent beyond margins of resection.
II	Tumor extended beyond kidney but is completely excised. Local extension into perirenal soft tissues, or periaortic lymph node involvement. No residual tumor apparent beyond margins of resection.
III	Residual nonhematogenous tumor confined to abdomen. Any of the following may occur: (a) tumor rupture before or during surgery; (b) implants on peritoneal surfaces; (c) lymph node involvement beyond abdominal periaortic chains; (d) incomplete tumor resection because of local infiltration into vital structures.
IV	Hematogenous metastases. Deposits are beyond Group III, affecting lung, liver, bone, and brain.
V	Bilateral renal involvement either initially or subsequently.

is inherited and loss of the second copy is likely. It is unclear how many cases involve autosomal dominant transmission, but it is frequent enough that Wilms' tumor in more than one child in a family is not unusual.

The tumor is also associated with certain congenital anomalies, including genitourinary malformations; hemihypertrophy of an organ or body part, alone or as a component of the Beckwith-Wiedemann syndrome; and aniridia. Several epidemiologic studies suggest an increased incidence in children of men exposed to lead and hydrocarbons, while other studies fail to confirm these findings.

Wilms' tumor is often discovered by a parent who notices an increase in the child's abdominal size or, on physical examination, as a nontender firm flank mass. The child may be asymptomatic or have additional signs and symptoms such as abdominal pain, vomiting, or gross or microscopic hematuria. Hypertension may be present due to tumor compression of the renal vasculature. Radiologic studies, abdominal **ultrasound,** abdominal **computerized tomography (CT),** and/or **magnetic resonance imaging (MRI)** are used to determine the location, extent, and stage of the primary tumor. Laboratory studies should include a CBC with differential, platelet count, liver function tests, renal function tests, serum calcium, and a urinalysis.

The most common metastatic site for Wilms' tumor is the lung; the disease may also spread to regional lymph nodes and the liver. The extent of disease is an important prognostic factor and is used to determine tumor stage (Table 36-2). Tumor **histology** is also of prognostic significance. Well-differentiated tumors are the most common and are associated with an excellent prognosis. Tumors of unfavorable histology, and accompanying poor prognosis, include those with anaplastic cytology and clear-cell sarcoma and rhabdoid tumors of the kidney.

Treatment

Nephrectomy is required for all patients with unilateral disease. Surgical treatment of patients with extensive bilateral disease involves excision of tumor with preservation of normal renal tissue if possible. Preoperative radiotherapy or chemotherapy to reduce tumor size is used only when surgical risk is high. Clinical trials conducted by the National Wilms' Tumor Study Group have led to significant strides in treatment. **Adjuvant** combination chemotherapy is recommended for Stage I and Stage II tumors; radiation to the tumor bed, in addition to chemotherapy, is recommended for Stage III and Stage IV tumors and for all tumors with unfavorable histology. Adjuvant chemotherapy for children with Stage I and Stage II favorable histology tumors involves vincristine and dactinomycin. A three-drug regimen with the addition of doxorubicin is used for Stage III tumors, and doxorubicin plus cyclophosphamide has been found to be beneficial in all Stage IV patients and for all tumors with unfavorable histology. With current therapy, the outlook for children with Wilms' tumor is excellent. Children with favorable histology and nonmetastatic disease have a 90% chance for long-term survival. Even those with advanced disease or unfavorable histology have an 80% survival rate. The most common site of disease recurrence is the lung. However, the tumor may also occur in the liver, opposite kidney, original tumor bed, and other intra-abdominal sites. After recurrence, approximately 50% of patients can be treated effectively with chemotherapy, radiation, and surgery.

NEUROBLASTOMA

Incidence

Neuroblastoma is the most common extracranial solid tumor in children and the most commonly diagnosed neoplasm during the first year of life. This tumor accounts for 10% of all pediatric cancers diagnosed annually in the United States. However, the incidence may be higher because of the phenomenon of spontaneous tumor regression and maturation. In this unique circumstance, neuroblastic tumor cells present in neonates and infants either disappear or develop into mature, normal neural cells. As a result, many of these cases go unreported because their presence was undetected.

Pathology

Neuroblastoma originates from neural crest cells that are normally the progenitors of the sympathetic nervous system. The precise cause(s) of the disease is unknown; however, chromosomal abnormalities and an increased number of copies of the *N-myc* **oncogene** have been found in some neuroblastoma cells. About 20% of cases are familial—again because of autosomal dominant gene transmission—with an increased incidence among siblings and identical twins.

Risk factors (parental and child) that contribute to the development of neuroblastoma remain unidentified, although many possibilities are being investigated.

Neuroblastoma can originate anywhere along the sympathetic nervous system. More than half the tumors occur in the retroperitoneal area and present as an abdominal mass. Other common sites include the posterior mediastinum, pelvis, and neck. The child should be evaluated using imaging studies (CT and/or MRI scan) to help clearly identify the location(s) of the solid tumor. A meta-iodobenzylguanidine (MIBG) bone scan can help determine bony and tissue involvement.

Nutritional problems, including weight loss, **anorexia, cachexia,** and diarrhea may be present at diagnosis. It is not uncommon for these children to require urgent nutritional interventions including, in some cases, the use of **total parenteral nutrition (TPN).** Urinary catecholamines are elevated in 80% of children with neuroblastoma. Symptoms related to increased catecholamines include hypertension, flushing, periods of excessive sweating, and irritability. Antihypertensive agents may be necessary to help stabilize the child's clinical condition.

A bone marrow aspirate is obtained for staging purposes. The **staging** for neuroblastoma proceeds from Stage I through Stage IV. If the bone marrow is involved, the child may experience bone pain and exhibit anemia, thrombocytopenia, and leukopenia. Spread to the orbits can cause ecchymosis and sometimes proptosis. Bluish, movable cutaneous or subcutaneous nodules are seen almost exclusively in infants.

Age at diagnosis, site of origin, and clinical stage of the disease affect survival. Age is the most important factor. Children under age 1 year have a 75% survival rate. Spontaneous remission without treatment can occur in infants, even with disease spread to other organ system(s). The survival rate for children diagnosed at age 2 years or older drops to 12%.

It would appear that early detection of neuroblastoma while a child is still young would help improve overall survival. However, mass screenings of infants for the detection of elevated urine catacholamines is plagued with enormous problems, including unreliable methods of urine collection, unreliability of test results, lack of access to all infants, infants lost to follow-up, consumption of expensive resources, and subjection of infants to treatment that may not be necessary. Mass **screening** trials continue despite these problems, but they have not become an established public health practice.

Children with an abdominal primary mass have a poorer survival record than those with a chest, neck, or pelvic primary tumor. Sites of metastatic spread include the lymph nodes, bone, bone marrow, liver, and subcutaneous tissue. Unfortunately, 50% of infants and 66% of older children have widespread metastatic disease at diagnosis. Children with advanced disease have the best prognosis if younger than 1 or older than 6 years of age, but the average age at diagnosis is 2 years. In addition, tumors often progress rapidly in patients with multiple copies of the N-myc oncogene in the neuroblastoma cells.

Treatment

Treatment for neuroblastoma involves surgery for staging and tumor removal and aggressive combination chemotherapy. Treatment regimens commonly use some combination of vincristine, etoposide, VM-26, ifosfamide, cyclophosphamide, cisplatin, caraboplatin, and doxorubicin. Radiation therapy to the primary tumor site may precede or follow surgery and chemotherapy. Children who are at risk for poor survival with conventional treatment alone may benefit from intensive short-term chemotherapy followed by **autologous bone marrow transplantation.**

RETINOBLASTOMA

Incidence

Retinoblastoma is the most common primary tumor of the eye in children. It occurs in approximately 1 in every 20,000 live births, and there are an estimated 200 to 300 new cases each year in the United States. The majority of tumors are diagnosed before the age of 5 years. The incidence in the United States is 10.42 cases per million children between birth and 4 years of age, 1.53 per million from 5 to 9 years of age, and 0.27 per million at ages 10 to 14 years.

Pathology

Approximately 70% of children present with a unilateral tumor, while 30% have bilateral disease. Risk factors for retinoblastoma are currently under investigation. In a recent epidemiologic study, five significant associations between occupation and retinoblastoma were identifed. The common factors across the identified occupations are thought to be metal and pesticide exposures prior to conception of the child, or during gestation or infancy.

Retinoblastoma can be hereditary or nonhereditary. The hereditary type is autosomal dominant with an 88% to 100% transmission rate. All bilateral tumors and 15% of unilateral tumors are hereditary. A deletion of band 14 on the long arm of chromosome 13 is seen in all cells of children with the hereditary form of the disease, but only in tumor cells in those with sporadic disease. Loss of the retinoblastoma gene results in unregulated cell proliferation and tumor development. Hereditary retinoblastoma also carries an increased risk for other malignancies.

The Reese-Ellsworth classification system is used for tumor staging, treatment, and prognosis. If the tumor is behind the equator and less than 4 (Group I) or no greater than 10 (Group II) optic disc diameters in size, survival is 85% to 100%. Larger lesions or those that extend anterior to the equator have a less favorable prognosis. Two types of growth patterns have been identified in retinoblastoma. Endophytic tumors grow mainly in the inner layers of the retina and fill the vitreous body. Exophytic tumors grow along the outer retinal layer and can spread to the subretinal space, causing retinal detachment. This commonly occurs with very large tumors, but it can be corrected after starting treatment. Most tumors are a combination of both growth patterns. Extraocular tumor growth usually occurs along the optic nerve. Invasion of the optic nerve with 10 to 15 mm of tumor growth can cause subarachnoid and intracranial spread. Optic nerve involvement carries a poor prognosis.

The tumor is usually painless. Symptoms include strabismus and leukokoria (white spots in the pupil of the eye). Leukokoria is the most common presenting symptom. Loss of vision also occurs, but it is difficult for small children to identify. Early tumor detection is critical. The extent to which vision is preserved is directly related to the size of the tumor at the start of therapy. If the tumor is detected early, cure is possible with radiation therapy alone, and the vision is preserved. Most cases of unilateral retinoblastoma are so far advanced that there is little or no hope of preserving vision. Enucleation is the treatment of choice.

Treatment

Bilateral disease treatment includes radiation and possible enucleation of one or both eyes if no vision can be saved. Chemotherapy is also used for extraocular disease or distant tumor spread. Finally, genetic counseling is recommended if a family history of retinoblastoma is identified. Nurses can emphasize to families the importance of monitoring siblings of affected children and also of monitoring a child with a history of retinoblastoma for a second malignancy.

RHABDOMYOSARCOMA

Incidence

Rhabdomyosarcoma is the most common soft tissue **sarcoma** and the seventh leading cause of cancer in children. The tumor, which is more prevalent in males than females, originates from the same embryonic cells that give rise to striated muscle. The peak incidence is between the ages of 2 and 5 years; a second peak occurs between the ages of 15 and 19 years. Its etiology remains unknown, but it can occur as a secondary malignancy after exposure to radiation and in children with the genetic form of retinoblastoma. Associations between the occurrence of this malignancy in the offspring of patients with cancer risk factors (smoking, chlorophenol exposure, breast cancer gene) are also being examined.

Pathology

The most common tumor sites are the head and neck, including the orbit (38%), the genitourinary tract (21%), and the extremities (18%). A painless mass is the major symptom at diagnosis. Specific symptoms present at diagnosis are usually related to the anatomical site of the tumor: nosebleeds, difficulty breathing, sinus congestion, and facial palsies from head and neck tumors; hematuria, urinary obstruction, and vaginal bleeding from genitourinary tumors; and an anatomical deformity from an extremity tumor. The diagnostic work-up should include an imaging scan of the suspected tumor area, as well as of distant organ systems (chest, abdomen, cranial spinal area) to evaluate for disease spread. A bone scan and bone marrow aspirate are also necessary.

Rhabdomyosarcoma is staged similarly to neuroblastoma. Stage I is localized and completely resectable. Disease with distant **metastasis** is categorized as Stage IV. Children without metastases at diagnosis have a much better prognosis.

Treatment

Treatment for rhabdomyosarcoma includes surgical removal (if possible), radiation, and chemotherapy. Chemotherapy can be administered before surgery to reduce the tumor size. Useful agents include vincristine, dactinomycin, cyclophosphamide, ifosfamide, and etoposide. With tumor shrinkage, less radical surgery is possible, resulting in less damage to adjacent tissues. Chemotherapy and radiation are used after surgery to eradicate any residual tumor cells. Chemotherapy is continued for 1 to 2 years, because the majority of patients relapse during this period. Patients who receive radiation for head, neck, and bladder tumors are at increased risk for late effects such as short stature (growth hormone impairment) and impaired secondary sexual development.

SUPPORTIVE CARE

The role of the nurse in supportive care is extensive in preventing and/or assessing and intervening to manage side effects of treatment. Children receiving treatment for cancer can experience numerous complications. Nausea and vomiting, infection, and pain are three complications that are most distressing for the child and, when poorly managed, can lead to physiologic harm. Nausea and vomiting are associated with chemotherapy and radiation therapy. The true vomiting center, located in the medulla of the brain, is stimulated by several sources including noxious substances, disagreeable tastes and smells, and psychogenic factors. Emphasis should be placed on prevention starting with the first course of therapy to minimize the development of anticipatory nausea and vomiting. Untreated, nausea and vomiting can lead to dehydration, electrolyte imbalance, and malnutrition. Most currently available antiemetic agents can be used safely in children. Dosages should be carefully calculated by body weight, and the child should be observed for any medication reactions. (Refer to Chapter 14 for antiemetic agents.)

Immunosuppression commonly occurs in children who receive dose-intensive therapy. Febrile **neutropenia** can occur when the absolute neutrophil count drops below 500/mm³. Bacterial infections occur most frequently and are usually attributed to gram-negative organisms, which have invaded the blood stream via the intestinal tract, or gram-positive organisms, which enter through breaks in the skin or through an indwelling catheter. Children are often treated with intravenous antibiotics for 10 to 14 days. They are at risk for development of new infections if the period of immunosuppression is prolonged. For these children, it maybe necessary to administer two to three different antibiotic agents.

The availability of colony-stimulating factors (CSFs) can help shorten the period of time the child is granulocytopenic. Granulocyte-CSF and granulocyte-monocyte-CSF are two agents that can expedite the production of white blood cells. These agents are administered on a daily basis following a course of chemotherapy and are discontinued once a desirable white blood cell count (WBC) is achieved. Viral infections, including cytomegalovirus (CMV) and the herpes virus group, can also occur. These viruses are especially dangerous, because there are few antiviral agents available to contain and treat them. Spread of viral infections to the lungs, liver, and CNS can be life threatening in children.

Pain in children with cancer can be tumor related, therapy related, or associated with invasive procedures. The frequency and degree of pain experienced by children is usually underestimated by healthcare providers. As a result, children are generally undermedicated, and their pain is poorly controlled. Medications useful in the management of tumor- and therapy-related pain include the nonopioid agents (acetaminophen, ibuprofen), opioids (codeine, morphine, fentanyl), and adjuvant agents (tricyclic antidepressants, corticosteroids). A carefully developed analgesia plan can integrate various agents to help control a child's pain. Tolerance to and dependence on opioids can develop in children, but addiction is extremely rare. Withholding analgesics based on fears of addiction is unwarranted.

Procedural pain is associated with invasive procedures, including bone marrow aspirates, lumbar punctures, and injections. Pharmacological sedation (midazolam, lorazepam) provides amnesia, but no analgesia. Opioids should be added to help maximize comfort and aid in the alleviation of distress. General anesthesia may be considered when the usual procedural sedation protocols fail. Nonpharmacologic techniques (e.g., hypnosis, imagery, relaxation, distraction) are also beneficial in decreasing the anxiety associated with procedures and increasing the child's ability to cooperate. (Refer to Chapter 14 for additional information on pain.)

PSYCHOSOCIAL IMPACT

The role of the nurse in psychosocial supportive care encompasses anticipatory guidance aimed at preventing emotional problems, as well as assessment and direct interventions to remedy problems. The vast majority of psychosocial care given to children with cancer and their families is provided by the professional nurse. Additionally, a great deal of nursing research has focused on the psychosocial impact of cancer in children.

Childhood cancer affects the entire family. An honest and open discussion of treatment, side effects of therapy, and psychosocial issues is an essential first step in family-centered care. It is important that the ill child and healthy siblings be given honest and developmentally appropriate information about the disease. Parents and other family members may need encouragement to ask questions about the child's cancer; parents may find it helpful to make a list of questions as they arise. Research has demonstrated that the first 6 months after diagnosis is the most critical time for providing education and emotional support.

Health care professionals can help parents by continually providing new information about the child's disease and therapy. Educational materials for families, children, and schoolteachers are available from the American Cancer Society and the National Cancer Institute. Resources for nurses are available from the Association of Pediatric Oncology Nurses. Support groups such as Candlelighters and family and sibling camps are also important resources for families.

Healthy siblings, in particular, experience a great deal of disruption as a result of their brother's or sister's illness. Siblings may feel isolated and abandoned, fear catching the disease, or resent the special attention given to the ill child. They may also feel guilty because of thoughts they once had about their ill brother or sister, or they may convince themselves that they are responsible for the illness. An age-appropriate discussion about the ill child's disease, treatment, and prognosis is recommended. Parents also need to prepare the healthy siblings for the physical changes that the ill child may experience as a result of therapy. Finally, parents are encouraged to spend special time or make frequent telephone contact with the healthy children and involve them in the care of their sick brother or sister.

The ill child's developmental level will influence his or her emotional response to the illness. The young child may experience separation anxiety from parents and fear of the hospital and medical procedures. Parents need to reassure their child that they will not be abandoned and that the medical procedures are not punishment for bad behavior. It is especially helpful to younger children if parents assume an active role in the child's care.

Older children also experience separation anxiety and threats to body integrity, as well as concerns about their independence, appearance, peer acceptance, sexuality, and future plans. Age-appropriate information about treatment and side effects, preparation for painful procedures, and emotional support during those procedures is essential for all children, regardless of age. In addition, the patient should be given ample opportunity to ask questions and participate in medical decisions, including the discussion of therapy options.

Prompt return to school and to extracurricular activities is crucial to the child's growth and development. Teachers need to be informed of the child's disease and treatment, as well as any special needs the child may have during school. Preparing peers for the child's return to school by discussing the disease, treatment, and physical changes such as hair loss will minimize isolation, teasing, and embarrassment. Finally, parents and teachers should be encouraged to continue to expect developmentally appropriate behavior and to maintain discipline.

DEALING WITH A LIFE-THREATENING ILLNESS AND BEREAVEMENT

The nurse's role in caring for children and families facing life-threatening illness or bereavement is aimed at facilitating the child's or the family member's coping and adaptation to the variety of stressors imposed by the diagnosis and treatment. Pediatric oncology nurses play a critical role in making developmentally appropriate explanations as well as advocating for the child's and family's best interests.

Religion, cultural background, previous experience with death and loss, communication and coping patterns within the family, and environmental factors can all influence the child's and family's response to life-threatening illness and death. Preparing the child for death is important, because it can help the child die more peacefully and help the family cope with the loss. The child should feel free to ask questions and express feelings of pain, fear, separation, and confusion, but not all children will choose to do so.

Children develop an understanding of death at different ages. Children with a life-threatening illness experience day-to-day physical changes that have a dramatic impact on their awareness of the seriousness of the situation. Children between the ages of 6 and 10 sense that their illness is not ordinary and that they may not get well. As the child's physical condition deteriorates, awareness of death increases.

Parents often need assistance in preparing the child and other family members for death. Families sometimes tend to avoid discussing death, because it can arouse intense emotions and feelings of discomfort. Pertinent books are helpful for both children and adults. Reading books with developmentally appropriate explanations and pictures is often a useful strategy, especially for young children.

Families experience intense feelings of grief and loss after a child's death. A bereavement follow-up by a healthcare professional who has already established a relationship with the family is recommended. Family members may also benefit from Candlelighters or other support groups, especially if they were involved with the group before the child's death.

LATE EFFECTS

Long-term survival of patients with childhood cancers continues to improve. It has been estimated that by the year 2010, 1 in 250 young adults will be survivors of childhood cancer. With increasing survival rates, the recognition of and concern about the late effects of disease and treatment have grown. The term *late effects* refers to the damaging effects of surgery, radiation, and chemotherapy on nonmalignant tissues and to the social, emotional, and economic consequences of survival. These effects appear months to years after treatment and can range in severity from subclinical to clinical to life threatening. Not all children experience such effects, but they are common enough to warrant study.

Late effects have been identified in almost every organ system. Treatments involving the central nervous system (CNS) can cause deficits in intelligence, hearing, and vision. Treatment involving the CNS, head and neck, or gonads can cause endocrine abnormalities such as short stature, hypothyroidism, or delayed secondary sexual development. Cardiomyopathy following anthracyclines can result in congestive heart failure. Surgery and radiation involving the musculoskeletal systems have been associated with defects such as kyphosis, scoliosis, and spinal shortening. Finally, although the incidence of multiple malignancies is low, the child who has received radiation and/or alkylating chemotherapy drugs for a first cancer has a 10 times greater risk of developing a secondary malignancy than children who have never had cancer treatment.

Long-term emotional problems—such as the inability to plan for the future or develop relationships—can interfere with the child's normal growth and development. The child who has residual physical effects may be at increased risk for emotional problems. The family may also experience emotional and economic consequences. Fears about disease recurrence and about the child's health in general may make it difficult for parents to permit age-appropriate independence. Difficulties obtaining health and life insurance for the cancer survivor are among the economic problems faced by the child and family.

Although the late effects discussed here are obviously distressing, it is important to remember that not all patients necessarily experience these effects and that positive long-term effects occur as well. Several authors have noted positive effects on these children and their families, such as increased maturity, resilience in coping with other life stressors, pride, increased sensitivity toward others, and greater closeness to family members.

Nursing Considerations

Nurses should stress the importance of regular health surveillance and prompt investigation of changes for former pediatric oncology patients. As these children reach adulthood, nurses in a variety of health care settings will have opportunities to assist with other concerns. For example, the college health or obstetrics and gynecology advanced practice nurse may assist with fertility and family planning concerns and can assure patients that most survivors can have healthy babies.

Long-term surveillance is important because late effects can occur many years after treatment. The effects of childhood cancer treatment on aging organs is still unknown. The child who was treated at an early age may have little understanding of the disease, its treatment, and implications for health maintenance. These are all important topics for discussion during off-therapy evaluations.

CONCLUSION

Advances in pediatric cancer have outpaced other areas of oncology. Significantly improved childhood survival rates are closely related to improved treatment, development of physical and psychosocial supportive modalities, and the pioneering utilization of the multidisciplinary team. Nurses in all settings are likely to be involved with bereaved parents and siblings or with former patients as they mature, enter the workforce, and begin their adult lives. Nurse-to-nurse consultation, especially between the generalist and the oncology specialist, can assist in promoting optimal outcomes for the children and their families.

BIBLIOGRAPHY

Bleyer, A. (1990). The impact of childhood cancer on the United States and the world. *CA—A Cancer Journal for Clinicians, 40*, 355–376.

Bunin, G. R., Petrakova, A., Meadows, A. T., et al. (1990). Occupations of parents of children with retinoblastoma: A report from the children's cancer study group. *Cancer Research, 50*, 7129–7133.

Fernbach, D. J., & Vietti, T. J. (1991). *Clinical pediatric oncology* (4th ed.). St. Louis: Mosby Year Book.

Foley, G. V., Fochtman, D., & Mooney, K. H. (1993). *Nursing care of the child with cancer* (2nd ed.). Philadelphia: W. B. Saunders.

Green, D. M., D'Angio, G. J., Beckwith, J. B. et al. (1996). Wilms tumor. *CA—A Cancer Journal for Clinicians, 46*, 46–63.

Noll, B., LeRoy, S., Bukowski, W. M., Rogosch, F. A., & Kulkarni, R. (1991). Peer relationships and adjustment in children with cancer. *Journal of Psychosocial Oncology, 16*(3), 307–326.

Shu, X. O., Reaman, G. H., Lampkin, B. et al. (1994). Association of paternal diagnostic x-ray exposure with risk of infant leukemia. *Cancer Epidemiology, Biomarkers & Prevention, 3*, 645–653.

Shu, X. O., Ross, J. A., & Pendergrass, T. W. (1996). Parental alcohol consumption, cigarette smoking, and risk of infant leukemia: A childrens cancer group study. *Journal of the National Cancer Institute, 88*(1), 24–31.

Walker, C., Wells, L., Heiney, S., Hymovich, D., & Weekes, D. (1993). Nursing management of psychosocial care needs. In G. V. Foley, D. Fotchman, & K. Mooney (Eds.), *Nursing care of the child with cancer* (2nd ed., pp. 397–434). Philadelphia: W. B. Saunders.

Yeazel, M. W., Buckley, J. D., Woods, W. G., et al. (1995). History of maternal fetal loss and increased risk of childhood acute leukemia at an early age. *Cancer, 75*(7), 1718–1727.

Zelter, K. L. (1993). Cancer in adolescents and young adults: Psychosocial aspects. *Cancer Supplement, 71*(10), 3463–3468.

Appendix I

Resources in Cancer Care

Marilyn Frank-Stromborg

The initial diagnosis of cancer is emotionally, financially, and socially devastating to patients and their families. Although there are multiple community-based resources available to assist the patient and family with treatment, rehabilitation, and financing, the patient and family are frequently unaware of the services that are offered. An important role of the nurse is to either supply the patient with information about cancer-related resources or to refer the patient to a structured agency that will supply this information (e.g., the hospital's social service department, local American Cancer Society unit, local public health agencies). Today the emphasis in health care is to reduce the time patients spend in the hospital, to deliver as much treatment as possible in an outpatient setting, and to keep the patient in the home setting. These trends have (a) decreased the time the nurse in the acute care setting has with the patient and family, and (b) increased the need for the patient and family to be familiar with community-based resources that will assist over trajectory of the illness. Thus, the nurse plays a crucial role in making sure that the patient is supplied with this information before discharge from the hospital.

ORGANIZATIONS SPONSORING SELF-HELP GROUPS, COUNSELING, SUPPORT, AND RELATED SERVICES FOR CANCER PATIENTS AND THEIR FAMILIES

Bone Marrow Transplant Family Support Network

P.O. Box 845
Avon, CT 06001
800-826-9376
800-MARROW2 (National Donor Line)

The Bone Marrow Transplant Family Support Network enables families to feel "connected" when coping with the decision to undergo a transplant. Patients and family are given information related to the daily routines both before and after the transplant and the required follow-up care.

Cancer Care, Inc.
and the National Cancer Care Foundation

1180 Avenue of the Americas
New York, NY 10036
212-302-2400
1-800-813-HOPE
212-719-0263 (Fax)
cancercare@aol.com (E-mail)

Cancer Care is a nonprofit, nonsectarian, East coast social service agency to help cancer patients and their families cope with the impact of cancer. It is the largest agency in the nation solely dedicated to providing psychological and financial support to cancer patients and their families and community education programs for the general public. Counseling is available on both a group and an individual basis.

The Candlelighters Childhood Cancer Foundation

7910 Woodmont Avenue, Suite 460
Bethesda, MD 20814
301-657-8401
800-366-2223 or 800-366-CCCF
301-718-2686 (Fax)
75717.3513@compuserve.com (E-mail)

Candlelighters has two primary goals: to obtain consistent and adequate federal support for cancer research and to help parents and other family members who share the particularly difficult experience of living with a child with cancer. Candlelighters maintains communications between parents and professionals through quarterly newsletters and among groups through quarterly newsletters. There are chapters in every state (over 400) and on every continent in the world. Contact the national office for the chapter nearest you. Candlelighters has an Ombudsman program that assists parents and adult survivors who are having difficulties with their health insurance and payment for medical expenses. They also have a program that assists in obtaining second medical opinions.

Encore Plus
YMCA of the USA Encore Plus

Office of Women's Health Initiatives
624 9th Street, NW
3rd Floor
Washington, DC 20001
202-628-3636
202-783-7123 (Fax)
hn2205@handsnet.org (E-mail)

The YWCA of the USA has a 20-year history of support for women with breast cancer. They have expanded this commitment to include breast and cervical cancer awareness, education, and referral to screening services and treatment links. Along with the breast and cervical education and referral program, there is postdiagnosis support that includes a specially designed exercise regimen and peer group support sessions.

Make-a-Wish Foundation of America

100 West Clarendon, Suite 2200
Phoenix, AZ 85013-3518
800-722-WISH or 602-279-WISH
602-279-0855 (Fax)
www.wish.org (E-mail)

This foundation grants wishes for people under the age of 18 who are suffering from life-threatening or terminal illnesses. The wish includes the immediate family and expenses. There are 82 chapters and 18 international affiliates. Contact the national office for a chapter near you.

Make Today Count

Connie Zimmerman, Director
Mid America Cancer Center
1235 East Cherokee
Springfield, MO 65804-2263
417-885-2273
800-432-2273
417-888-7426 (Fax)

Make Today Count is a mutual support group for persons with life-threatening illnesses. It provides support groups and educational programs as well as brochures and handouts. The purpose of the support groups is to allow people to discuss their personal concerns so that they may deal with them in a positive way. There are chapters in the United States, Canada, and Europe. Contact the national headquarters for the chapter near you.

National Coalition for Cancer Survivorship (NCCS)

1010 Wayne Avenue, 5th Floor
Silver Spring, MD 20910
301-650-8868
301-565-9670 (Fax)

NCCS represents grassroots organizations throughout the United States. The primary goal of NCCS is to generate a national awareness of survivorship, demonstrating that there can be a vibrant productive life after a cancer diagnosis. NCCS provides a national communication network between people and organizations involved with survivorship; facilitates communication among people involved with cancer survivorship; promotes peer support; and serves as an information clearinghouse.

The Oley Foundation

214 Hun Memorial, A23
Albany Medical Center
Albany, NY 12208
518-262-5079
800-776-OLEY
518-262-5528 (Fax)

The foundation offers support to consumers of home parenteral or enteral nutrition (PEN) therapy and their families. The foundation provides patient/family support group meetings in multiple locations across the United States. Their bi-monthly newsletter, *Lifeline Letter*, includes articles contributed by home PEN consumers, families, clinicians, researchers, and home healthcare services. As part of Oley's education and outreach effort, the newsletter is provided at no charge to consumers and consumers' families.

US TOO International, Inc.

930 North York Road
Suite 50
Hinsdale, IL 60521-2993
800-80-USTOO or 800-808-7866
708-323-1002
708-323-1003 (Fax)

US TOO is a nonprofit organization that provides support for survivors of and patients with prostate cancer. This organization offers information and counseling and conducts educational meetings to assist patients in the decision-making process. There are chapters throughout the United States, and they hold monthly meetings for individuals with prostate cancer and their families. The American Cancer Society recognizes US TOO as a national support group for individuals who have (or had) prostate cancer and their families.

Y-ME National Breast Cancer Organization, Inc.

212 West Van Buren
4th Floor
Chicago, IL 60607-3908
312-986-8338
312-986-9505 (Hispanic hotline)
312-986-8228 (24-hour hotline)
800-221-2141 (Toll-free hotline, 9 A.M. to 5 P.M. Central time, weekdays)
312-986-0020 (Fax)
http:\\www.y-me.org (E-mail; Click on through Home Page)

Y-ME has become the largest breast cancer support program in the United States. It provides hotlines staffed by trained professionals and volunteers who have personally experienced breast cancer. There is a medical advisory board that monitors the medical information that is provided the public. Y-ME offers preoperative counseling, open-door meetings, early detection workshops, a speakers bureau, a resource library, a wigs and prosthesis bank, and inservice workshops for health professionals.

NATIONAL ORGANIZATIONS PROVIDING INFORMATION AND OTHER SERVICES FOR CANCER PATIENTS AND THEIR FAMILIES

American Cancer Society (ACS)

800-ACS-2345 (for cancer information)
(Check your local directory for the Unit or Division nearest you.)

ACS offers programs of cancer research, education, and patient service and rehabilitation. The ACS is organized into the national office, state or division offices, and local units. Many ACS Units provide equipment and supplies to make home care as comfortable as possible. Both large items such as beds and wheelchairs and smaller items such as walkers are available in many areas. Transportation to and from cancer treatments is also supplied by many local units. Local staff and volunteers can answer questions about cancer and assist patients with getting the help they need from organizations in their community. The ACS has extensive free professional and patient education materials including films, videotapes, booklets, pamphlets, books, national conference proceedings, and posters. The ACS also sponsors many valuable patient and family support and educational groups. Following is a list of some of the programs and services the ACS·offers:

CanSurmount This is a one-to-one patient visitor program, broader in scope than Reach to Recovery, encompassing colon, prostate, and other cancers. CanSurmount provides a patient-to-patient or family member-to-family member support system.

Laryngectomy Visitors This program is designed to help give the cancer patient the support and skills needed to communicate and continue with normal life.

Ostomy Visitors The American Cancer Society also works closely with the United Ostomy Association to jointly produce educational materials for ostomy patients nd to offer an ostomy visitation program.

Housing Housing for patients and families traveling to treatment centers may be provided by American Cancer Society Divisions in the cities where the centers are located. The Divisions have worked out agreements with local hotels and motels to provide free rooms on a rotating basis. In some areas, Divisions operate their own housing, either in the Division's headquarters or in separate buildings called Hope Lodges.

Camps for Children A number of Divisions of the American Cancer Society operate camps for children with cancer. They are usually offered free, and they are staffed by volunteers, including on-site doctors and nurses.

Road to Recovery Road to Recovery is offered in many American Cancer Society Divisions. The program is completely managed by volunteers, and 95% of the trips to treatment are provided by volunteers in their own vehicles.

I Can Cope I Can Cope is an education program designed to clarify facts and myths about cancer. It helps patients and their families cope with the problems of living with this disease. Information is given about cancer, its treatment, and the possible side effects of both.

International Association of Laryngectomees ACS sponsors this voluntary organization that promotes and supports the total rehabilitation of people with laryngectomies. Members who are themselves laryngectomees call on hospitalized patients to offer moral support and encouragement. For the location of the Lost Chord, New Voice, or Anamile club nearest a patient, contact the local Unit of the ACS. The goals of the Lost Chord clubs are to help new patients make early adjustments to the loss of voice and to over-come psychosocial problems.

Man to Man   This program offers group education, discussion, and support for men with prostate cancer and their wives.

Look Good . . . Feel Better   Patients can use this program to look better during treat-ment using the services of cosmetologists to teach them cosmetic techniques that are designed to improve their appearance. This program is a joint venture of the Cosmetic, Toiletry, and Fragrance Association Foundation, the ACS, and the National Cosmetology Association. For more information, call 800-395-LOOK or the local ACS.

Reach to Recovery   This is one of the best known self-help groups. Reach to Recovery provides rehabilitation support for women who have had breast cancer. Designed to meet physical, psychological, and cosmetic needs, the program works through volunteer visitors who have adjusted successfully to their surgery. A trained volunteer who has had breast cancer offers emotional support and information to both the pre- and postdiagnosed patient, as well as to the patient experiencing a recurrence.

Consult your telephone directory for the number of your local Unit for complete infor-mation about all programs. A listing of Division offices follows this chapter.

American Brain Tumor Association (ABTA)

2720 River Road
Suite 146
Des Plaines, IL 60018
847-827-9910
800-886-2282 (Patient line)
847-827-9918 (Fax)
ABTA @ aol.com (E-mail)

ABTA is a national organization that provides written information about brain tumors and their treatment. Services include patient education materials, listings of brain tumor support groups, referrals to support organizations, and information about treatment facil-ities. A biannual newsletter, *The Message Line,* describes research advances and announces updates to publications. Services of this association include listings of brain tumor support groups, a CONNECTIONS Pen-Pal program, and information about treat-ment facilities.

Cancer Information Service (CIS)

Attn: Chris Thomsen
National Cancer Institute
Building 31, Room 10A16
Bethesda, MD 20892
800-4-CANCER or 800-422-6237
301-496-8664

CIS, a program of the National Cancer Institute, is a network of regional offices with trained staff and volunteers who provide accurate and confidential telephone information to questions concerning cancer rehabilitation, research, causes, prevention and detection, diagnosis, treatment, support services, and so forth. Information can be supplied in English and Spanish. CIS serves as a resource for state and regional organizations by providing printed materials and technical assistance for cancer education, media campaigns, and community programs.

Choice in Dying (CID)

(formerly Concern for Dying and the Society for the Right to Die)
Karen Orloff Kaplan, M.Ph., Sc.D., Executive Director
200 Varick Street
10th Floor
New York, NY 10014-4810
212-366-5540 or 800-989-WILL (9455)
212-366-5337 (Fax)
72420.1653@ compuserve.com (E-mail)

This is a national nonprofit organization that pursues a program on several fronts: legal services, legislation, and promotion of citizens' rights. The organization provides members and nonmembers with a *Living Will Declaration* and a state-specific *Statutory Short Form Power of Attorney for Health Care*. It is the nation's largest provider of state-specific *advance directives*—the general term for two types of legal documents: a living will and a durable power of attorney for health care. A nominal annual membership fee provides the latest information on right-to-die developments, including any changes in the law. This is the only organization that deals broadly and practically with end-of-life issues and provides free public and professional education and counseling about the preparation and use of advance directives.

Corporate Angel Network, Inc.

Westchester County Airport
Building 1
White Plains, NY 10604
914-328-1313
914-328-3938 (Fax)
corpangl@ix.netcom.com (E-mail)

This is a nonprofit organization that arranges free air transportation for cancer patients going to and from health care centers for recognized treatments, consultations, or check-ups. The program utilizes available seats on corporate aircraft and is free of charge for both the ambulatory patient and one attendant or family member. Financial need is not a requirement.

Susan G. Komen Breast Cancer Foundation

5005 LBJ Freeway
Suite 370
Dallas, TX 75244
214-450-1777
800-I'M AWARE or 800-462-9273 (National helpline)
214-450-1710 (Fax)
SGK.WORLDLINK@NOTES.compuserve.com (E-mail)

This is a national volunteer organization working through local chapters and Race for the Cure events across the country. Its mission is to eradicate breast cancer as a life-threatening disease by advancing research, education, screening, and treatment. The national helpline is answered by trained volunteers who provide information to callers with breast cancer or breast health concerns.

Leukemia Society of America, Inc. (L.S.A.)

600 Third Avenue
New York, NY 10016
212-573-8484
800-955-4LSA (Call to get number of chapter nearest you.)

L.S.A. offers financial assistance and consultations about referrals to cancer patients with leukemia and related disorders (lymphoma and multiple myeloma). Financial coverage is reserved for outpatient care. The program includes payment for drugs used in the cure, treatment, and/or control of leukemia; laboratory costs associated with blood transfusion; transportation; radiotherapy in the first stages of Hodgkin's disease; and prophylactic radiation for children with acute leukemia. There are 57 chapters throughout the United States.

National Hospice Organization (NHO)

1901 North Moore Street
Suite 901
Arlington, VA 22209
703-243-5900
800-658-8898 (Hospice helpline)
703-525-5762 (Fax)
drsnho@cais.com (E-mail)

NHO is a nonprofit organization promoting quality care to the terminally ill and their significant others. There are several different membership categories to meet the diverse needs of people working with hospice. Members receive *The Hospice Journal*, among numerous other publications and workshops. NHO has worked over the past decade to establish hospice as a part of the health care delivery system in the United States. As a result of its efforts, hospice is now included as a Medicare/Medicaid benefit and as an employee benefit for 66% of American workers. Most hospices are part of NHO and receive NHO's technical assistance, education programs and events, publications, and advocacy and referral services.

National Marrow Donor Program (NMDP)

Coordinating Center
3433 Broadway Street, NE
Suite 400
Minneapolis, MN 55413
612-627-5844
800-627-7692 or 800-MARROW-2
612-627-5877 and 612-627-5899 (Fax)

The NMDP is a computerized registry of unrelated potential volunteer marrow donors. It provides information on how to be listed as a potential donor along with transplant information for patients with leukemia, aplastic anemia, or any other life-threatening disease.

Because the need for minority donors is especially great, NMDP provides funding for testing for minority donors. Business hours are Monday through Friday from 8 A.M. to 6 P.M. (CST).

Ronald McDonald House Charities

Grants Manager
McDonald's Office Campus
Kroc Drive
Oak Brook, IL 60521
630-575-3571
630-575-7488 (Fax)

Ronald McDonald House is a "home away from home," a temporary lodging facility for the families of seriously ill children being treated at nearby hospitals. There are Ronald McDonald Houses throughout the world. The Houses provide an environment for emotional support to parents and siblings of sick children through a loving, caring, stable place they can call home.

United Ostomy Association (UOA)

36 Executive Park
Suite 120
Irvine, CA 92714
714-660-8624
800-826-0826
714-660-9262 (Fax)
uoa@deltanet.com (E-mail)

Local chapters of UOA are composed of ostomates who provide mutual aid, moral support, and education to those who have had colostomy, ileostomy, or urostomy surgery. All local chapters are volunteer organizations; a list of them is available from the UOA. UOA publishes a magazine, *Ostomy Quarterly*, and has publications and slide programs that cover every aspect of ostomies.

NATIONAL PROFESSIONAL AND RELATED ORGANIZATIONS

American Association for Cancer Education (AACE)

Robert M. Chamberlain, Ph.D., Secretary
University of Texas
M. D. Anderson Cancer Center
Box 189
1515 Holcombe Boulevard
Houston, TX 77030
713-792-3020
713-792-0807 (Fax)

The purpose of AACE is to provide a forum for health professionals concerned with the study and improvement of cancer education at all levels (undergraduate, graduate, continuing education, and paraprofessional). It is a multidisciplinary organization that holds an annual fall meeting. The official journal of AACE is the *Journal of Cancer Education*.

Association of Pediatric Oncology Nurses (APON)

4700 West Lake Avenue
Glenview, IL 60025-1485
847-375-4700
847-375-4777 (Fax)
assnmgmt@dial.cic.net (E-mail)

Membership in APON is open to all registered nurses who are either interested in or engaged in pediatrics or pediatric oncology. Members received a copy of the quarterly journal, *Journal of the Association of Pediatric Oncology Nurses*, the APON *Newsletter*, and other related publications. APON holds an annual conference. APON offers certification in pediatric oncology nursing.

Hospice Nurses Association (HNA)

5512 Northumberland Street
Pittsburgh, PA 15217-1131
412-687-3231
412-687-9095 (Fax)

HNA's purpose is to exchange information, experiences, and ideas; to promote understanding of the specialty of hospice nursing; and to study and promote hospice nursing research. Members receive a newsletter, *FANFARE*, a discount on their certification examination, educational programs and an opportunity to participate on HNA committees.

International Society of Nurses in Cancer Care

The Royal College of Nursing
20 Cavendish Square
London W1M OAB
071-495-6119
071-495-6104 (Fax)

The society's goal is to enable cancer nurses to share their knowledge and problems on a worldwide basis. Membership in the society is open to cancer nursing societies, universities, and institutions involved in cancer care and other entities whose work affects or involves the care of people with cancer. Members receive the newsletter *International Cancer Nursing News*. The society has attained advisory status with the United Nations, the World Health Organization, and the International Council of Nurses. A conference is held every 2 years and is attended by nurses from around the world.

Intravenous Nurses Society (INS)

Fresh Pond Square
10 Fawcett Street
Cambridge, MA 02138
617-441-3008
617-441-3009 (Fax)

INS is a national nonprofit professional association for nurses involved in the delivery of intravenous therapies. The purpose of INS is to upgrade intravenous therapy nursing practice through continuing education, professional certification, and the development of standards of practice. INS's official publications are the *Journal of Intravenous Nursing* and the newsletter *Newsline*. The society holds two major educational meetings each year, in May and November.

Oncology Nursing Society (ONS)

501 Holiday Drive
Pittsburgh, PA 15220-2749
412-921-7373
412-921-6565 (Fax)
412-921-7373, press 1 then 6 (Fast Fax)
member@nauticom.net

The purpose of ONS is to promote the highest professional standards of oncology nursing; research and exchange information, experiences, and ideas leading to improved oncology nursing; encourage nurses to specialize in the practice of oncology nursing; identify resources within the group; and establish guidelines of nursing care for patients with cancer. In addition to guidelines and standards for oncology nursing practice and education, the society publishes a journal, the *Oncology Nursing Forum*, and a newsletter, the *ONS News*, which are provided to members. ONS also holds a national Congress and Fall Institute, and there are chapters throughout the county. ONS offers certification as a generalist oncology nurse (OCN) and as an advanced oncology nurse (AOCN). The society is an ANA-accredited approver and provider of continuing education.

FEDERAL AND OTHER AGENCIES THAT RELATE TO ONCOLOGY

Food and Drug Administration (FDA)
Office of Consumer Affairs, HFE-88
5600 Fishers Lane
Rockville, MD 20857
301-443-3170
301-443-9767 (Fax)

FDA is a consumer source of publications dealing with food-related subjects, FDA regulations, cosmetics, general medical drug information, medical devices, radiologic health, and health fraud.

Office of Minority Health Resource Center (MHRC)

U.S. Department of Health and Human Services
P.O. Box 37337
Washington, DC 20013-7337
800-444-6472
301-589-0884 (Fax)

The activities of the MHRC include a bilingually staffed toll-free number to provide minority health information and referrals to health professionals; a computerized database of materials, organizations, and programs; and a resource persons network of professionals active in the field. They provide health-related resources targeting Asians, Pacific Islanders, African Americans, Hispanics/Latinos, and Native Americans at the federal, state, and local levels.

U.S. Department of Labor Occupational Safety and Health Administration (OSHA)

Directorate of Technical Support
200 Constitution Avenue, NW
Washington, DC 20210
202-219-7047

OSHA is involved in the development and enforcement of occupational safety and health standards and works to ensure safe and healthful working conditions for every worker in the country. Information on work-related hazards and occupational injuries and illnesses, including radiation safety and chemotherapy administration safety, is available upon request.

NATIONAL FINANCIAL RESOURCES FOR ONCOLOGY PATIENTS AND THEIR FAMILIES[1]

American Cancer Society

1-800-ACS-2345

Divisions at the state level offer direct services that may include financial assistance. (See listing of Division office addresses and telephone numbers following this section.)

American Kidney Fund

6110 Executive Boulevard
Suite 1010
Rockville, MD 20852
301-881-3052
800-638-8299

Applications can be secured from local dialysis social workers. This fund provides support for medications, transportation, and special diets required by dialysis.

Cancer Care, Inc.

1180 Avenue of the Americas
New York, NY 10036
212-302-2400
1-800-813-HOPE

[1](*Source:* Hartung article listed in Bibliography.)

Financial assistance for home care, transportation, pain medication, and limited funds for cancer treatments in New York, New Jersey, and Connecticut.

Directory of Pharmaceutical Manufacturers' Indigent Programs

800-PMA-INF0 (762-4636)

Reimbursement support program to assist health care providers and patients with claims and coverage issues.

Leukemia Research Foundation

Attn: Janie Weisenberg, Executive Director
4761 West Touhy
Suite 211
Lincolnwood, IL 60646
708-982-1480

Provides funds to persons within a 100-mile radius for treatment-related costs up to $750 a year.

Leukemia Society of America

Program Services Department
600 Third Avenue
New York, NY 10016
212-573-8484 Ext. 159

Provides funding for treatment-related costs and transportation. Applications available from local Leukemia Society chapter or national headquarters in New York.

National Bone Marrow Transplant Link

29209 Northwestern Highway
Room #624
Southfield, MI 48034
810-932-8483

Provides links between individuals and sources of financial assistance and fundraising.

National Leukemia Research Association, Inc.

Attn: Kay Ruggerio, Patient Aid Director
585 Stewart Avenue
Suite 536
Garden City, NY 11530
516-222-1944

Provides funds for drugs, diagnostic costs and laboratory fees not covered by insurance. Applications from national office in New York.

Organ Transplant Fund, Inc.

Donna Noelker, Director of Services
1027 South Yates Road
Memphis, TN 38119
901-684-1697
800-489-3863 (National office)
800-798-3863 (Illinois office)

Bone marrow transplants and solid organs are covered.

Transplant Foundation

Attn: Debbie Hopkins, MSW, Executive Director
8002 Discovery Drive
Suite 310
Richmond, VA 23229
804-285-5115

Provides money for immunosuppressive drugs.

YMCA of the USA-Encore Plus

624 9th Street, NW
3rd Floor
Washington, DC 20001
202-628-3636

Local offices provide funding for early detection, screening, outreach, education, and postdiagnostic support.

BIBLIOGRAPHY

Each listed article contains an extensive listing of organizations and government agencies that are helpful to the health professional seeking cancer-related resources for oncology patients and their families.

Hartung, P. (1996). Financial resources for adults with cancer. *Cancer Practice*, 4(2), 105–108.
Kinsey, R., & Doty, T. (1995). Cancer resources in the United States. *Oncology Nursing Forum*, 22(9), 1421–1432.
Frank-Stromborg, M., & Barhamand, B. (1993). Yellow pages: Cancer nursing resources. In S. Groenwald, M. Frogge, M. Goodman, & C. Yarbro (Eds.), *Cancer nursing: Principles and practice* (3rd ed., pp. 1631–1672). Boston: Jones and Bartlett.

Appendix II

The American Cancer Society: Who We Are and What We Do

Terri B. Ades

The American Cancer Society is the nationwide, community-based, voluntary health organization dedicated to eliminating cancer as a major health problem by preventing cancer, saving lives, and diminishing suffering from cancer, through research, education, advocacy, and service.

When the American Society for the Control of Cancer (ASCC), forerunner of the American Cancer Society, was founded in New York City in 1913, the word *cancer* was seldom spoken in public. The organization was begun by 10 doctors and 5 laymen who saw a need to educate the public about the benefits of finding and treating cancer early, and one of their daughters took on the task of raising the money the new organization needed to begin its task. About $10,000 was raised the first year, and a pamphlet, *Facts about Cancer*, was published to educate the public.

After 2 decades of sporadic local public education, the Society concentrated its educational efforts on physicians. In 1937, through its Women's Field Army, it launched its first nationwide public education program. In 1945, the Society's leadership reorganized the ASCC into the American Cancer Society, expanding its programs and giving lay individuals a voice on the volunteer board. That year, the American Cancer Society conducted its first major, national fundraising campaign, raising $4 million, with $1 million earmarked to support its research program. Since then, the Society has invested over $1 billion in research. Its educational and patient service programs have greatly expanded and today reach into nearly every community in the United States.

With an office in nearly every county in the United States, the American Cancer Society is led by volunteers locally, at the state level, and nationally. The national headquarters are in Atlanta, Georgia. At each level, a volunteer board of directors governs the organization, setting policy and administering budgets. A professional staff comprising a fraction of the Society's nearly 2 million volunteers supports the volunteer's programming and fundraising efforts.

The Society's major programs include research, patient services, prevention, detection and treatment, advocacy, and fighting cancer worldwide.

RESEARCH

The American Cancer Society is the largest private source of cancer research funds in the United States. About $90 million is spent every year supporting the research program, which consists of three components: extramural grants and clinical awards, intramural epidemiology and surveillance research, and intramural behavioral research.

The extramural program supports investigator-initiated projects taking place in leading centers across the country. Applications for grants are subjected to a rigorous external peer review, which ensures that only the highest-quality applications receive funding. Through the clinical award component of the program, health professionals receive support for education and training.

PATIENT SERVICES

The American Cancer Society's service programs help cancer patients and their families cope with cancer. Through the Resources, Information, and Guidance program, callers receive information about cancer, Society services, and other resources in the community to help meet the needs of cancer patients and others coping with cancer. In some communities, volunteers transport patients to and from treatment.

Other programs include I Can Cope, an educational program for patients and their families; Man to Man, a prostate cancer education and support program; and programs to support laryngectomy and ostomy patients.

For over 25 years, the American Cancer Society's Reach to Recovery volunteers have helped women deal with breast cancer, assuring them that there can be life after breast cancer. Look Good . . . Feel Better helps women manage physical changes in their appearance caused by treatment, such as skin problems and hair loss.

PREVENTION

Healthcare professionals and the public look to the American Cancer Society for information and education on ways to prevent cancer and to reduce the risk of developing cancer. To accomplish its prevention goals, the Society focuses on tobacco control, the relationship between diet and cancer, comprehensive school health education, and the prevention of skin cancer. Volunteers are recruited and trained to promote and deliver programs aimed at reaching specific audiences, either adults or children.

The American Cancer Society has joined with other health, education, and social service agencies to promote delivery of a planned health education program in the schools that teaches school-age children from preschool through grade 12 how to reduce their cancer risks.

DETECTION AND TREATMENT

Health providers and the public look to the American Cancer Society for guidelines to help find cancer at the earliest possible stage. The Society publicizes recommendations for men and women.

The Society provides information and publications about cancer treatment and symptom management, including pain control, and sponsors continuing-education conferences for healthcare professionals.

ADVOCACY

The American Cancer Society recognizes that cancer is a political, as well as a medical, social, psychological, and economic issue. A small government-relations staff actively seeks to educate policymakers at all levels of government who make decisions impacting the lives of millions of Americans with a history of cancer and their families, as well as millions of potential cancer patients.

The Society is organized to mobilize thousands of volunteers across the country to advocate for public policy initiatives affecting the welfare of cancer patients and their families, protection from cancer risks for potential cancer patients, and cancer research funding and direction. In support of its cancer educational and service programs, the American Cancer Society seeks to influence public policy on such issues as tobacco control, access to health care, employment discrimination against cancer patients, and environmental cancer issues.

FIGHTING CANCER WORLDWIDE

The American Cancer Society collaborates with more than 5,000 cancer control organizations around the world to fight this disease, providing expertise in the form of informational materials and volunteer faculty, both scientific and lay. As a leader in tobacco control, voluntarism/organizational issues, and breast cancer awareness efforts, the Society serves as a model and resource for other, often less-developed, international counterpart agencies.

Glossary

Linda Yoder

Absolute neutrophil count (ANC)   The actual count of the neutrophils in the blood. Segmented neutrophils + band neutrophils = total neutrophils × WBC.

Addiction   A combination of physical and psychological dependence on a drug; a behavioral pattern of compulsive drug use.

Adenocarcinoma   A malignant neoplasm of epithelial cells in glandular pattern.

Adjuvant therapy   A therapy that aids another, such as chemotherapy after surgery.

Adrenocorticotropic hormone (ACTH)   A hormone secreted by the anterior pituitary gland that has a stimulating effect on the adrenal cortex.

Age-adjusted incidence/mortality rate   A cancer incidence or mortality rate that has been mathematically adjusted to account for the difference in the age distributions of the populations that are being compared.

Ageism   Prejudice against a person because of his or her age.

Allogeneic bone marrow transplants   Transplants of bone marrow from one person to another person who is of the same tissue type.

Alopecia   Loss of hair resulting from the destruction of the hair follicle. Sometimes a side effect of chemotherapy or radiation therapy to the head. May be transient or permanent, depending on course of treatment.

Alpha-fetoprotein (AFP)   An antigen tumor marker associated with testicular germ-cell tumors, liver cancers, and gastric malignancies.

Alternative therapies   Unproven or disproven methods of cancer treatment.

Anemia   Having less than the normal amount of hemoglobin or red blood cells.

Anorexia   Loss of appetite.

Antibody   Proteins produced by B-lymphocytes in response to an antigen. Important components in humoral immunity. Also called *immunoglobulins*.

Anticipatory nausea   The inclination or desire to vomit due to the sight or odor of a substance that stimulates a mental image of a distressing situation that has occurred previously; occurs in about 25% of cancer patients as a result of classic operant conditioning from stimuli associated with chemotherapy, most commonly when efforts to control vomiting related to the therapy have been unsuccessful.

Antigen A molecule that stimulates an immune response and is capable of reacting with antibodies or other sensitized cells of the immune system, such as T-lymphocytes.

Anti-oncogenes Genes having the ability to regulate growth and inhibit carcinogenesis.

Astrocytoma A tumor composed of neuroglial cells of ectodermal origin, characterized by fibrous or protoplasmic processes. This tumor is classified in order of malignancy as Grade I (consists of fibrillary or protoplasmic astrocytes), Grade II (astroblastoma), or Grades 111 or IV (glioblastoma multiforme).

Autologous bone marrow transplantation (ABMT) Transplanting the patient's own bone marrow after ablative treatment.

B-cells Another term for a B-lymphocyte (bursa-equivalent lymphocyte). These cells develop from the stem cell and are involved in humoral immunity and the secretion of antibodies.

Bence-Jones protein A low-molecular-weight, heat-sensitive protein found in patients with multiple myeloma. The presence of these proteins in the urine may lead to the formation of precipitates in the tubules, resulting in tubular obstruction, foreign body reaction, and tubular degeneration.

Benign Not malignant; not recurrent; favorable for recovery.

Biological response modifiers (BRMs) Agents or approaches that modify the host's own biologic response to a tumor in an attempt to treat the cancer by changing one of the body systems involved in cancer growth; sometimes referred to as the fourth cancer treatment, with the other three being surgery, radiotherapy, and chemotherapy.

Biotherapy The use of agents derived from biological sources or of agents or approaches that affect the body's biological responses.

Blast crisis A sudden, severe change in the course of chronic myelocytic leukemia, in which the clinical picture resembles that seen in acute myelogenous leukemia with an increase in the proportion of myloblasts.

Blocks Devices used in radiotherapy to prevent radiation beams from striking areas of the body that do not require treatment or require shielding, such as the heart.

Body surface area Calculation of area of body mass expressed in square meters (m²); determination is usually accomplished with the use of a nomogram (body surface calculator).

Brachytherapy Radiation from a source placed within the body or a body cavity.

BRCA1 and BRCA2 genes Breast cancer susceptibility genes identified, in 1994, on chromosome 17q21. Their significance is yet to be fully defined. Currently thought to be responsible for 5% to 10% of inherited forms of breast cancer.

Breast self-examination (BSE) Visual and manual examination of the breast, which should be done after menstruation when the breasts are normally soft. A physician should be contacted if any lump in the breast can be felt.

Cachexia A condition of severe malnutrition, emaciation, and debility.

Cancer Encompasses a group of neoplastic diseases in which there is a transformation of normal body cells into malignant ones, with uncontrolled proliferation.

Carcinoembryonic antigen (CEA) A tumor marker associated with malignancies of the gastrointestinal tract.

Carcinogen A substance that causes cancer.

Carcinogenesis Production of cancer.

Carcinoma A malignant growth consisting of epithelial cells tending to infiltrate surrounding tissues and give rise to metastases.

Basal cell carcinoma An epithelial tumor of the skin that seldom metastasizes, but has the potential for local invasion and destruction.

Carcinoma in situ Neoplastic activity in which the tumor cells have not yet invaded the basement membrane but are still confined to the epithelium of origin; a lesion with all the histological characteristics of malignancies except invasion.

Squamous cell carcinoma Neoplastic cells arising from the squamous epithelium and having cuboid cells.

Cardiac tamponade Compression of the heart due to critically increased volume of fluid in the pericardium.

Cell cycle Sequence of steps through which cells grow and replicate.

Cell cycle specific Drugs (chemotherapeutic) that exert their effect during a particular phase of the cell cycle; for example, antimetabolites exert their effect during the S phase by interfering with RNA and DNA synthesis. Most effective against cells when they are rapidly dividing.

Cell cycle nonspecific Drugs that exert their effect on the cell without regard to a particular phase of the cell cycle; for example, antitumor antibiotics interfere with DNA function; they act on both proliferating and nonproliferating cells.

Cell-mediated immunity Type of immune response dependent on T-lymphocytes, which are primarily concerned with a type of delayed immune response.

Central nervous system prophylaxis Administration of intrathecal chemotherapy and cranial irradiation, designed to eradicate leukemic cells that may sequester themselves behind the blood-brain barrier, thus out of reach of most chemotherapy.

Chemopreventive agents Drugs, vitamins, or micronutrients used in the prevention of cancer.

Chemotherapy The systemic treatment of illness by medication. The term was first applied to the treatment of infectious diseases, but now is used primarily in context with treatment of cancer.

Chondrosarcoma A malignant tumor derived from cartilage cells or their precursors.

Choriocarcinoma A malignant neoplasm of trophoblastic cells formed by the abnormal proliferation of the placental epithelium, without the production of chorionic villi.

Citrovorum factor Folinic acid. Also called *leucovorin*. A metabolically active derivative of folic acid used to treat folic acid deficiency and as an antidote to folic acid antagonists, such as methotrexate.

Clinical trial Rigorous evaluation to determine the effectiveness and safety of a specific intervention, especially therapeutic interventions; the procedure by which new cancer treatments are tested in humans.

Colony-stimulating factor (CSF) Soluble protein factors that stimulate division and maturation of bone marrow stem cells. All CSFs are named as a function of the cell most responsive to the factor (e.g., granulocyte-stimulating factor).

Colposcopy The process of examining the vagina and cervix by means of a speculum and a magnifying lens; procedure used for the early detection of malignant changes on the cervix/vaginal cuff.

Complement cascade   Series of steps or stages within the immune system that, once initiated, continues to the final steps of complement activation, resulting in the formation of many biologically active complement fragments that act as anaphylatoxins, opsonins, or chemotactic factors. There are two classic pathways in the complement system; both play a vital role in immunity.

Complementary therapies   Supportive therapies that are used to complement standard treatment.

Computerized tomography   A radiologic imaging technique that produces images of "slices" 1 cm thick through a patient's body. Also referred to as *computerized axial tomography, CAT scan,* or *CT scan.*

Conditioning or preparative regimen   Doses of chemotherapy and/or total body irradiation lethal to bone marrow given in an effort to eradicate the population of tumor cells in the body. Commonly used in the treatment of leukemia.

Congenital melanocytic nevi   A mole present since birth that is composed of melanocytes; usually pigmented.

Conization   The removal of a "cone" of tissue as a partial excision of the cervix. This can be done with a scalpel or electrocautery. The scalpel technique preserves the histologic elements of the tissue better.

Consolidation chemotherapy   A phase of treatment in leukemia consisting of one to three intensive cycles of chemotherapy designed to bring together the gains made during remission-induction therapy. This therapy begins as soon as a complete remission is documented, to ensure that any remaining leukemic cells will be eradicated. Doses of chemotherapy drugs are administered to induce an anticipated marrow hypoplasia, from which the patient will recover in 7 to 14 days.

Continent urinary reservoir   Also called the *Kock pouch;* a surgical procedure that provides an intra-abdominal pouch that stores urine and has two nipple valves that maintain continence and prevent ureteral reflux.

Cure rate   Percentage of patients with cancer who are treated and then have a survival that matches the survival of other people in the same age group.

Cytokines   Cell products used as biologic response modifiers. These soluble proteins have a variety of activities that may alter the growth and metastasis of cancer cells by enhancing the immune responsiveness of noncancerous cells. Most are still highly experimental and are undergoing clinical trials.

Cytoreductive surgery   Surgery to reduce the bulk of the malignant tumor.

Cytotoxic agent   An agent capable of specific destructive action on certain cells; usually used in reference to antineoplastic drugs that selectively kill dividing cells.

Debulking   Surgery to reduce tumor burden to aggregates of 2 cm or less; improves the response to postoperative chemotherapy.

Detection   Finding or discovering the existence of disease. In relation to cancer, this can occur via screening methods or tests such as breast self-examination or mammography.

Diagnosis   A concise, technical description of the cause, nature, or manifestations of a condition, situation, or problem.

Diethylstilbestrol (DES)   A synthetic nonsteroidal estrogen used to relieve vasomotor symptoms associated with menopause; also used for female hypogonadism, atrophic vaginitis, primary ovarian failure, palliative treatment for female breast carcinoma, and to relieve the symptoms of prostatic cancer.

Differentiated Fully matured; ready to perform the specific function unique to its cell type.

Differentiation The act or process of having recognizable, specialized structures and functions; usually refers to a cellular process that causes an increase in morphological heterogeneity.

Diffuse histiocytic lymphoma Characterized by the presence of huge tumor cells that resemble histiocytes morphologically but are considered to be of lymphoid origin. The neoplastic cells infiltrate the entire lymph node without any organized pattern.

Digital rectal examination (DRE) An examination of the rectum performed with the examiner's fingers. Used to check the rectum for masses and to ascertain the size of the prostate.

Disseminated intravascular coagulation (DIC) Widespread formation of clots (thromboses) in the microcirculation, mainly within the capillaries. This intravascular clotting ultimately produces hemorrhage because of the rapid consumption of fibrinogen, platelets, prothrombin, and clotting factors V, VIII, and X. It is a secondary complication of a diverse group of hemolytic and neoplastic disorders that in some way activate the intrinsic coagulation sequence.

Duke's staging A system of staging colorectal tumors based on an assessment of the depth of invasion of the carcinoma and the absence or presence of metastasis.

Dumping syndrome A complex reaction resulting from excessive, rapid emptying of the contents of the GI tract.

Dyspareunia Painful intercourse experienced by women.

Dysphagia Difficulty in swallowing.

Dysplastic nevi Moles that have a greater tendency to be malignant; they differ from regular moles in that they are irregular in shape, variably pigmented, larger in size, and located in unusual places (scalp, buttocks, breasts).

Dyspnea Shortness of breath; difficulty breathing.

Endoscopic laser therapy Laser therapy administered via visual examination of interior structures of the body using an endoscope.

Enteral feeding Nutrition administered directly to the stomach or small intestine.

Epidemiology The science concerned with the study of factors determining and influencing the frequency and distribution of disease, injury, and other health-related events.

Equianalgesic Having equal pain killing effect; morphine sulfate, 10 mg intramuscularly, is generally used for opioid comparisons.

Ewing's sarcoma Marrow-originating bone cancer seen primarily in children and adolescents.

Extravasation Escape from the blood vessel into the tissue; term used to describe chemotherapy escaping from a blood vessel into the tissue, resulting in tissue damage.

FAB morphology The French-American-British morphologic classification system used to describe cellular morphology.

Familial adenomatous polyposis A hereditary condition marked by many polyps with high malignancy potential lining the intestinal tract, especially the colon; usually begins around the time of puberty.

Fecal occult blood test A test of feces to determine the presence of hidden (occult) blood. This test is indicated when intestinal bleeding is suspected but the stool does not appear to contain blood upon gross examination.

Flexible sigmoidoscopy A procedure using a hollow lighted tube to visually inspect the wall of the rectum and distal colon.

Flow cytometry The characterization and measurement of cells and cellular constituents by suspending cells in a fluid flow one at a time through a focus of exciting light, which is scattered in patterns characteristic of the cells and their components. A sensor detecting the scattered light measures the size and molecular characteristics of individual cells; tens of thousands of cells can be examined this way per minute because the data are processed by computer.

Fractions Divisions of the total dose of radiation into small doses given at intervals.

Gene therapy A form of biotherapy that attempts to alter patients' genetic material in order to fight or prevent disease.

Gestational trophoblastic disease (GTD) A neoplasm that occurs as the result of the excessive proliferation of chorionic epithelium during very early pregnancy.

Glioblastoma multiforme Astrocytoma Grade III or IV; a rapidly growing tumor, usually of the cerebral hemispheres, composed of spongioblasts, astroblasts, and astrocytes.

Glioma A tumor composed of neuroglia in any state of development; sometimes extended to include all intrinsic neoplasms of the brain and spinal cord, such as astrocytomas.

Gonadotropin-releasing hormone (GnRH) A decapeptide hormone of the hypothalamus that stimulates the release of follicle-stimulating hormone and luteinizing hormone from the pituitary gland; used in the differential diagnosis of hypothalamic, pituitary, and gonadal dysfunction.

Graft-versus-host disease (GVHD) A frequent complication of allogenic bone marrow transplant. Immunocompetent T-lymphocytes derived from the donor tissue recognize the recipient's tissue as foreign and react to it, producing clinical manifestations that include edema, erythema, ulceration, loss of hair, and heart and joint lesions similar to those occurring in connective tissue disorders.

Granulocytopenia A decrease in white blood cells.

Gray The Sl (Système International d'Unites) unit of absorbed radiation dose, defined as the transfer of 1 joule of energy per Kg of absorbing material. 1 Gray = 100 rads.

Gynecomastia Abnormally large mammary glands in the male; may secrete "milk."

Hematopoiesis The process by which all formed elements of the blood are produced in the bone marrow.

Hematopoietic growth factors Natural body proteins that regulate the growth, differentiation, and biological activity of hematopoietic cells.

Hereditary nonpolyposis cancers Types of colorectal cancers that run in families that are not associated with the formation of polyps in the intestinal tract; associated with a specific genetic defect; accounts for only 5% of colon cancers.

Histology Examination of tissue dealing with the minute structure, composition, and function of tissues as seen through a microscope.

Hodgkin's disease A specific type of lymphoma, differing from all other lymphomas in its predictability of spread, microscopic characteristics, and occurrence of extranodal tumors. The Reed-Sternberg cell is essential to the diagnosis. The accepted histopathologic classification distinguishes four different disease patterns:

    Nodular sclerosing Characterized by the lymph node's being divided into nodules by sclerosing bands of collagen. The lymphocytes in the collagen-bound nodules may be of various types, from predominantly small lymphocytes to the large histiocytic forms.

    Lymphocyte-predominant Characterized by sheets of mature-appearing small lymphocytes with few Reed-Sternberg cells; has a good prognosis.

    Lymphocyte-depleted Characterized by a small quantity of the small lymphocytes, a large number of Reed-Sternberg cells, and a predominance of histiocytes; has a poor prognosis.

    Mixed cellularity Characterized by a histology between lymphocyte-predominant and lymphocyte-depleted.

Hormone receptor assay A laboratory test used to determine the quantity of autoantibodies to the particular hormone receptor in question and to identify those tumors that are endocrine sensitive. Used commonly in breast cancer, this information is used for planning treatment.

Hospice An organized institution designed to provide palliative and supportive care to terminally ill patients and their families.

Human chorionic gonadotropin (hCG) A glycopeptide hormone produced by the fetal placenta that is thought to maintain the function of the corpus luteum during the first few weeks of pregnancy. It is also present in certain neoplastic conditions; used as a tumor marker in choriocarcinoma and testicular cancer

Human-leukocyte antigen (HLA) The human major histocompatibility complex located on the short arm of chromosome number 6. Transplants, platelet, and leukocyte transfusions are least likely to be rejected by the recipient when the donor and the recipient are HLA-identical.

Humoral immunity A response that begins as soon as a substance enters the body and is interpreted as being foreign. Antibodies are released from plasma cells and enter the body fluids, where they can react with the specific antigens for which they were formed. This release of antibodies is stimulated by antigen-specific groups of B-lymphocytes.

Hydatiform mole An abnormal pregnancy resulting from a pathologic ovum, with proliferation of the epithelial covering of the chorionic villi. It results in a mass of cysts resembling a bunch of grapes. Also called *hydatid mole*.

Hyperalimentation Nutritional supplementation of calories, protein, lipids, and other nutritional elements.

Hypercalcemia Excessive quantity of serum calcium. Weakness, confusion, and possible ventricular dysrhythmias are classic symptoms and require immediate intervention.

Hyperviscosity syndrome Any syndrome associated with the effects of exaggeration of adhesive properties of the blood.

Immunotherapy Passive immunization of an individual by administration of preformed antibodies actively produced in another individual (serum or gamma globulins). The term has also come to include the use of immunopotentiators, replacement of immunocompetent tissue (bone marrow), and infusion of specialty treated white blood cells.

Incidence   The rate at which a certain event occurs, such as the number of new cases of a specific disease occurring during a certain time period.

Incidence rate   The number of new cases of cancer divided by the number of people in the population during a given period of time (usually 1 year). The results are usually multiplied by 100,000 to express the rate more conveniently.

Incidence rate epidemiology   The science concerned with the study of the factors determining and influencing the frequency and distribution of disease.

Induction chemotherapy   The initial chemotherapy regimen used in the treatment of leukemia, when the greatest number of leukemic cells are affected. The combination of drugs is designed to cause severe bone marrow depression, and the goal of treatment is remission of the disease.

In situ   Confined to the site of origin.

Intensification therapy (also called reintensification therapy)   This therapy has been proposed to prevent the return of the leukemic cell population. After 1 year of sustained, complete remission, the person undergoes the same intensive induction therapy as in the initial treatment period. The objective is bone marrow depression. After recovery from the bone marrow depression, the person continues on maintenance therapy for another year.

Interferons   Natural glycoproteins released by cells invaded by viruses or certain infectious agents; act as stimulants to noninfected cells, causing them to synthesize another protein with antiviral capabilities. Interferons are divided into three subsets, with each originating from a different cell and having distinctive chemical and biologic properties:

  Alpha   Produced by leukocytes in response to a viral infection.

  Beta   Produced by fibroblasts in response to a viral infection.

  Gamma   Produced by lymphoid cells in culture that are stimulated by a mitogen.

Interleukins   A group of cytokines that aid in the control of specific immune responses; over 15 interleukins have been identified.

Interleukin-2   A glycoprotein produced by helper T-cells that is an essential factor in the growth of T-cells and seems to induce the production of interferon. It is used as an anticancer drug in the treatment of a wide variety of solid tumors.

Intraperitoneal implanted port   A hollow housing containing a compressed latex septum over a portal chamber that is connected via a tube of silicone or a polyurethane catheter that is inserted into the peritoneal cavity; peritoneal ports usually have catheters with larger lumens and multiple exit sites to allow for rapid infusion of fluids; usually placed on the lower rib cage, but could be in a pocket of the lower abdomen; used to administer intermittent intraperitoneal chemotherapy for colon or ovarian cancer.

Intrathecal chemotherapy   Cytotoxic drugs injected into the cerebrospinal fluid (CSF), thereby bypassing the blood-brain barrier.

Intravenous hyperalimentation   Nutritional supplementation by peripheral intravenous or central intravenous line infusion; also known as *total parenteral nutrition (TPN)*.

Intravesical chemotherapy   Chemotherapy administered via a Foley catheter for the treatment of bladder cancer. The Foley is then usually clamped for a period of time and then emptied. This procedure delivers a high local concentration to the tumor area. Patients receiving this therapy require life-long cytoscopic surveillance for recurrent disease.

Invasive mole (chorioadenoma destruens)   A form of hydatidiform mole in which molecular chorionic villi penetrate into the myometrium and may invade the parametrium. Hydropic villi may be transported to distant sites, most often the lungs, but they do not grow as metastases.

Leukemia   A progressive disease of the blood-forming organs, marked by distorted proliferation and development of leukocytes and their precursors in the blood and the bone marrow. It is accompanied by a reduced number of red blood cells and platelets, resulting in anemia and increased susceptibility to infection and bleeding. Leukemia is classified on the basis of duration and character of the disease—acute or chronic; the cell type—myelocytic, lymphoid, or monocytic; and increase in or maintenance of the number of abnormal cells in the blood.

> **Acute lymphocytic leukemia (ALL)**   Most common type of pediatric leukemia. Infiltration and accumulation of immature lymphoblasts occurs within the bone marrow, as well as the extramedullary lymphatic tissue, causing painful lymphadenopathy and hepatosplenomegaly.

> **Acute nonlymphocytic leukemia (ANLL)**   A broad term referring to all leukemias that are not lymphocytic. This leukemia occurs most commonly after treatment with alkylating agents and is characterized by pancytopenia, megablastic bone marrow, nucleated red cells in the peripheral marrow, and refractoriness to treatment, with a short survival time. Most patients have chromosomal abnormalities in marrow cells.

> **Acute myelocytic leukemia (AML)**   A subtype of ANLL. This type of childhood leukemia encompasses various subtypes, with myloblastic leukemia being the most common type. This type of leukemia is rare.

> **Chronic myelocytic leukemia (CML)**   May occur in older adults as well as in children. The onset is insidious, and the leukocytosis consists of predominantly mature white blood cells.

> **Hairy-cell leukemia (HCL)**   An adult leukemia marked by splenomegaly and by an abundance of large, mononuclear, abnormal cells with numerous irregular cytoplasmic projections that give them a flagellated or hairy appearance in the bone marrow, spleen, liver, and peripheral blood.

> **Chronic lymphocytic leukemia (CLL)**   An adult onset form of leukemia in which the leukemic cells have T-cell properties, with frequent dermal involvement, lymphadenopathy, hepatosplenomegaly, and a subacute or chronic course. It is associated with the human T-cell leukemia-lymphoma virus.

Leukophoresis   Removing white blood cells from the patient; usually used in leukemic patients when the white blood cell count gets too high. Can be accomplished by continuous-flow cell separators or filtration techniques.

Leukoplakia   The development of white, thickened patches on the mucous membranes of the cheeks, gums, or tongue. These patches have a tendency to fissure and become malignant. They tend to grow into larger patches, or they may take the form of ulcers. Those in the mouth may cause pain during swallowing, eating, or talking.

Leukostasis   Occurs as a result of leukemic blast cells accumulating and invading vessel walls, causing rupture and bleeding.

Leutinizing hormone-releasing hormone (LHRH) agonist   Newer pharmacologic agent that stimulates the pituitary to increase leutinizing hormone (LH), thereby stimulating testosterone production. Used to treat prostate cancer.

Limb perfusion   Used in the treatment of malignant melanoma, where certain chemotherapeutic drugs (usually L-phenylalanine and DTIC) are instilled into the affected extremity by arterial perfusion. A pump system counteracts the normal arterial pressure, permitting a steady state of infusion, allowing the drugs to have the greatest effect at the disease site. Usually performed after surgical removal of the bulk of the tumor mass.

Lymphadenectomy   Surgical excision of one or more lymph nodes.

Lymphangiogram   The film produced by lymphangiography, which is an x-ray of the lymphatic channels after introduction of a contrast medium.

Lymphocyte   Any of the mononuclear, nonphagocytic leukocytes found in the blood, lymph, and lymphoid tissue. Divided into two classes, B- and T-lymphocytes, which are responsible for humoral and cellular immunity, respectively.

Lymphokines   Cytokines produced by lymphocytes and capable of regulating the immune response. Examples are interleukin-2 and interferon.

Lymphokine-activated killer (LAK) cells   Cells that are produced in the laboratory by incubating human lymphocytes with interleukin-2. These cells selectively lyse tumor cells that are resistant to natural killer cells, without affecting normal cells. They are part of a class of anticancer agents known as *biologic response modifiers*.

Lymphoma   Any neoplastic disorder of the lymphoid tissue, including Hodgkin's disease. Classifications are based on predominant cell type and degree of differentiation. Various categories may be subdivided into nodular and diffuse types, depending on the predominant pattern of cell arrangement.

Macrophage   Any of the large, mononuclear, highly phagocytic cells derived from monocytes that occur in the walls of the blood vessels and in loose connective tissue. They are usually immobile, but become mobile when stimulated by inflammation. They have a vital role in the immune system.

Magnetic resonance imaging (MRI)   A noninvasive nuclear procedure for imaging tissues of high fat and water content that cannot be seen with other radiologic techniques. Provides information that allows the distinction between normal tissues versus cancerous, atherosclerotic, or traumatized tissues.

Maintenance chemotherapy   This leukemia therapy begins when the marrow and peripheral blood have recovered, after either induction or consolidation therapy. Drug doses are chosen to cause significant, but not life-threatening, cytopenias.

Malignant   Having the properties of anaplasia, invasiveness, and metastasis.

Malignant melanoma   Least common form of malignant skin cancer, usually developing from a nevus and consisting of black masses of cells with a marked tendency to metastasis.

Malignant transformation   Cellular transformation whereby the cells take on properties of anaplasia, invasiveness, and metastasis; term used in conjunction with tumor development.

Meningioma   A hard, usually vascular tumor occurring mainly along the meningeal vessels and superior longitudinal sinus, invading the aura and skull, which leads to the erosion and thinning of the skull.

Metastasis   Secondary malignant lesions originating from the primary tumor but located in anatomically distant places.

Metastatic cascade   A series of steps that, once initiated, continue to the end result of the transfer of abnormal cells to a site in the body that is distant from the site initially affected. The end result is the formation of a new focus of disease in a distant part of the body.

Micrometastases Tumor cells escaping into the smaller sections of the lymphatic or vascular flow where they can travel to other parts of the body.

Mohs surgery A technique for microscopically controlled serial excisions of fresh tissue used for microscopic analysis in the diagnosis and treatment of skin cancer.

Monoclonal antibodies (MoAbs) Antibodies formed through a special process of immunizing mice with a desired antigen, removing immunized lymphocytes from the mice, and fusing the lymphocytes with mouse myeloma cells to form a hybridoma, which is capable of unlimited cell division. Cells that produce the desired antibody are selected, and those are cloned to produce large amounts of uniform antibodies specific to the target antigen. These antibodies are still being tested in an attempt to find antibodies which are tumor-cell specific for various cancers.

Monoclonal gammopathy of unknown significance (MGUS) Pathologic condition of plasma cells. Benign monoclonal gammopathy exists when there is the presence of a serum M-component without signs and symptoms of multiple myeloma.

Monokines Cytokines produced by macrophages and other cells that are capable of regulating the immune response.

Mortality The number of deaths due to a disease, in this case, cancer.

Mortality rate The death rate; the ratio of total number of deaths from a particular disease (cancer) divided by the total number of people in the population during a given period of time (usually 1 year). The results are usually multiplied by 100,000 to express the rate more conveniently.

Mucosal erythroplasia A condition of the mucous membranes characterized by erythematous papular lesions.

Mucositis Inflammation of a mucous membrane. Oral mucositis is a common side effect of some types of chemotherapy.

Myelosuppression A reduction in bone marrow function, resulting in a reduced release of erythrocytes, leukocytes, and platelets into the peripheral circulation and/or the release of immature cells into the circulating blood.

Nadir The period of time when an antineoplastic drug has its most profound effects on the bone marrow.

Natural killer cells A group of large, granular lymphocytes that have the intrinsic ability to recognize and destroy some virally infected cells and some tumor cells.

Neo-adjuvant therapy Preliminary cancer therapy (usually chemotherapy or radiation therapy) that precedes a necessary second modality of treatment.

Neuroblastoma Most common extracranial solid tumor in children; originates from neural crest cells of the sympathetic nervous system.

Neutropenia Abnormally low number of white blood cells (neutrophils) in the blood.

Nonseminomatous tumors A histologic type of testicular cancer consisting of the embryonal (including yolk sac), teratocarcinoma, teratoma, and choriocarcinoma tumors, which can produce human chorionic gonadotropins, causing gynecomastia.

Non-small-cell carcinoma of the lung A broad term referring to all bronchogenic cancers that are not small-cell; includes large-cell, adenocarcinoma, and epidermoid lung cancers.

Observed survival rate The proportion of a cohort of persons with cancer that are still alive after a given time interval.

Odynophagia Painful swallowing of food.

Oligodendroglioma   A neoplasm derived from and composed of non-neural cells of ecto-dermal origin forming part of the adventitial structure of the central nervous system.

Ommaya reservoir   This device is a subcutaneous cerebrospinal fluid (CSF) reservoir that is implanted surgically under the scalp and provides access to the CSF through a burr hole in the scalp. Drugs are injected into the reservoir with a syringe, and the domed reservoir is then depressed manually to mix the drug within the CSF. This device eliminates the need for multiple lumbar punctures in the repeated administration of intrathecal chemotherapy.

Oncogenes   Genes whose protein products may be involved in the processes of transformation of a normal cell to a malignant state. Classically, it is a normal cellular gene that has been incorporated into an RNA virus and causes the transformation when the virus infects the cell.

Orchiectomy   Surgical removal of one or both testes.

Osteoblast cells   A cell arising from a fibroblast, which, as it matures, is associated with bone production.

Osteoclast-activating factor (OAF)   A lymphokine that stimulates the proliferation of large multinuclear cells (osteoclasts) frequently associated with the resorption of bone, severe bone pain, and pathologic fractures; usually found in multiple myeloma.

Osteoradionecrosis   Necrosis of bone as a result of excessive exposure to radiation.

Osteosarcoma   Most common primary bone cancer.

Papanicolaou (Pap) smear   A technique that uses exfoliated cells and subjects them to cytologic staining for the purpose of detecting abnormal cells. Most commonly used to detect cancer of the cervix and uterus, but may also be used in the diagnosis of lung, stomach, and bladder cancers.

Paraneoplastic syndrome   A collective term for disorders arising from metabolic effects of cancer on tissues remote from the tumor. These disorders may appear as primary endocrine, hematologic, or neuromuscular problems.

Pelvic exenteration   Total pelvic exenteration includes a radical hysterectomy, pelvic lymph node dissection, and removal of the bladder and rectosigmoid. Occasionally a posterior exenteration, which preserves the bladder, or an anterior exenteration, which preserves the rectum, can be performed.

Pericardial effusion   Accumulation of fluid in the pericardial sac.

Peripheral blood stem cell transplants   Transplants of stem cells taken from the peripheral blood, as compared to a bone marrow transplant in which stem cells are obtained from the bone marrow and used for transplanting.

Pheochromocytoma   A usually benign tumor of the sympatho-adrenal system that produces catecholamines; produces a hypertension that may be sudden in nature.

Philadelphia chromosome (Ph^1)   An abnormality of chromosome 22, characterized by shortening of its long arms. This chromosome is seen in the marrow cells of most patients with chronic myelogenous leukemia.

Plasma cells   Descendants of B-cells that are capable of producing antibodies.

Plasmacytoma   A malignant tumor of plasma cells; usually a discrete, presumably solitary, plasma cell tumor mass.

Pluripotent stem cell   The cell that can generate all cell lineages in the bone marrow, such as red blood cells, white blood cells, and platelets. (See *Stem cell.*)

Polyp Any growth or mass protruding from a mucous membrane. Polyps are usually an overgrowth of normal tissue, but sometimes they are true tumors.

Predictive value The percentage of persons with a positive screening test who actually have cancer.

Prevalence The number of existing cases of a disease in a given population at a specific time.

Primary prevention Interventions aimed at protecting individuals from cancer before pathological changes have begun; includes both general health promotion and specific measures.

Procedural pain A feeling of distress, suffering, or agony caused by the stimulation of nerve endings during a medical procedure. The distress may also be psychological in nature due to fear of the known or unknown.

Prostate-specific antigen (PSA) A tumor marker that has been used to monitor tumor activity of prostate carcinomas. An elevation of this enzyme is thought to indicate advanced disease regardless of whether the metastatic sites are obvious.

Proto-oncogenes Genes in normal cells similar to viral-transforming genes. Some proto-oncogenes encode proteins that influence the controlled cellular proliferation and differentiation. Mutations, amplifications, and rearrangements of proto-oncogenes allow them to function as oncogenes.

Purged bone marrow Bone marrow that has had tumor cells removed by a chemical treatment (purge) or by a mechanical removal (usually using a magnet that pulls off tumor cells that have attached to monoclonal antibodies), or a combination of both methods.

Radionuclide A type of atom that is radioactive and disintegrates with the emission of corpuscular or electromagnetic radiations; used in nuclear medicine scanning for diagnostic and evaluative purposes.

Relative risk A ratio comparing the rate of disease among exposed individuals with the rate of disease among unexposed individuals. This risk does not reveal probability of disease occurrence; it measures the strength of the association between a factor and the outcome. The higher the relative risk, the greater the evidence for causation.

Relative survival rate The observed survival rate in the cancer cohort divided by the expected survival rate in the general population. This rate reflects the fact that some cancer patients die of causes other than their cancer.

Response rate Percentage of patients showing some evidence of improvement following an intervention.

Retinoblastoma A malignant, congenital hereditary blastoma composed of retinal cells arising from the nuclear layers.

Retroviruses RNA viruses that propogates via conversion into duplex DNA.

Risk The probability that an individual member of the population will develop or die from cancer in a given period of time. Estimated by incidence and mortality rates.

Risk factor An element of personal behavior, genetic make-up, or exposure to a known cancer-causing agent that increases a person's chances of developing a particular form of cancer.

Sarcoma A tumor that is often highly malignant, composed of cells derived from connective tissue such as bone and cartilage, muscle, blood vessel, or lymphoid tissue. These tumors usually develop rapidly and metastasize through the lymph channels. The different types of sarcomas are named for the different types of tissues they affect:

Ewing's sarcoma   A malignant tumor of bone that arises in medullary tissue, occurring more often in cylindrical bones, with pain, fever, and leukocytosis as prominent symptoms.

Fibrosarcoma   A sarcoma arising from collagen-producing fibroblasts.

Kaposi's sarcoma   Malignant neoplastic vascular proliferation characterized by the development of bluish red cutaneous nodules, usually on the lower extremities, which spread slowly, increase in size and number, and spread to more proximal sites. The tumors often remain confined to the skin and subcutaneous tissue, but widespread visceral involvement may occur.

Osteogenic sarcoma   Malignant primary tumor of the bone composed of a malignant connective tissue stroma with evidence of osteoid, bone, and/ or cartilage formation.

Schwannomas   A neoplasm originating from Schwann cells (of the myelin sheath) of neurons. These neoplasms include neurofibromas and neurilemomas.

Screening   Tests that are systematically applied to defined populations for the detection of early and asymptomatic disease.

Secondary prevention   Interventions aimed at detecting cancer early and treating it promptly.

SEER   Surveillance, Epidemiology, and End Results Program of the National Cancer Institute. Maintains the statistical database of cancer in the United States.

Seminoma   A malignant tumor of the testes thought to arise from the primordial germ cells of the sexually undifferentiated embryonic gonad.

Sensitivity   The probability that a screening test will correctly classify an individual as positive for cancer when the individual has the disease.

Serotherapy   The treatment of infectious disease by the injection of immune serum or antitoxin. In cancer research, the ability to deliver a treatment or label to tumor cells by binding with the surface antigens on tumor cells; a form of biotherapy using the principles of humoral immunity.

Sexuality   A broad concept referring to the physical, psychological, social emotional, and spiritual makeup of an individual.

Small-cell carcinoma of the lung   A radiosensitive tumor composed of small, undifferentiated cells. Also called oat-cell carcinoma.

Specificity   The probability that a person not having a disease will be correctly identified by a clinical/diagnostic test. The number of true negatives divided by the number of true negatives and false positives.

Specific immunity   Response wherein an antigen is recognized by the lymphocytes, triggering a cascade of events to destroy the invader.

Spinal cord compression (SCC)   Pressure on the spinal cord by a tumor, causing a medical emergency that can lead to paraplegia, quadraplegia, loss of bowel and bladder function, and possibly death. Usually seen in cancers that have a tendency toward bony metastasis, such as breast cancer.

Staging   The classification of the severity of disease in distinct stages on the basis of established criteria.

Stem cell   The hematopoietic pluripotent stem cell is the source of new cells in the blood. Stem cells are capable of self-replication and differentiation. Daughter cells of the pluripotent stem cell divide and differentiate to become lymphocytes, neutrophils, monocytes, macrophages, eosinophils, basophils, erythrocytes, and platelets.

Stereotactic surgery   A surgical technique used in neurology in which precise localization of the target tissue is possible through use of three-dimensional coordinates. Also known as *stereotaxic surgery*.

Superior vena cava syndrome (SVCS)   An oncologic emergency that occurs when tumors of the superior mediastinum on the right obstruct the return of blood to the heart by the superior vena cava. This produces a characteristic syndrome of edema of the upper half of the body associated with prominent collateral circulation. This condition necessitates prompt therapy aimed at relieving the pressure on the superior vena cava.

Support   Usually used in the term *social support*, defined as that situation in which ill persons believe that they are loved, that they are an important part of a network of communication, that they are esteemed and valued, and that a network of mutual obligations exists exclusive of tangible or material aid.

Survival rate   Percentage of survivors with no trace of disease within a specific time frame after diagnosis or treatment; for example 5-year survival rate.

Survivorship   The state of living with cancer in remission or having obtained a prognosis of "cured."

Syndrome of inappropriate secretion of antidiuretic hormone (SIADH)   A disorder in which antidiuretic hormone is continually released despite a plasma osmolality below normal, leading to weakness, confusion, nausea, and vomiting. Treatment aims to remove the underlying cause (the tumor), restrict fluid intake/output, and protect patients from injury.

Syngeneic bone marrow transplantation   Transplanting bone marrow cells from an identical twin.

T-cells   Thymus-dependent lymphocytes, also called **T-lymphocytes,** which originate from stem cells and undergo differentiation in the thymus when triggered by thymin and thymopoietin. A type of white blood cell that produces lymphokines and is involved in cell mediated immunity. Differentiated T-cells play important roles in the immune system:

> **Cytotoxic T-cells**   A subset of T-cells capable of direct destruction of foreign cells.

> **Helper T-cells**   A subset of T-cells that stimulates other T-cells and B-cells.

Tertiary prevention   Interventions aimed at limitation of disability and rehabilitation of those with disability.

Thermography   A technique wherein an infrared camera photographically portrays the body's surface temperature, based on self-emanating infrared radiations; used as a diagnostic aid.

Therapies   Procedures designed to treat disease, illness, or disability.

Thrombocytopenia   An abnormally low quantity of platelets in the circulating blood.

Thyroid cancer   Because the thyroid contains a variety of cells, malignant tumors may arise within the thyroid from any of the following cells:

> **Anaplastic thyroid carcinoma**   Resembles a variety of other tumors such as sarcoma. Highly malignant and locally invasive. Invasion beyond the thyroid usually present at the time of diagnosis. Often presents with compression of the esophagus and trachea.

> **Follicular thyroid carcinoma**   Usually solitary and encapsulated. May be well circumscribed and well differentiated. Uncommon as pure follicular.

> **Medullary thyroid carcinoma**   Tends to be unencapsulated. Cells vary in morphology, but do not contain papillary or follicular cells.

Papillary thyroid carcinoma   Usually multifocal and unencapsulated. Pure papillary is uncommon; usually mixed with follicular.

TNM staging classification   A system of cancer staging where T stands for the primary tumor growth, N stands for spread to primary lymph nodes, and M stands for metastasis. This is the staging system recommended by the American Joint Committee on Cancer.

Tolerance   A reduced responsiveness to any effect of any drug as a consequence of prior administration of that drug, necessitating larger doses of the drug to produce an equivalent effect to that of the initial dose.

Total parenteral nutrition (TPN)   Nutritional supplementation by peripheral intravenous or central intravenous line infusion; also known as *intravenous hyperalimentation*.

Transcutaneous electrical nerve stimulation (TENS)   Mild electrical stimulation applied by electrodes in contact with the skin over a painful area. The stimulation interferes with the transmission of pain signals and helps to suppress the sensation of pain in the area; current is supplied by a hand-held battery-operated pulse generator.

Tumor   Neoplasm; a new growth of tissue in which cell growth is uncontrolled and progressive.

Tumor-infiltrating lymphocytes (TILs)   Lymphocytes collected from the site of a tumor and exposed to IL-2 in vitro. When these cells are injected back into the tumor-bearing host, they will kill the specific tumor from which they originated.

Tumor lysis syndrome (TLS)   Severe hyperphosphatemia, hyperkalemia, hyperuricemia, and hypocalcemia occurring after effective induction therapy of rapidly growing malignant tumors; thought to be due to release of intracellular products after cell lysis.

Tumor markers   Abnormal proteins on the surface of some malignant cells; sometimes used to monitor recurrence or response to treatment.

Tumor necrosis factor (TNF)   Produced primarily by activated macrophages, TNF is cytotoxic for some neoplastic cells. This factor induces hemorrhagic necrosis in some tumors and is similar to interleukin-1 in the inducement of acute phase reaction. This factor is also known as *cachectin*.

Tumor-suppressor genes   Also known as *anti-oncogenes*; genes coding for proteins that "turn off" malignant growth.

Tumorocidal   Destructive to cancer cells.

Ultrasound   Radiologic technique in which deep structures of the body are visualized by recording the reflections of ultrasonic waves into the tissues; uterine tumors and other pelvic masses can be detected using this technique.

Ultraviolet radiation (UVR)   The type of light that consists of electromagnetic radiation of wavelength shorter than that of the violet end of the spectrum, having wavelengths of 4 to 400 nanometers. It is used in the treatment of various diseases, particularly those affecting the skin, but is also thought to be a causative agent in some types of skin cancer.

Underserved populations   Populations of individuals who not receive adequate services, in this case healthcare services. This term is used in relation to people in certain geographic regions, individuals of low socioeconomic status, individuals of various racial/ethnic groups, or a combination of these characteristics.

Undifferentiated or anaplastic   Characterized by a loss of differentiation of cells, an irreversible alteration in adult cells toward more primitive cell types. A characteristic of tumor cells.

Vascular access device (VAD)   A device that provides intravascular access in the care of individuals with cancer:

> **Tunneled catheter**   Single-, double-, or triple-lumen catheter with dacron cuff that secures catheter within the SQ tissue and minimizes the risk of ascending bacteria within the tunnel; peripherally inserted catheter.

> **PICC**   Single- or double-lumen catheters inserted intravenously, usually in the antecubital area.

> **Implantable port**   Provides access to peritoneal, arterial, venous, or epidural body systems through a portal septum.

Vector   A plasmid or viral chromosome into whose genome a fragment of foreign DNA is inserted, used to introduce the foreign DNA into a host cell in the cloning of DNA.

Veno-occlusive disease   An acute or chronic disease of the liver characterized by partial or complete occlusion of the branches of the hepatic veins by endophlebitis and thrombosis, leading to centrilobular necrosis, fibrosis, and ascites.

Wilms' tumor   A rapidly developing malignant mixed tumor of the kidneys, comprised of embryonal elements, usually occurring before the age of 5.

Xeroderma pigmentosa   A rare and frequently fatal pigmentary and atrophic disease in which the skin and eyes are extremely sensitive to light. It begins in childhood and progresses to early development of excessive freckling, keratosis, papillomas, carcinoma, and melanoma.

Xerostomia   Dryness of the mouth from salivary gland dysfunction.

Index

Addiction, 175, 457
Adjuvant therapy, 85, 175, 457
Age
    cancer risk and, 15, 17t, 63, 307; carcino-
    genesis and, 423–424; prostate cancer and,
    327
Aged patients. *See* Elderly patients
Airway obstructions
    head and neck cancer and, 278–279; lung
    cancer and, 292–293
Alcohol
    breast cancer and, 296; cancer risk and, 37,
    40, 273
Alkylating agents, 106, 106t, 108f
Allogeneic transplants
    description of, 140, 45t; HLA typing in,
    141; leukemia and, 384–385. *See also*
    Hematopoietic stem cell transplantation
Alpha interferon, 124t, 126, 130t–131t
Alternative therapies, 152–157
    categories of, 153–154; definition of,
    152–153; evaluation of, 153t; nurse's role
    in, 155–156, 156f; for pain, 177–178; rea-
    sons for use of, 154f, 154–155
Ambulatory pumps, 197, 198t. *See also* Vascular
    access devices
American Association for Cancer Education,
    447–448
American Brain Tumor Association, 444
American Cancer Society
    address and phone numbers of, 443, 450;
    breast cancer and, 297, 298, 298t; cervical
    cancer and, 338; colorectal cancer and,
    308; description of, 453–455; educational
    materials and, 8; head and neck cancer
    and, 282; programs and services of,
    443–444; prostate cancer and, 328; rehabil-
    itation and, 257, 259; screening recommen-
    dations of, 44, 45t; skin cancer and, 362,
    364f–365f
American Kidney Fund, 450
Americans with Disabilities Act, 256

Amyloidosis, 404
Analgesics, 175–177
Anaplastic cells, 27
Anemia, 457
    assessment of, 164–165, 166, 167; causes of,
    164, 387; erythropoietin for, 127, 171; nurs-
    ing interventions for, 168t–170t
Anorexia, 100f, 113t, 200, 212, 457. *See also*
    Nutrition
Antibodies, 123, 402t, 457
Anticonvulsants, 354, 356
Antidiuretic hormone, 215t, 217t, 221–224,
    224t
Antiemetic therapy, 178t, 179–180
Antimetabolites, 106–107, 108f
Antineoplastic agents. *See* Chemotherapeutic
    agents
Antitumor antibiotics, 106t, 107, 108f
Astrocytoma, 350, 351, 351t, 352t, 458
Autologous bone marrow transplantation. *See*
    Hematopoietic stem cell transplanta-
    tion

Behavioral techniques, 281
Beta interferon, 124t, 126, 130t–131t
Biliary cancer, 417–418
Biological response modifiers. *See* Biotherapy
Biopsy
    in diagnosis of disease, 81–84, 82t–83t;
    guidelines for, 81; pain and, 175f
Biotherapy, 122–137, 458
    cytokines as, 127–132; definition of, 122;
    gene therapy as, 134, 136; history of,
    122–123; list of approved agents, 124t;
    monoclonal antibodies as, 132, 134; for
    multiple myeloma, 407; nursing challenges
    in, 136–137; for renal cell cancer, 325; side
    effects in, 130t–131t; for skin cancer, 369
Bladder cancer, 316–322
    diagnosis and staging of, 316–317, 317t,
    318t; treatment of, 317–322
Bladder dysfunction, 116t

Blood cell count, 162t
Blood disorders
    leukemia causing, 387; surgery and, 87;
    thrombocytopenia-related, 167
B-lymphocytes, 402
Body image, 89, 302
Bone cancer, 372–378
    clinical manifestations of, 373; diagnosis
    and evaluation of, 373; incidence of, 372;
    metastatic, 376; nursing considerations in,
    376–377; risk factors for, 372–373; types of,
    373
Bone marrow depression, 403, 404, 408
Bone marrow harvest, 143
Bone Marrow Transplant Family Support
    Network, 439–440
Bone marrow transplants. See Hematopoietic
    stem cell transplantation
Bone metastasis pain, 175, 177
Bowel dysfunction, 113t–114t, 116t, 180–181
Brachytherapy
    for brain tumors, 355; description of, 96,
    458; for head and neck cancer, 276; precau-
    tions in, 94, 97
Brain tumors. See Central nervous system can-
    cers
Breast cancer, 295–306
    combination therapy for, 105–106; diagno-
    sis and staging of, 299, 300t; early detection
    of, 46, 51–52, 297–298, 298t, 458; inci-
    dence of, 14, 16f, 295; long-term sequelae
    of, 305, 305t; myelosuppression and, 162;
    nursing considerations in, 306; prevention
    of, 296–297; prognostic factors in, 301; risk
    factors for, 39t, 295–296; treatment of,
    301–305; types of, 299–301
Breast self-examination, 298, 298t

Cachexia, 279, 458. See also Nutrition
Calcitonin, 376
Cancer Care, Inc., 450–451440
Cancer care settings, 5–6
Cancer cells, characteristics of, 27–29, 28t
Cancer center program, 71, 73
Cancer Information Service, 444–445
Cancer resources. See Resources in cancer care
Candlelighters Childhood Cancer Foundation,
    440
CanSurmount, 443
Carcinogenesis, 458
    age and, 423–424; factors related to, 38–41;
    process of, 29–32, 30f
Carcinogen(s), 459
    alcohol as, 29t, 37, 40, 273; chemical, 29t,
    38, 41; industrial and environmental, 284;
    radiation as, 29t, 38, 381; tobacco as, 29t,
    38–40, 273
Cardiac tamponade, 215t, 217t, 219–221, 220t,
    459
Cardiovascular system, chemotherapy and, 115t
Catheters. See Vascular access devices

Cell cycle, 105, 105f, 459
Cell cycle phase nonspecific drugs, 105, 106,
    106t, 107, 459
Cell cycle phase specific drugs, 105, 106t, 107,
    459
Central nervous system, lymphoma and,
    396–399
Central nervous system cancers, 349–358
    classification of, 350t, 350–352, 351t; clini-
    cal presentation of, 353–354; diagnosis of,
    354; incidence of, 349–350; long-term
    sequelae in, 357; nursing considerations in,
    357–358; risk factors for, 352–353; side
    effects and complications of, 356–357;
    treatment of, 354–356
Cerebellar astrocytoma, 351, 352t
Cervical cancer, 337–340, 339t
    early detection of, 46, 53, 337–338
Chemical carcinogens, 38, 41
Chemotherapy, 103–120, 459
    administration of, 107–108, 119f; assess-
    ment guide for, 109; for bladder cancer,
    317–318, 319, 322; for bone cancer,
    374–375; bowel dysfunction and, 180; for
    brain tumors, 355–356, 357; for breast can-
    cer, 297, 303–304; for cervical cancer, 339;
    classifications in, 105; for CNS lymphoma,
    398–399; for colorectal cancer, 311–312,
    313; in combination therapy, 105–106; con-
    solidation, 383, 425; for endometrial cancer,
    337; for esophageal cancer, 411–412; for
    gestational trophoblastic disease, 347; hair
    loss and, 183; for head and neck cancer,
    276–277; hematopoietic stem cell trans-
    plantation and, 145; history of, 103; for
    Hodgkin's disease, 392–393; induction, 383,
    425; for leukemia, 383–384, 386, 425, 426t;
    leukostasis and, 221; list of agents, 104f; for
    liver cancer, 417; lung cancer and, 288,
    290, 290f; maintenance, 384, 425; mecha-
    nisms of action for, 106–107, 108f; mucosi-
    tis and, 181; for multiple myeloma, 406;
    myelosuppression and, 161–162, 164t; nau-
    sea and vomiting and, 179; for neuroblas-
    toma, 430; for non-Hodgkin's lymphoma,
    396, 398–399; nursing management of, 109,
    111; nutrition and, 204; for ovarian cancer,
    341, 343; pain and, 175f; prechemotherapy
    assessment guide, 112t–118t; radiation ther-
    apy and, 93; rationale for, 103, 105–106; for
    rhabdomyosarcoma, 432; safe handling of,
    119f–120f; side effects of, 109, 112t–118t;
    for skin cancer, 367, 368, 370; for stomach
    cancer, 413; superior vena cava syndrome
    and, 216–217; during surgery, 87–88; for
    unknown primary cancer, 421; for Wilms'
    tumor, 428
Childhood cancers, 423–437
    acute leukemia, 424–425; bone, 373–374;
    central nervous system, 349, 351–352, 352t,
    354, 357; coping strategies in, 434–435; late

effects of, 435–436; neuroblastoma, 428–430; nursing considerations in, 436; psychosocial impact of, 433–434; retinoblastoma, 430–431; rhabdomyosarcoma, 431–432; sexuality and, 239–240; supportive care in, 432–433; Wilms' tumor, 426–428, 427t

Children
    camps for, 443; grief and, 251–252; pain management for, 179
Choice in Dying, 445
Cholangiocarcinoma, 417–418
Chondrosarcoma, 375, 459
Chromosome evaluation, 32, 33f, 383
Clinical trials, 69–79, 459
    challenges in, 78–79; current programs, 71, 73, 73f; drug development and, 73; ethical issues in, 76–78; history of, 69–70; nursing research in, 7, 73–74; obstacles to participation in, 75–76; phases of, 70–71, 72t; role for nurses in, 74–75
Clustering, familial, 33–34
CMF protocol, 105–106
Coagulation, disseminated intravascular, 215t, 217t, 225, 228f, 229–230
Colony-stimulating factors, 460
    administration and toxicities of, 127; biologic activity of, 127; childhood cancers and, 432–433; descriptions of, 128t–129t; indications for, 124t, 128t; lymphoma and, 396, 399; side effects of, 129t, 130t–131t
Colorectal cancer, 307–315
    diagnosis of, 308–309; early detection of, 46, 53–54, 308; incidence of, 307; long-term sequelae in, 313; nursing considerations in, 313–315; pathophysiology of, 310–311; prevention of, 308; prognosis in, 312; risk factors for, 39t, 307–308; side effects and complications in, 312–313; staging of, 309, 310t; treatment of, 311–312
Colostomies, 311
Combination therapy, 85–86, 87–88, 93, 105–106
Community Clinical Oncology Program, 73
Complementary therapies. See Alternative therapies
Compression
    cardiac tamponade and, 219–221, 220t; spinal cord, 215t, 217t, 218–219
Confidentiality, 77
Constipation, 114t, 180–181
Cooperative Group Outreach Program, 73
Cooperative Oncology Groups, 71, 73f
Corporate Angel Network, Inc., 445
Corticosteroids, 354, 356
Cough, 101f, 293
Cryosurgery, 85, 275–276
Cultural beliefs and values
    cancer risk and, 17; sensitivity to, 63, 281–282
Cushing's syndrome, 289t

Cystectomy, 319, 321
Cytokines
    definition of, 126, 460; examples of, 126–127, 132; indications for, 124t; multiple myeloma and, 403; side effects of, 130t–131t
Cytosine arabinoside, 387
Cytotoxic agents. See Chemotherapy

Death and dying
    attitudes toward, 260–261; childhood cancers and, 434–435; right-to-die organizations, 445. See also Mortality
Decision-making, patient participation in, 156
Detection. See Screening
Dexamethasone, 407t
Diagnosis, 461
    history and physical examination in, 46–47, 47f; psychosocial responses to, 247–248; screening tests or procedures in, 45t; surgery in, 81–84, 82t–83t
Diarrhea, 101f, 113t, 180
Diet. See Nutrition
Digital rectal examination, 52, 54, 309, 328, 461
Disseminated intravascular coagulation, 215t, 217t, 225, 228f, 229–230, 387, 461
DNA
    carcinogenesis and, 29–30; chemotherapy and, 106–107, 108f; gene therapy and, 136, 137f; radiation therapy and, 91
Doxorubicin, side effects of, 407t
Dumping syndrome, 202, 413, 461
Dysplastic nevi, 360–361
Dyspnea, 183–184, 292, 461

Education
    minority-based, 62; nursing, 7, 8; in prevention of cancer, 41–42; resources for, 173, 439–450. See also Patient teaching
Elderly patients
    altered protective mechanisms in, 64t; cancer in, 63–66; cancer screening in, barriers to, 65; nursing practices and, 65–66; screening of, barriers to, 63
Electrosurgery, 85
Encore Plus, 440–441, 452
Endocrine cancers, 418
Endometrial cancer, 39t, 335–337, 336f
Enteral feeding, 209, 461
Ependymoma, 352, 352t
Epilepsy Foundation, 357–358
Epoetin alfa (Epogen; erythropoietin), 124t, 127, 128t–131t, 171
Epstein-Barr virus, 273, 397
Esophageal cancer, 410–412
Esophagitis, 101f
Estrogen, endometrial cancer and, 40
Ethical issues
    in biomedical research, 77, 77f; palliative care and, 267

Ethnic groups. *See* Racial/ethnic group(s)
Ewing's sarcoma, 375, 462, 470
Extravasation, 109, 462

Fallopian tube cancer, 346–347
Familial clustering, 33–34
Families
    childhood cancers and, 433–434; rehabilitation and, 253–254, 256
Family Leave Act, 256
Fatigue
    anemia-related, 167; causes of, 182; nursing management of, 182–183; radiation therapy causing, 100f, 303
Fecal occult blood testing, 54, 309, 462
Fetal development, 118t
Fever, septic shock and, 229
Fibrosarcoma, 375, 470
Filgrastim (G-CSF), 128t–129t, 171, 172f
Food and Drug Administration, 449

Gamma interferon, 124t, 126, 130t–131t
Gastric cancer, 412–414
Gender differences
    in cancer risk, 14, 14t, 15t, 16f; in cancer sites, 14, 16f, 307
Gene therapy, 134, 136, 136f, 137f, 462
Genetics
    breast cancer and, 296, 297; in cancer development, 32–34, 38; leukemia and, 382–383
Geographical differences, 17, 20f
Gestational trophoblastic disease, 347, 347t, 462
Graft-versus-host disease, 140, 141, 146, 147t, 149, 150t, 180
Granulocyte colony-stimulating factor (G-CSF), 124t, 127, 128t–131t, 171, 172f
Granulocyte macrophage colony-stimulating factor (GM-CSF), 124t, 127, 128t–131t, 171, 399
Granulocytopenia, 164, 462
Grief
    children and, 251–252; palliative care and, 266
Growth, tumor, 28–32
Growth factors. *See* Colony-stimulating factors
Gynecologic cancers, 39t, 335–348

Hair loss, 183
Head and neck cancers, 271–283
    detection of, 273–274; diagnosis of, 274; incidence of, 271–272; nursing considerations in, 277–282; primary sites for, 271, 272f; rehabilitation in, 277; risk factors for, 273; staging of, 274; treatment of, 274–277, 276t
Headache, central nervous system cancers and, 353

Health care system, changes in, 5
Health insurance
    for cancer survivors, 249; palliative care and, 267–268
Health promotion, as primary prevention, 35–36
Hematopoiesis
    chemotherapy and, 112t; definition, 462; normal blood values and, 162t; process of, 161, 163f; role of colony-stimulating factors in, 127
Hematopoietic growth factors
    definition, 463; leukemia and, 385–386; lymphoma and, 396, 399; for myelosuppression, 171
Hematopoietic stem cell transplantation, 139–150
    admission phase in, 144; for breast cancer, 305; collection of cells in, 143–144; complications of, 146, 147t, 149, 150t; conditioning regimen for, 145; discharge phase in, 148; HLA typing in, 141; Hodgkin's disease and, 393; indications for, 141, 142t, 143f; infusion of cells in, 145–146; leukemia and, 384–385, 386; for multiple myeloma, 407–408; non-Hodgkin's lymphoma and, 396; nursing care in, 148, 149; patient evaluation and preparation in, 142–143; process of, 142–149; purging in, 144; rationale for, 140; recovery phase in, 146, 148; rehabilitation in, 149; types of, 140–141
Hepatitis, liver cancer and, 416
Hepatocellular carcinoma, 415–417
Herbal alternative therapies, 153
Hereditary factors. *See* Genetics
History taking, in screening, 46, 47f
HIV/AIDS
    Kaposi's sarcoma and, 359–360, 369–370; lymphoma and, 396–399
HLA system, 141
Hodgkin's disease, 390–394, 463
    clinical presentation of, 391; diagnosis and staging of, 391, 392t; etiology of, 390–391; incidence of, 390; nursing considerations in, 394; treatment of, 106, 392–393, 393f
Home care, 5, 254
Hormones
    breast cancer and, 296, 297, 304; as chemotherapeutic agents, 107, 108f; gynecologic cancers and, 335, 337, 341; prostate cancer and, 328–329
Hospice care
    concept and goals of, 261–262, 262f, 463; issues in, 267–268; primary unit in, 262–263; quality of life and, 252; spirituality and, 263–264, 265–266; team approach in, 263
Hospice Organization, National, 446
Housing programs, 443

Human immunodeficiency virus infection. *See* HIV/AIDS
Human-leukocyte antigen system, 141, 463
Hybridoma technique, 133–134, 135f
Hydatiform mole, 347, 463
Hyperalimentation, 209, 212, 212f, 463
Hypercalcemia, 408, 464
Hyperviscosity syndrome, 404, 464

I Can Cope, 258, 282, 443
Immune system
    humoral and cell mediation in, 125f; overview of, 123, 126; septic shock and, 229–230
Immunoglobulins, 123, 402t
Immunotherapy. *See* Biotherapy
Implantable ports. *See* Vascular access devices
Incidence
    by age, 15, 17t; definition of, 13–14; by gender, 14, 14t, 16f; by race, 14t; by site, 14, 16f, 22f; socioeconomic status and, 62; trends in, 17, 21, 22f; in United States, 17, 20f
Infections
    assessment of, 166–167; childhood cancers and, 432–433; liver cancer and, 416; multiple myeloma and, 404, 408–409; neutropenia and, 164, 165t, 166; in transplant recipients, 147t, 149, 150t; vascular access devices and, 192–193, 194t
Informed consent, 78, 111
Infusion pumps, 197, 198t
Interferon
    administration and toxicities of, 126–127; biologic activity of, 126; indications for, 124t, 126; for multiple myeloma, 407; side effects of, 127, 130t–131t, 407t
Interleukin-2 (IL-2), 124t, 130t–131t, 132, 133t, 464
    for renal cell cancer, 325
Interleukin-6 (IL-6), multiple myeloma and, 403
Interleukins
    administration and toxicity of, 132; biologic activity of, 127, 132; definition, 464; indications for, 124t; names and functions of, 132, 133t; side effects of, 130t–131t
International Association of Laryngectomees, 443–444
Intraoperative radiation therapy, 95–96
Intrathecal chemotherapy, 425, 465
Intravascular coagulation, disseminated, 215t, 217t, 225, 228f, 229–230
Intravesical chemotherapy, 317–318, 319, 465
Ionizing radiation, 38, 381

Japan, stomach cancer in, 412

Kidney. *See* Renal *entries*
Kock pouch, 321f

Laryngectomy, 275, 276–277, 280–281
Laryngectomy visitation program, 443
Larynx, cancer sites in, 271. *See also* Head and neck cancers
Laser surgery, 85, 276
Leukemia, 379–389, 424–425, 465
    in children, 424–425, 426t; classification of, 379–381, 380f, 465; diagnosis of, 382–383; early detection of, 382; evaluation and staging of, 383, 384t, 385t; Hodgkin's disease therapy and, 393; incidence of, 381, 424; long-term sequelae in, 388; myelosuppression and, 162; nursing considerations in, 388; relapse in, 385; risk factors for, 381–382; side effects of, 386–387; treatment of, 383–386, 425, 426t
Leukemia Society of America, Inc., 446, 451
Leukine (GM-CSF), 128t–129t, 171
Leukostasis, 215t, 217t, 221, 386, 466
Levamisole, side effects of, 130t–131t
Limb perfusion, 368–369, 466
Liver cancer, 415–417
Liver metastasis, 312
Look Good...Feel Better, 302, 304, 444
Lost Chord Club, 281, 443–444
Lung cancer, 284–294
    advanced, nursing management of, 292–293; diagnosis and staging of, 285f, 285–288, 286t, 287t, 289t; early detection of, 285; incidence of, 14, 16f, 17, 21; long-term sequelae of, 290–291; myelosuppression and, 162; non-small-cell, 285, 286t, 286–288; nursing considerations in, 291–292; prevention of, 284–285; risk factors for, 37, 38–39, 39t, 284; small-cell, 285, 286t, 287–288, 289t, 290; treatment of, 288, 290
Lymphadenopathy, 391
Lymphedema, 89, 302
Lymphocytes, function of, 123, 402t, 466
Lymphokines, 126, 466
Lymphomas, 390–400, 466
    AIDS-related, 396–399; Hodgkin's disease, 390–394, 392t, 393f; myelosuppression and, 162; non-Hodgkin's, 394–396, 395t

Macrophages, 126, 466
Make Today Count, 441
Make-a-Wish Foundation of America, 441
Male patients
    genital cancers in, 327–334; sexuality education tool for, 241f–242f
Malnutrition. *See* Nutrition
Mammography, 297–298, 298t
    recommendations on, 44, 52
Man to Man, 444
Marrow Donor Program, National, 446–447
Massage therapy, for pain, 177
Medulloblastoma, 351, 352t
Megesterol acetate, 212

Melanoma
    incidence of, 40; malignant, 367–369, 368t
Melphalan, side effects of, 407t
Meningioma, 351, 467
Metastasis, process of, 31–32, 467
Metastatic brain tumors, 356
Methotrexate, 374
Minorities. See Racial/ethnic group(s)
Minority Health Resource Center, 449–450
Mohs surgery, 366–367, 467
Monoclonal antibodies
    administration and toxicities of, 134; defini-
    tion, 467; hybridoma technique for,
    133–134, 135f; indications for, 124t; side
    effects of, 130t–131t
Monoclonal gammopathy, 403, 467
MOPP protocol, 106
Mortality
    by age, 15, 17t, 65; definition of, 14, 467;
    by gender, 14, 15t, 16f; by race, 14, 15, 15t,
    17, 18t–19t; by racial/ethnic group,
    58t–59t; by site, 14, 15, 16f, 17, 18t–19t;
    trends in, 17, 21, 23f
Mourning, 251–252, 266
Mucositis, 181–182
Multiple myeloma, 401–409
    clinical features of, 403–405; diagnosis of,
    405t, 405–406, 406t; epidemiology of, 401;
    etiology of, 402; nursing considerations in,
    408–409; pathophysiology of, 402–403;
    treatment of, 406–409, 407t
Myelosuppression, 161–173
    assessment of, 165–167, 168t; causes of,
    161–162; chemotherapy and, 161–162,
    164t; complications from, 162, 164–165;
    definition of, 161, 467; nursing manage-
    ment of, 165–173, 168t–170t; patient edu-
    cation in, 169t–170t, 172–173; radiation
    therapy and, 162; treatment of, 167,
    171–172

National Bone Marrow Transplant Link, 451
National Cancer Care Foundation, 440
National Cancer Institute (NCI), Cooperative
    Oncology Groups of, 71, 73f
National Coalition for Cancer Survivorship,
    249, 259, 442
National Hospice Organization, 446
National Leukemia Research Association, Inc.,
    451
National Marrow Donor Program, 446–447
Nausea and vomiting
    antiemetic agents for, 178t, 179–180;
    chemotherapy causing, 113t, 179; child-
    hood cancers and, 432; nursing manage-
    ment of, 179–180; radiation therapy caus-
    ing, 101f, 179
Nephrectomy, 323–324
Nervous system, chemotherapy and, 116t
Neupogen (G-CSF), 128t–129t, 171, 172f
Neuroblastoma, 428–430, 468

Neuropathy, 116t
Neutropenia
    colony-stimulating factors for, 127, 171; def-
    inition, 468; infections and, 164; leukemia
    causing, 386; nursing interventions for,
    168t–170t
Neutrophil count, 164, 165t
Nitrosoureas, 106, 106t, 108f
Non-Hodgkin's lymphoma, 394–396, 395t
    AIDS-related, 396–399; staging of, 395,
    395t; treatment of, 395–396
Nonsteroidal anti-inflammatory drugs
    (NSAIDs), 175
Nursing associations, 448–449
Nutrition, 200–213
    assessment of, 204–206, 205t, 207f; breast
    cancer and, 296, 297; cancer risk and, 37,
    40, 154, 273; chemotherapy and, 204;
    development of care plan for, 204–206,
    205t, 207f; effects of cancer on, 200–202,
    201f; effects of treatment on, 202–204;
    enteral, 209; esophageal cancer and, 411;
    head and neck cancer and, 279; interven-
    tion and counseling in, 206, 208f, 209,
    210t–211t; neuroblastoma and, 429; pancre-
    atic cancer and, 414, 415; parenteral, 209,
    212, 212f; pharmacological management of,
    212; radiation therapy and, 203–204; stom-
    ach cancer and, 412–413, 414; surgery and,
    87, 202–203, 203f

Obstruction
    lung cancer and, 292; superior vena cava
    syndrome and, 216–217
Oley Foundation, 442
Oligodendroglioma, 351
Oncogenes, 32, 38, 134, 136f, 468
Oncologic emergencies, 214–230
    hematolic or immunologic disorders, 225,
    228f, 229–230; metabolic disorders,
    221–225, 223t, 224t, 226t–227t; nursing
    considerations in, 214, 216, 217t; obstruc-
    tive or compressive disorders, 218–221,
    220t; radiation therapy for, 94; surgery for,
    86; tumor type and, 215t
Oncology nursing, 3–10
    challenges and rewards of, 9–10; clinical tri-
    als and, 73–75; opportunities in, 4–6; prepa-
    ration for, 8; roles in, 6–7
Oncology Nursing Society, 8
Oncoscint, 124t, 134
Opiods, 175, 176t, 177
Oral cancer, 39t, 39–40, 273. See also Head and
    neck cancers
Oral cavity, 271, 272f
Oral mucositis, 181–182
Osteoclast-activating factors, 403, 468
Osteosarcoma, 373–374, 468
Ostomy Association, 447
Ostomy visitation program, 443
Ovarian cancer, 340–343, 342t

Pain
  assessment of, 174–175, 179; bone, 175, 177, 403, 404, 408; bone cancer and, 373, 374, 377; causes of, 174, 175f; fatigue and, 182; head and neck cancer and, 279–280; lung cancer and, 291; management of, 175–179; multiple myeloma and, 403, 404, 408; palliative care and, 265; pediatric, 179, 433; phantom, 374, 377; procedural, 175f, 177; rehabilitation and, 255

Palliation, 260–268
  bereavement and, 266–277; hospice care and, 261–263, 262f; issues in, 267–268; for lung cancer, 288, 290; nursing and, 264–267; radiation therapy as, 93–94; spirituality and, 263–264, 265–266; surgery as, 85

Pancreatic cancer, 414–415
Papanicolaou smear, 44, 46, 53, 337–338, 468
Paraneoplastic syndromes, 288, 289t, 468
Parenteral nutrition, 209, 212, 212f

Patient teaching
  chemotherapy and, 111; clinical trials and, 74, 76, 78; colorectal cancer and, 314–315; myelosuppression and, 169t–170t, 172–173; nutrition and, 173, 206–207; postoperative, 88; preoperative, 87; radiation therapy and, 97; sexuality and, 241f–244f, 244; for transplant recipients, 148; vascular access devices and, 197. See also Education

Pelvic examination, 53
Pelvic exenteration, 339, 469
Penile cancer, 333
Pericardial effusion, 219–221, 220t, 469
Peripheral blood stem cell transplantation, 141, 469. See also Hematopoietic stem cell transplantation
Peripheral blood stem cells, collection and mobilization of, 144
Pharyngitis, 101f
Pharynx, 271, 272f. See also Head and neck cancers
Philadelphia chromosome, 32, 33f, 383, 469
Plant alkaloids, 107, 108f
Plasma cells, 402–403, 469
Plasmacytoma, 404, 469
PLISSIT model, 234, 239f
Poverty, cancer and, 62, 65
Prednisone, 407t

Prevention of cancer, 35–42
  alcohol and, 40; approaches to, 41–42; diet and, 40; early detection and, 43–55; in elderly, 63–65; ethnic/racial barriers to, 60t–61t; hormones and, 40; levels of, 35–36; nurses and, 4, 41t, 41–42, 43, 54–55, 62–63, 65–66; occupational regulations and, 41, 285; radiation therapy for, 94; socioeconomic status and, 62; sunlight and, 40; surgery and, 84; tobacco and, 38–40, 284

Proctosigmoidoscopy, 54

Prostate cancer, 327–330, 329f
  early detection of, 52–53; incidence of, 14, 16f; risk factors for, 39t
Prostate-specific antigen test, 52, 328
Prosthesis, breast, 301, 302
Proteinuria, Bence-Jones, 403, 404
Psychological therapies, 154

Psychosocial responses, 245–252
  assessment of, 246–247; of cancer survivors, 248–250; to childhood cancer, 433–434; to diagnosis, 247–248; to head and neck cancer, 281–282; to recurrence, 250; during terminal phase, 251–252; to treatment, 248
Pulmonary fibrosis, 114t–115t
Purging, in hematopoietic stem cell transplantation, 144

Quality of life
  focus on, 245; hospice care and, 252; palliative care and, 264–265

Racial/ethnic group(s)
  breast cancer and, 295; cancer and, 57–62, 58t–59t, 60t–61t; cancer incidence and, 14t; cancer mortality and, 14, 15, 15t, 17, 18t–19t; cancer survival and, 21, 24t–25t; esophageal cancer and, 410; multiple myeloma and, 401; prostate cancer and, 327; stomach cancer and, 412
Radiation exposure, 29t, 38, 381

Radiation therapy, 91–102
  administration of, 94–96; biologic effects of, 91; for bladder cancer, 322; for bone cancer, 375; bowel dysfunction and, 180, 181; for brain tumors, 355, 356–357; for breast cancer, 303; for cervical cancer, 338–339; chemotherapy and, 93; for CNS lymphoma, 398; for colorectal cancer, 311, 313; in combination treatment, 93; doses for, 92; for endometrial cancer, 337; for esophageal cancer, 412; external, 94–95, 95f, 96; hair loss and, 183; for head and neck cancer, 203–204, 276; hematopoietic stem cell transplantation and, 145; for Hodgkin's disease, 392, 393f; internal, 94, 96, 97, 276, 355; intraoperative, 95–96; for lung cancer, 288, 290, 291–292; machines for, 94–95, 95f; mucositis and, 181; for multiple myeloma, 406–407, 407t; myelosuppression and, 162; nausea and vomiting and, 179; for non-Hodgkin's lymphoma, 396, 398; nursing considerations in, 97–102; nursing management of, 100f–101f; nutrition and, 203–204; for oncologic emergencies, 84; for ovarian cancer, 343; pain and, 175f; as palliative treatment, 93–94; in prevention of disease, 94; as primary treatment, 92; principles of, 91–92; for prostate cancer, 328; for renal cell cancer, 324; side effects of, 97, 98t–99t, 100f–101f, 407t; for skin cancer, 367, 370; spinal cord compression and,

Radiation therapy, *Cont.*
    218–219; stereotactic, 95; simulation and
    treatment planning in, 96; for stomach can-
    cer, 413, 414; superior vena cava syndrome
    and, 216; surgery and, 87–88, 92, 93; thy-
    roid cancer and, 418, 419; uses of, 92–94
Radioactive isotopes, 96
Radiosensitivity of tumor cells, 92, 93t
Radiosurgery, 355
Reach to Recovery, 258, 302, 444
Rectal cancer. *See* Colorectal cancer
Recurrence of cancer, psychosocial responses
    to, 250
Rehabilitation, 253–259
    barriers to, 254–255; breast cancer and,
    302–303; families and, 253–254; nursing
    management of, 5, 257–259; site-specific,
    256–257, 258t; team approach to, 255–256,
    257t; work and identity during, 256
Religion, spirituality and, 263
Renal cell cancer, 322–325
    diagnosis and staging of, 322–323, 323t,
    324t; treatment of, 323–325; Wilms' tumor,
    426–428, 427t
Renal system
    chemotherapy and, 115t; multiple myeloma
    and, 404, 404f, 409; surgery and, 88–89
Reproductive system, 116t–118t
Research
    ethics in, 77, 77f; nurses and, 74–75. *See
    also* Clinical trials
Resources in cancer care, 439–452
    for cancer patients and families, 439–447;
    financial, 450–452; government, 449–450;
    professional, 8, 447–449
Respiratory system, 114t–115t
Retinoblastoma, 430–431, 470
Rhabdomyosarcoma, 431–432
Risk assessment, 37
Risk factor(s)
    age as, 63; definition of, 37, 470; environ-
    mental, 38; genetic, 38; lifestyle as, 38;
    occupational, 41; types of, 36–38
Road to Recovery, 443
Ronald-McDonald House Charities, 447

Sargramostim (GM-CSF), 128t–129t, 171
Screening
    for breast cancer, 51–52, 297–298, 298t; for
    cervical cancer, 53, 337–338; for colorectal
    cancer, 53–54, 308; definition, 470; for
    endometrial cancer, 335–336; issues in,
    44–47; nursing role in, 4, 47, 48t–49t, 50,
    54–55; for ovarian cancer, 341; participa-
    tion in, factors influencing, 48t–49t; physi-
    cal examination and, 46–47; for prostate
    cancer, 52–53, 328; recommendations for,
    44, 45t; as secondary prevention, 36, 43; for
    skin cancer, 50–51; for testicular cancer,
    330, 331
Self-care, culture and, 281–282

Self-examination
    of breast, 51, 297, 298t; compliance in, 50;
    factors influencing, 48t–49t; of skin, 50–51,
    362, 364f–365f; of testicles, 330, 331
Septic shock, 215t, 217t, 229–230
Serotherapy, 123, 132, 134, 471
Sexuality, 231–244
    assessment of, 232–233, 233f, 234, 239,
    240f; chemotherapy affecting, 116t–118t;
    childhood cancers and, 239–240; definition
    of, 231, 471; effects of cancer on, 233–234,
    235t–238t, 239–240; male genital cancers
    and, 329, 332, 333; nursing interventions
    related to, 234, 235t–238t, 239, 239f;
    patient education on, 241f–244f, 244;
    surgery affecting, 89, 321
Skin, radiation therapy and, 100f
Skin Cancer Foundation, 362, 363f
Skin cancers, 359–371
    basal cell and squamous cell, 361t, 366–367;
    characteristics and sites of, 361t; incidence
    of, 359–360, 361t; Kaposi's sarcoma,
    359–360, 369–370; malignant melanoma,
    367–369, 368t; nursing considerations in,
    370; prevention and early detection of,
    50–51, 362, 363f, 364f–365f; risk factors for,
    37, 39t, 360, 362; ultraviolet radiation and,
    29t, 37, 40, 360
Smoking
    as carcinogen, 39, 273; lung cancer and,
    38–41, 39t, 284; pancreatic cancer and,
    414; renal cell cancer and, 322
Socioeconomic status, 17, 62, 65
Specific immunity, 123, 471
Spinal cord compression, 215t, 217t, 218–219,
    471
Spine tumors, 356
Spirituality, 263–264, 265–266
Staging
    of bladder cancer, 317, 317t, 318t; of breast
    cancer, 299, 300t; of colorectal cancer, 309,
    310t; definition, 471; of gynecologic can-
    cers, 336t, 339t, 342t, 345t, 346t, 347t; of
    head and neck cancers, 274; of Hodgkin's
    disease, 391, 392t; of leukemias, 383, 384t;
    of lung cancer, 285–288, 286t, 287t, 289t;
    of male genital cancers, 329t, 332t; of
    melanoma, 367, 368t; of multiple myeloma,
    405t, 405–406; of neuroblastoma, 429; of
    non-Hodgkin's lymphoma, 395, 395t, 398;
    of renal cell cancer, 323, 323t, 324t; of
    retinoblastoma, 430; surgical, 83t, 84; of
    Wilms' tumor, 427, 427t
Stereotactic radiosurgery, 95, 471
Sterility, testicular cancer and, 331–332
Stomach cancer, 412–414
Stomatitis, oral, 100f
Stress-reducing techniques, 177
Strontium-89, 94, 94f, 376
Subjective Global Assessment (SGA) of nutri-
    tional status, 206, 207f

Sunlight, cancer risk and, 273
Sunscreens, 362, 363f
Superior vena cava syndrome, 215t, 216, 217t, 471
Suppressor genes, 38
Surgery, 80–89
as adjuvant therapy, 85; for bladder cancer, 317–318, 319, 321; blood disorders and, 87; for bone cancer, 374, 375; for brain tumors, 355, 356; for breast cancer, 301–303; chemotherapy during, 87–88; for CNS lymphoma, 398; for colorectal cancer, 311, 313; in combination treatment, 85–86, 87–88; in diagnosis of disease, 81–84, 82t–83t; for endometrial cancer, 336–337; for esophageal cancer, 411; for head and neck cancer, 275–276, 276t; for insertion of therapeutic devices, 86; late effects of, 88–89; for liver cancer, 416; for lung cancer, 288, 290; lymphedema from, 89; for non-Hodgkin's lymphoma, 395, 398; nursing considerations in, 86–88; nutrition and, 87, 202–203, 203f; for oncologic emergencies, 86; for ovarian cancer, 341–342; pain and, 175f; as palliative treatment, 85; for pancreatic cancer, 415; physical asymmetry and, 88; in prevention of disease, 84; as primary treatment, 84–85; principles of, 80–81; for prostate cancer, 328; radiation therapy during, 87–88, 95–96; radical, 203t; reconstructive, 86; for renal cell cancer, 323–324; renal effects of, 88–89; as salvage treatment, 85; sexuality and, 89; for skin cancer, 366–367, 368; spinal cord compression and, 219; in staging of disease, 83t, 84; for stomach cancer, 413; techniques in, 85; for thyroid cancer, 419; for vulvar cancer, 344; for Wilms' tumor, 428
Survival rates, 21, 471
race and, 21, 24t–25t; socioeconomic status and, 62
Survivorship, 248–250, 259, 471
Susan G. Komen Breast Cancer Foundation, 445
Syndrome of inappropriate secretion of antidiuretic hormone (SIADH), 215t, 217t, 221–224, 224t, 471
lung cancer and, 289t
Syngeneic transplants, 141, 471. See also Hematopoietic stem cell transplantation

Tamoxifen, breast cancer and, 297, 304
Taste changes, 100f
Terminal phase
insurance benefits during, 267–268; psychosocial responses during, 251–252
Testicular cancer, 330–333, 332t
Thrombocytopenia
assessment of, 165, 167; defintion, 472; nursing interventions for, 168t–170t; treatment of, 171–172

Thrombopoietin, 172
Thyroid cancer, 418–420, 472
Time trends
in cancer incidence and mortality, 17, 21, 22f, 23f; in cancer survival, race and, 21, 24t–25t
T-lymphocytes, 123, 125f, 126, 402
Tobacco. See Smoking
Tolerance, 175, 472
Total body irradiation (TBI), 145
Total parenteral nutrition, 209, 212, 212f, 472
Toxoplasmosis, CNS lymphoma and, 397
Transcutaneous electrical nerve stimulation (TENS), 177, 472
Transportation programs, 443, 445
Transurethral resection, 317–318
Tricyclic antidepressants, 175
Tumor angiogenesis factor, 31
Tumor lysis syndrome, 215t, 217t, 224–225, 226t–227t, 387, 472
Tumor markers, 28, 309, 420, 472
Tumor necrosis factor, 130t–131t, 403, 473
Tumor-node-metastasis (TNM) system, 274
Tumors
grading of, 317, 350–351, 351t; growth of, 28–32, 30f; heredity and, 32–34; oncogenes and, 32, 38; radiosensitivity of, 92, 93t
Tumor-suppressor gene, 134, 136f, 473

Ultraviolet radiation, 29t, 37, 40, 360, 473
United Ostomy Association, 447
Urinary diversions, 319–321, 321f, 329f
Urinary tract cancers, 316–326
U.S. Department of Health and Human Services, 449–450
U.S. Department of Labor, Occupational Safety and Health Administration, 450
US TOO International, Inc., 442

VAD regimen, side effects of, 407t
Vaginal cancer, 344, 346, 346t
Vaginal mucositis, 182
Vascular access devices, 185–198, 473
advantages and disadvantages of, 186t; ambulatory pumps, 197, 198t; blood withdrawal and, 192; care of, 190–192, 191t; complications of, 192–197, 194t, 195f–196f; implantable ports, 188–189, 473; insertion of, 86; occlusion and, 193, 195f–196f, 197; overview of, 185–189; patient education regarding, 197; peripherally inserted catheters, 187–188; placement of, 187f; selection of, 189–190; tunneled catheters, 188, 473
Vincristine, side effects of, 407t
Viruses, carcinogenic, 29t
Vitamin therapies, 154
Vulvar cancer, 344, 345t

Warning signs for cancer, 46, 47f
We Can Weekend, 282

Weight loss, 200–201, 201f
Wilms' tumor, 426–428, 427t, 473
Women, sexuality education tool for, 243f–244f
Workplace discrimination, 249, 254–255, 256

Xerostomia, 101f, 182, 279, 473

YMCA of the USA-Encore Plus, 440–441, 452
Y-ME National Breast Cancer Organization, Inc., 442

THANK YOU!

Thank you for taking the time to review this new edition from the American Cancer Society and Jones and Bartlett Publishers. We hope you found it to be a welcome addition to your bookshelf! Please take the time to tell your colleagues about this exciting new resource and offer the attached order form as an easy way to share this valuable information with them, or to inquire about other publications by Jones and Bartlett.

☐ YES! Please rush me_____copy(ies) of *A Cancer Source Book for Nurses, Seventh Edition* (0-7637-0242-0) for $32.50 list*. If not completely satisfied, I may return the book within 30 days for a full refund. (*Prices subject to change.)

☐ YES! Please rush my copy of the Jones and Bartlett Oncology Nursing catalog.

☐ YES! Please contact me with information on volume discounts for my institution.

☐ Bill me later

☐ Check enclosed   ☐ VISA   ☐ MasterCard

Exp date:_____

Card Number: _____

Signature: _____

Name:_____Title:_____

Institution:_____

Address:_____

City:_____State:_____Zip:_____

Telephone: (   )_____

E-mail address:_____

Source: ACSORD

JONES AND BARTLETT PUBLISHERS
40 Tall Pine Drive, Sudbury, MA 01776
Phone: 800.832.0034 / 508.443.5000   FAX: 508.443.8000
info@jbpub.com   *Your Oncology Nursing Connection*
http://www.jbpub.com/oncology/